ORTHOPAEDIC PHYSIOTHERAPY

ARIAN TIDSWELL

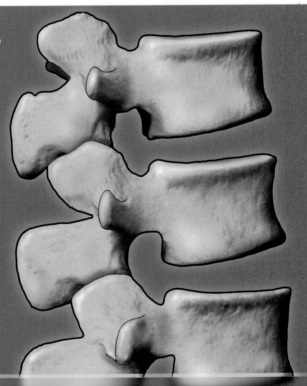

Orthopaedics (or:tho:pe:dix). That part of surgery which deals with the abnormnalities, diseases and injuries of the locomotor system.

ORTHOPAEDIC
PHYSIOTHERAPY

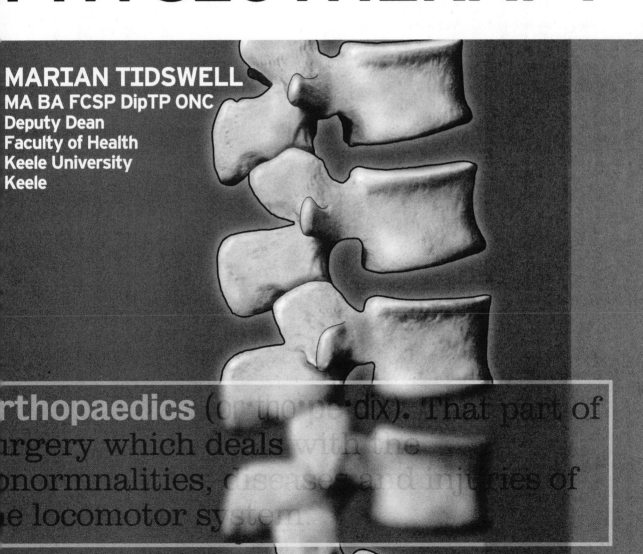

MARIAN TIDSWELL
MA BA FCSP DipTP ONC
Deputy Dean
Faculty of Health
Keele University
Keele

rthopaedics (orthop dix). That part of
rgery which deals with the
bnormmalities, disease and injuries of
e locomotor system

Mosby
London Philadelphia St Louis Sydney Tokyo

Publisher	**Jill Northcott**
Development Editor	**Gillian Harris**
Project Manager	**Claire Brewer**
Design	**Greg Smith**
Layout	**Rob Curran**
Cover Design	**Greg Smith**
Illustration Manager	**Danny Payne**
Cover Manager	**Mike Saiz**
Illustrators	**Mike Saiz**
	Robin Dean
	Paul Bernson
Production	**Hamish Adamson**
Indexer	**Anita Reid**

Copyright © 1998 Mosby International Limited

Published by Mosby, an imprint of Mosby International Limited, Lynton House, 7-12 Tavistock Square, London WC1H 9LB, UK

ISBN 0 7234 2592 2

Printed by Printer Trento s.r.l., Trento, Italy

Set in: Scala: Fontworks. Interstate: Font Bureau. (Supplied by Fontworks UK)

For full details of all Mosby titles, please write to Mosby International Publishers Limited, Lynton House, 7-12 Tavistock Square, London WC1H 9LB, UK.

A CIP catalogue record for this book is available from the British Library.

CONTENTS

Having used the original textbooks written by Joan Cash as a student physiotherapist, I later was involved in both the Orthopaedics and Rheumatology for Physiotherapists books as author or editor and now complete the cycle by editing the first edition of Orthopaedic Physiotherapy.

The disciplines of medicine and science which underpin the practice of physiotherapy continue to develop and the contribution they make to the knowledge base encompassed by the two major sub-disciplines of Orthopaedics and Rheumatology within physiotherapy is such that it is no longer possible to give each area the required individual attention in a shared text. The decision was taken therefore, for this edition to separate the texts to ensure a more realistic coverage for each topic area. It would have been thought that if the text was to cover Orthopaedics alone, that the selection of content would be facilitated, however, that is not the case and the choice as to what is to be included or excluded is as difficult as ever. It is hoped that the final choice will give the reader sufficient knowledge to approach the challenge of patient management in the field of orthopaedics with enthusiasm and stimulate interest for continued contact with this important area of a physiotherapist's responsibility.

Recent changes in the pattern of delivery of health care and the implementation of clinical audit and evidence based care as routine tools for the monitoring of the effectiveness of therapeutic interventions have contributed significantly to a diversification of the role and responsibilities of practising physiotherapists. A team approach to the management of patients' problems reflected in chapters in this text is an essential feature of the therapeutic relationship. This has produced more effective care packages for patients who benefit from the input of the most appropriate professional expertise at each stage of recovery.

Another significant change that has affected attitudes and orientation for practitioners was the achievement of graduate entry to the profession for all physiotherapists qualifying from British based courses from 1994. This, combined with the right to generate their own work load as they were, in 1977, removed from the need to receive patients only by referral from doctors, dentists or veterinary surgeons has enabled expansion of practice into areas where the physiotherapist's particular knowledge of disorders of function can be explored. The development of therapeutic concepts which rely on this knowledge and expertise has been encouraged and it has been possible to include some of these innovations in this text. Although many of the authors are employed in the National Health Service, chapters have been included from others with practice bases outside the NHS, illustrating the variety of practice opportunity that is available to practitioners.

In their enthusiasm to explore new frontiers, physiotherapists have not ignored their responsibilities to other disciplines involved in patient care and the close working relationships with the medical profession continues to be a feature of practice within the orthopaedic field. The nature of the relationship has changed over the years and physiotherapists are now not only implementing predetermined therapeutic management programmes, but also diversifying practice and developing their own management strategies particularly with regard to long term pain and disability.

This edition is aimed at the honours-level undergraduate and newly qualified physiotherapist who will be practising in a patient focused environment that demands effective use of scarce resources and competent ethical practice. In addition to providing a guide for implementation of competent practice in orthopaedic physiotherapy, it is hoped the text will stimulate the reader to search for more specialised literature in the areas of interest and develop the clinical reasoning and reflective practice essential to all practitioners approaching the millennium.

The final text is the product of the contributions of a great number of people who have devoted considerable time and effort to the project and I thank the authors for their contributions.

My grateful thanks are also given to the Mosby team, particularly to Jill Northcott and Gillian Harris, whose enthusiasm, support and expertise have brought the book to publication.

Marian E Tidswell MA, BA, FCSP, Dip TP, ONC
Deputy Dean of the Faculty of Health, Keele University
(formerly Head of the Department of Physiotherapy Studies, Keele University)

Karen Barker Msc MCSP SRP
Superintendent Physiotherapist, Nuffield Orthopaedic
Centre NHS Trust, Windmill Road, Headington, Oxford.
Chapter 8

Alyson Biggs MCSP
Senior Physiotherapist in Orthopaedics,
Wrexham Maelor Hospital, Croesnewydd Road,
Wrexham, Clwyd. Chapter 6

Mr Andrew J Carr ChM FRCS
Consultant Orthopaedic Surgeon, Upper Limb Unit,
Nuffield Orthopaedic Centre NHS Trust, Windmill Road,
Headington, Oxford. Chapter 7

Dr Alan J Darby MB BS FRCPath
Consultant Histopathologist, Robert Jones and Agnes
Hunt Orthopaedic and District Hospital NHS Trust,
Oswestry, Shropshire. Chapter 1

Dr Michael Davie MD FRCP
Medical Director, Charles Salt Research Unit,
Robert Jones and Agnes Hunt Orthopaedic and District
Hospital NHS Trust, Oswestry,Shropshire. Chapter 9

Mr Stephen Eisenstein MB Bch PhD FRCS(Ed)
Director, Centre for Spinal Studies,
Robert Jones and Agnes Hunt Orthopaedic Hospital
NHS Trust, Oswestry, Shropshire. Chapters 4 & 13

Mr Gwyn A Evans MB BS FRCS FRCS(Orth)
Consultant Orthopaedic Surgeon, Children's
Orthopaedic Unit, Robert Jones and Agnes Hunt
Orthopaedic and District Hospital NHS Trust, Oswestry,
Shropshire. Chapter 10

Kirstie L Haywood BSC Hons MCSP SRP
Postgraduate Research Student, Department of Health
and Sciences and Clinical Evaluation, University of York,
Heslington, York. Chapter 14

**Barbara J Hollins MSc MCSP MMACP CertEd DipTP
SRP**
Lecturer, Department of Physiotherapy Studies, Mackay
Building, Keele University, Keele, Staffordshire.
Chapters 14 & 15

Mr David C Jaffray MB ChB FRCS(Ed)
Consultant Orthopaedic Surgeon, Robert Jones and
Agnes Hunt Orthopaedic and District Hospital NHS
Trust, Oswestry, Shropshire. Chapter 12

Kim Jones MSc MCSP DipTP CertEd CMS
Honorary Research Fellow,School of Physiotherapy
University of West of England, Bristol. Chapter 18

Rachel Jones MCSP ONC
Senior Paediatric Physiotherapist, Robert Jones and
Agnes Hunt Orthopaedic and District Hospital NHS
Trust, Oswestry, Shropshire. Chapters 10, 11 & 13

Alan J Leigh MSc GDAMT(NZ) MMACP MCSP SRP
Lifestyle Physiotherapy Clinic, Radbrook Professional
Centre, Bank Farm Road, Radbrook Green, Shrewsbury.
Chapter 20

Richard E Major BSc GradCertEd CEng MIPEM
Head of Bioengineering, Regional Medical Physics
Department, Newcastle General Hospital, Newcastle
upon Tyne. Chapter 3

Else Mellor MCSP
Innishale, Clachan Seil, Isle of Seil, Nr Oban, Argyll.
Chapter 16

**Mr Michael D Northmore-Ball MA MB BChir FRCS
CI Mech E**
Consultant Orthopaedic Surgeon, Robert Jones and
Agnes Hunt Orthopaedic and District Hospital NHS
Trust, Oswestry, Shropshire. Chapter 5

Senior Clinical Lecturer, Department of Orthopaedic
Surgery, School of Postgraduate Medicine, Keele
University, Keele, Staffordshire.

Judith Pitt-Brooke MSC MCSP CertEd DipTP
Lecturer, Division of Physiotherapy Education, Faculty
of Medicine and Health Sciences, University of
Nottingham, Nottingham. Chapter 17

East Midlands Physiotherapy Clinic, Loughborough,
Leicester.

Mr Andrew H Roberts MBChB DM FRCS
Consultant Orthopaedic Surgeon, Children's
Orthopaedic Unit, Robert Jones and Agnes Hunt
Orthopaedic and District Hospital NHS Trust, Oswestry,
Shropshire. Chapter 11

Senior Clinical Lecturer, Department of Orthopaedic
Surgery, School of Postgraduate Medicine,
Keele University, Keele, Staffordshire.

**Graham N Smith GradDipPhys MCSP DipTP CertEd
SRP**
Chartered Physiotherapist, Rehabilitation and Sports
Injury Consultant, 45c Carrick Street, Glasgow.
Chapter 19

John Stallard BTech CEng FIMechE FIPEM,
Technical Director, Orthotic Research and Locomotor
Assessment Unit, Robert Jones and Agnes Hunt
Orthopaedic and District Hospital NHS Trust, Oswestry,
Shropshire. Chapter 3

Mr Peter BM Thomas MB BS FRCS(Ed) FRCS(Lond)
Consultant Orthopaedic Surgeon, Royal Infirmary
Princes Road, Hartshill, Stoke-on-Trent. Chapter 2

SECTION 1

GENERAL TOPICS

thopaedics (orthopædix). That part of
rgery which deals with the
normalities, diseases and injuries of
e locomotor system.

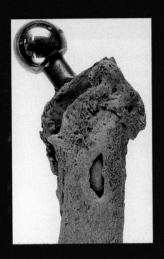

1 A J Darby

BONE AND JOINT PATHOLOGY

CHAPTER OUTLINE

- Congenital disorders of bone
- Metabolic bone disease
- Tumours of bone
- Osteoarthritis

- Rheumatoid arthritis
- Infective arthritis
- Metabolic arthritis

The first section of this chapter considers the development of bone and its growth, adaptation to function, stress modelling and renewal, before leading on to the pathological processes affecting bone tissue. This is followed by a description of the congenital disorders that affect bone, and the effects of injury, infection, metabolic disorders, vascular disturbances and tumours on the structure and functioning of bone. Those diseases that commonly affect joints, i.e. osteoarthritis, rheumatoid arthritis, infective arthritis and metabolic arthritis, are presented, and the chapter concludes with a brief consideration of the effect of joint replacement on the quality of bone.

BONE

Bone is a uniquely versatile tissue combining strength, elasticity and adaptability. In the fetus, bones develop in two ways. Firstly, the skull and some other bones, e.g. the scapula, are formed by intramembranous ossification, i.e. the direct transformation of primitive fibrous tissue into bone. The rest of the skeleton comes into being by a process known as endochondral ossification, where the bones are formed initially as cartilaginous models which are then converted into bone by a specialised structure called the growth plate. The growth plate also controls the increase in the length of the bones in both the fetus and the growing child (Cormack, 1987).

As well as being able to change its overall size and shape, bone can also mould its internal structure to accommodate long-term mechanical stresses (Figure 1.1) (Lanyon, 1992). Indeed, throughout life, bone is continually remodelling and renewing itself by the action of specialised cells, the osteoclasts and osteoblasts. Resorption of bone by osteoclasts and formation of bone by osteoblasts are united in discrete spatial and temporal units known as bone remodelling units (MacDonald & Gowen, 1993). It is the manipulation of these opposing cellular processes that enables the skeleton to repair itself after injury and to undergo its necessary dimensional changes during childhood. Failure of the normal controlling mechanisms for resorption and formation leads to osteoporosis, the commonest disease of bone, and is also involved in a number of other congenital and acquired disorders (Eriksen & Langdahl, 1995). In addition, bone acts as a reservoir for calcium and certain ions essential for the function of other body organs.

In spite of its strength and versatility, bone is subject to all the various pathological processes that affect the other tissues of the body. These may be grouped into:
- Congenital disorders of bone.
- Injury.
- Infections.
- Metabolic bone disease.
- Vascular disorders.
- Tumours.

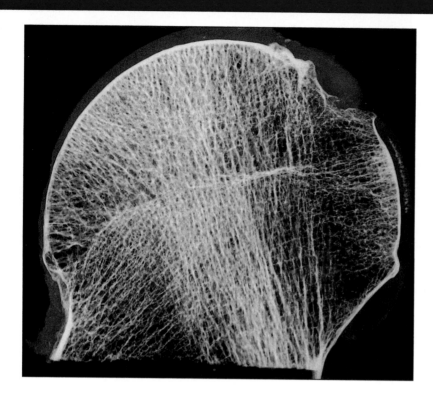

Figure 1.1 X-ray film of a slice through a femoral head, showing the stress-oriented pattern of the trabecular bone.

CONGENITAL DISORDERS OF BONE

Congenital disorders of bone may be generalised, known as the skeletal dysplasias, or localised to a specific part of the body. There are over 200 types of skeletal dysplasia (Beighton *et al.*, 1992), many of which cause death *in utero* or in early childhood. Two of the commonest forms of skeletal dysplasia associated with survival into adult life are achondroplasia and osteogenesis imperfecta.

Achondroplasia

In achondroplasia, the inherited defect prevents the normal functioning of chondrocytes in the growth plate. This causes the long bones of the arms and legs to be shorter than normal, resulting in short-limb dwarfism. Many patients with achondroplasia are able to lead a full and active life, although complications include spinal stenosis and spinal cord compression.

Osteogenesis Imperfecta

Osteogenesis imperfecta results from a mutation in the gene encoding collagen type I. Because of this, the osteoblasts are unable to form bone of sufficient strength and quantity, and the patients suffer repeated fractures from an early age.

INJURY

The type of injury of most concern in orthopaedics is mechanical, particularly when bones become fractured. The healing of fractures progresses through several stages (Sevitt, 1981). Immediately after the injury there is haemorrhage, closely followed by inflammation. During the next few days, young fibrous tissue rich in blood vessels, the granulation tissue, grows from the raw bone ends. At the same time, a collar of cartilage and immature bone called the callus is produced by the periosteum and laid down around the shaft of each bone. During the next few days or weeks this external callus proliferates to bridge the gap between the bone ends. Lagging behind this is the formation of internal callus in the medullary cavity of the bone. With time this immature callus is remodelled and replaced by mature bone. In the growing child the whole process is completed after a few weeks, but in the adult it may take many months. Sometimes, children, athletes or adults taking unaccustomed exercise may sustain stress fractures. These are small incomplete fractures involving just the cortex, and not the full thickness of the bone.

Fracture healing may be delayed, or even prevented, if the bone ends are too widely displaced, the fracture is inadequately immobilised, the blood supply is impaired or infection supervenes.

INFECTIONS
Pyogenic Osteomyelitis

Osteomyelitis is most commonly caused by infection with the bacterium *Staphylococcus aureus*. Bacteria reach the bone either by the bloodstream or by the direct bacterial contamination of bone during surgery or after severe trauma. In children, acute osteomyelitis commonly occurs in the metaphyseal region, because this is the most vascular part of the growing bone. In adults, infection of the spine is not uncommon and is often associated with urinary tract infection, which, in men, may follow prostatectomy. Patients who are receiving steroids or immunosuppressive therapy are particularly prone to osteomyelitis. Joint replacement surgery also leads to infection in a small percentage of cases (Figure 1.2).

Bacterial proliferation starts in the bone marrow of the medullary cavity. The ensuing inflammatory reaction, together with the production of bacterial toxins, causes the death of both soft tissues and bone. Pain and pyrexia are early features of the disease; the other signs of inflammation—swelling and redness—develop later, if at all, depending on the site of the lesion and the virulence of the organism.

The diagnosis of osteomyelitis may often be made confidently by a combination of clinical and radiological signs, but biopsy is essential to confirm the diagnosis. In a readily accessible site this may be by curettage to remove all the affected tissue, but in areas such as the vertebral column, needle biopsy under X-ray guidance is quicker and easier. Antibiotic treatment can be started immediately after the biopsy and altered, if necessary, on the basis of sensitivity tests on the bacteria isolated in the laboratory.

In the absence of prompt antibiotic treatment, chronic osteomyelitis develops, with the formation of an abscess cavity. Pus may track along the marrow cavity; in children, the growth plate usually acts as a barrier, preventing spread into the epiphysis and the joint cavity. Pus may also travel through the vascular channels of the cortex to the periosteal surface. Here it lifts the periosteum and stimulates it to form a shell of new bone called the involucrum. Later the periosteum itself is breached and a sinus may develop, communicating between the medullary cavity of the bone and the skin surface and causing a persistent purulent discharge. Areas of necrotic bone are recognised by the body, and certain processes are initiated to remove the dead tissue. Osteoclasts are attracted from neighbouring viable bone and begin to resorb the dead bone. As this process of resorption continues, the dead bone becomes separated from the living bone, known as a sequestrum. With continuing osteoclastic activity, the sequestrum is often divided into smaller fragments, which may be extruded through the sinuses to the skin surface. The surgical removal of sequestra greatly improves the rate of healing of osteomyelitis.

At any stage of pyogenic osteomyelitis, the patient is at risk of developing septicaemia. Established chronic osteomyelitis may be very resistant to treatment, and two other serious complications may result. One is the development of secondary amyloidosis with involvement of the kidneys, resulting in chronic renal failure. The other is the presence of squamous cell carcinoma in the chronically irritated skin around the edge of a sinus. Fortunately, both of these complications are now rare.

Tuberculous Osteomyelitis

Following the advent of antituberculous drugs and BCG vaccination, tuberculosis had become uncommon in developed countries. However, with the spread of AIDS and the emergence of resistant strains of mycobacteria, tuberculosis is

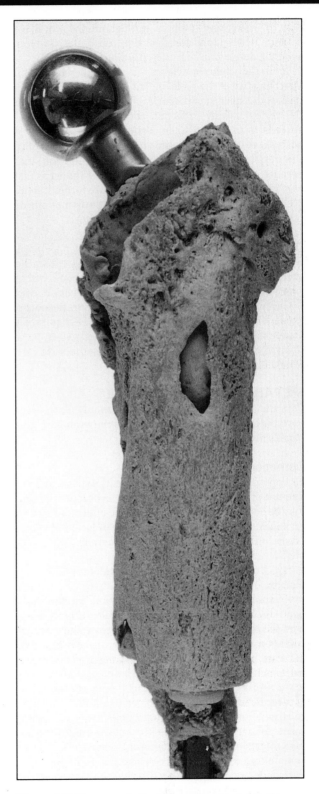

Figure 1.2 Upper end of a femur showing chronic osteomyelitis caused by infection of a joint prosthesis. The granular surface is the involucrum, consisting of bone formed by the periosteum in response to the infection. Part of a sequestrum can be seen at the base of the hole in the involucrum.

now an increasing problem throughout the world. In Britain, mostly adults are affected by tuberculosis, whereas in the developing countries and among immigrants, it is commonly children who are affected. Tuberculosis can affect any part of the skeleton, but nearly half of the cases involve the spine, a condition known as Pott's disease. In the vertebral body, infection starts near the disc and spreads to involve adjacent vertebrae. A paravertebral abscess results, which can be seen on X-ray film. Progression is slower than in pyogenic infection and, because the necrotic bone can be resorbed almost as fast as it is produced, only small sequestra are formed. Bone destruction and collapse of the anterior portion of one or more vertebral bodies leads to angular kyphosis.

Other Infections
Syphilis, both congenital and acquired, may affect the skeleton. In syphilis, there is irregular new bone formation, often periosteal, and patchy destruction and replacement of bone by fibrous granulation tissue. In sheep-farming areas, hydatid disease of bone is still seen occasionally. Immunocompromised patients are subject to a variety of infections, including the otherwise rare fungal diseases of bone.

METABOLIC BONE DISEASE
Four metabolic bone diseases are commonly recognised: osteoporosis, osteomalacia, hyperparathyroidism and Paget's disease.

Osteoporosis
Osteoporosis is a reduction in the density of bone, and the amount of both cancellous (soft) and cortical (hard) bone may be decreased. Osteoporosis may be either localised or generalised. The most common cause of localised osteoporosis is immobility after fracture. It may also occur secondary to joint inflammation.

Generalised osteoporosis is the commonest of all bone diseases. It is caused by an imbalance between the normal processes of bone resorption and formation. All adults lose bone slowly with age, but this loss is accelerated in women after the menopause because of the decrease and eventual cessation of oestrogen production by the ovaries. The decrease in bone density is accompanied by a decline in bone strength, which, in a high proportion of women, leads to fractures. Vertebral collapse fractures account for most of the loss of height in elderly women (Figure 1.3). Anterior collapse of the thoracic vertebrae causes kyphosis, the so-called dowager's hump. More important is fracture of the neck of the femur—the combination of blood loss, surgery and prolonged immobility is a major cause of morbidity in the elderly, and many patients die within a year of fracture.

In men, osteoporosis tends to occur at a more advanced age, probably due to a more gradual decline in the levels of male sex hormones. In younger people, steroid therapy is an important iatrogenic cause of osteoporosis, but the mechanism for this is poorly understood. Thyrotoxicosis is another hormonally mediated cause of osteoporosis.

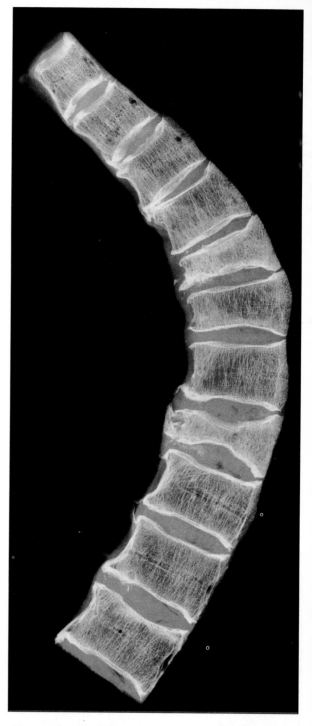

Figure 1.3 X-ray film of a slice through the spine of a patient with osteoporosis. There is collapse fracture of several vertebrae with angulation, causing a kyphosis.

Treatment of osteoporosis is as yet controversial and largely unsatisfactory, but most cases of postmenopausal osteoporosis could probably be prevented by hormone replacement therapy.

Osteomalacia

Osteomalacia, known as rickets in children, results from a lack of the active metabolite of vitamin D—1,25-dihydroxy-cholecalciferol [1,25(OH)$_2$D](1,25-dihydroxyvitamin D)—which is necessary for bone to mineralise properly as well as enhancing calcium absorption from the gut. There are two sources of vitamin D, from the skin by the action of ultraviolet irradiation in sunlight, and from the diet. 1,25(OH)$_2$D is formed by further metabolism in the liver and kidney. In children, 1,25(OH)$_2$D is necessary for calcification of the growth plate, without which longitudinal growth of bones cannot occur. In both children and adults, 1,25(OH)$_2$D is needed for the mineralisation of bone produced by osteoblasts. In children, who are making bone rapidly, a disruption to this mineralisation may lead to bending and deformity of the bones as well as short stature. In adults, the poorly calcified bone is weak and results in multiple microfractures which cause pain—and sometimes complete fracture. The diagnosis of inadequate mineralisation of bone is usually possible by biochemical tests that show high levels of serum alkaline phosphatase and low levels of calcium. In more problematic cases, bone biopsy may be necessary (Figure 1.4).

Hyperparathyroidism

Parathyroid hormone (PTH) helps maintain the level of serum calcium in two ways. Firstly, it increases the amount of osteoclastic activity relative to osteoblastic activity in bone, thus releasing some of the skeleton's calcium stores into the blood. Less directly, it increases calcium absorption from the gut by facilitating renal production of 1,25(OH)$_2$D. Excess production of PTH is usually caused by a benign tumour (adenoma) of one of the four parathyroid glands. This condition is called primary hyperparathyroidism. Less commonly, secondary hyperparathyroidism results from an attempt by all four parathyroid glands to counteract calcium depletion caused by chronic renal failure.

In both cases the effect on the skeleton is to increase the amount of skeletal remodelling. Although regional variations occur, in severe hyperparathyroidism there is an overall tendency towards osteoporosis. Early diagnosis and treatment means that severe hyperparathyroidism is now rare; previously it was an important cause of renal stones from the prolonged hypercalcaemia. Treatment is directed at the cause of the disease, i.e. either surgery to the parathyroid glands or medical treatment of the hypercalcaemia and/or renal disease.

Paget's Disease

Although Paget's disease is usually included with the metabolic bone disorders, it is not a generalised disorder of bone and there is increasing evidence that it may be of viral aetiology. Its incidence varies widely throughout the world. Paget's disease is almost unknown in Asiatic countries, but affects about 10% of the elderly population in Britain. Fortunately, in most people the disease is asymptomatic and is diagnosed by a chance finding on X-ray examination. The pelvis and lumbar vertebrae are most commonly involved. Usually only a part of one bone is affected and the abnormal area gradually increases in extent over the years. In severe cases there may be gross deformity and involvement of many bones.

The disorder starts as an area of intense but unco-ordinated bone remodelling. Giant osteoclasts are found on microscopic examination of the bone, and the lesion is predominantly lytic on X-ray film. As the disease progresses, the lytic areas become filled by an excess of bone that is

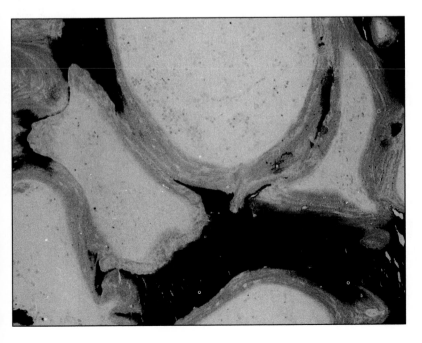

Figure 1.4 Photomicrograph of trabecular bone from a patient with osteomalacia. The mineralised bone is stained black. There is a great increase in the extent and thickness of grey unmineralised osteoid tissue. Normally, only a thin layer of osteoid covers about 20% of the bone surface.

irregularly laid down—this appears sclerotic on X-ray film—and new areas of lysis develop in the adjacent bone. The disorganised remodelling process often leads to expansion and deformity of the affected bone and an abnormal bony architecture (Figure 1.5). The remodelling disorder is reflected histologically by a mosaic pattern of cement lines (Figure 1.6). The normal demarcation between cortical and cancellous bone is lost, and, because much of the new tissue (woven bone) is weak, bowing and fracture of long bones may occur. Even without fracture the affected area may be the source of persistent pain. The most serious, but rare, complication is the development of a sarcoma in the pagetic bone. Such tumours are usually highly malignant, and survival is seldom longer than a year.

Treatment of Paget's disease is directed at stopping the abnormal osteoclastic activity. If this can be achieved, the remaining abnormal remodelling is usually prevented and the disease progression may be halted or even partially reversed. Drugs used in treatment include the hormone calcitonin and the group of agents known as bisphosphonates.

VASCULAR DISORDERS

Infarction, also termed avascular necrosis, is the most important vascular disorder of bone. It consists of the death of a region of bone following the interruption of its blood supply. In some cases, e.g. fracture of the femoral neck or sickle cell disease, there is a clear mechanism for

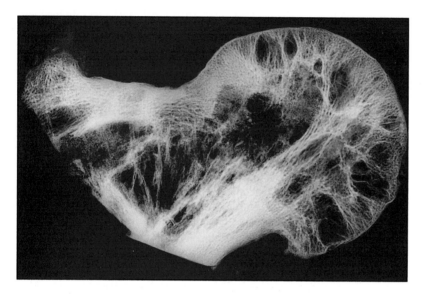

Figure 1.5 X-ray film of a slice through a femoral head in Paget's disease of bone. There is gross distortion of the trabecular bone architecture caused by the anarchic remodelling activity of Paget's disease.

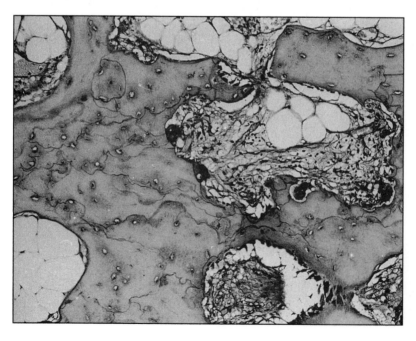

Figure 1.6 Photomicrograph of a bone biopsy from a patient with Paget's disease of bone. The five prominent black blobs on the bone surface represent abnormally large osteoclasts. The bone itself is crisscrossed by an irregular mosaic pattern of dark cement lines resulting from successive waves of bone resorption and formation.

the loss of blood supply; this also applies to tunnellers and divers, who may suffer multiple bone infarcts. In many patients, however, the pathogenesis is unknown, even though there may be a recognised association with other conditions, e.g. alcoholism or steroid treatment.

Many cases involving the shaft of the bone are asymptomatic and only discovered as incidental findings on X-ray examination. When the end of a bone, such as the femoral head, is affected, the necrotic bone collapses and, if untreated, secondary osteoarthritis may develop (Figure 1.7). A much rarer complication is the development of a sarcoma at the site of infarction.

TUMOURS OF BONE

By far the commonest form of tumour involving bone is metastatic carcinoma. This often involves multiple sites, and radioisotope scanning is the most efficient method of detecting the bone metastases. The most common primary sites for tumours metastatic to bone are breast, lung, thyroid, kidney and prostate. Most metastases destroy bone and appear lytic on X-ray film. Occasionally other tumours, but particularly prostatic metastases, cause bone sclerosis (Figure 1.8A and B).

Primary tumours of bone may be either benign or malignant and are classified according to their presumed cell of origin (Table 1.1). However, in some cases this may be uncertain and any classification will reflect areas of ignorance and controversy. Table 1.1 is by no means complete, but includes most of the important categories of bone tumour.

Most benign tumours tend to affect children and young adults. Malignant tumours, however, arise in middle-aged and elderly patients, except for Ewing's sarcoma, which is commonest in childhood, and osteosarcoma, which affects teenagers and young adults. Only a brief description of selected tumours follows.

Osteoblastic Tumours

Osteoid Osteoma

Osteoid osteoma produces a rounded mass of poorly formed osteoid trabeculae which never exceeds 2 cm in diameter. The tumour is often associated with persistent nagging pain. The surrounding bone reacts by becoming sclerosed; this may obscure the lesion on plain X-ray film, but shows as an intense hot spot on isotope scanning.

Benign Osteoblastoma

Benign osteoblastoma is similar in histology to the osteoid osteoma but is larger and lacks a sclerotic reaction. It occurs most frequently in the vertebral column, and complete removal may be difficult. Although benign, tumour recurrence following inadequate surgery may cause serious local problems.

Osteosarcoma

Osteosarcoma is the most important of the bone-forming tumours. It arises in the metaphyseal region of long bones, particularly the distal femur and proximal tibia (Figure 1.9). Although a tumour of osteoblasts, the amount of mineralised bone produced is variable and X-ray films show a

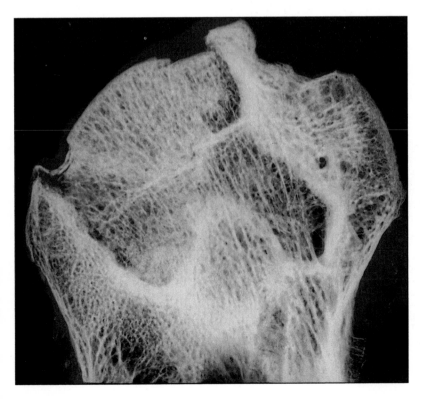

Figure 1.7 X-ray film of a slice through a femoral head affected by avascular necrosis. The area of infarction is bordered by a broad white zone of reactive, sclerotic, new bone formation. The necrotic bone has collapsed, causing discontinuity of the articular surface. This would have led to osteoarthritis if left undisturbed.

mixed pattern of lysis and sclerosis. Tumour growth is rapid and aggressive, and early invasion through the cortex produces a soft tissue mass. Even when impalpable on clinical examination, this soft tissue extension is usually visible on X-ray film and is well seen on magnetic resonance scanning images.

Although osteosarcoma may present at any age, it is predominantly a tumour of teenagers and young adults. Most such tumours arise spontaneously, but in older people osteosarcoma may arise following radiotherapy to the affected site or as a complication of Paget's disease of bone (see page 7). The long-term prognosis is not good, but 5-year survival has improved with a combination of aggressive chemotherapy and either amputation or prosthetic replacement of the affected bone.

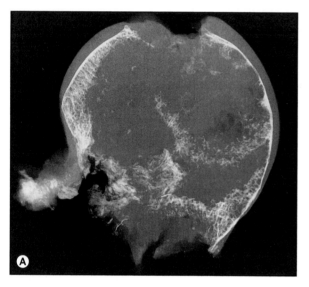 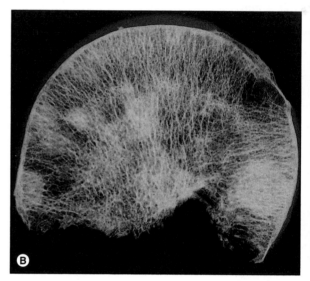

Figure 1.8 X-ray films of slices through two femoral heads with lytic (A) and sclerotic (B) metastases. Both patients suffered from carcinoma of the breast.

Table 1.1 Classification of primary bone tumours.

Classification of primary bone tumours		
Cell type	**Benign**	**Malignant**
Osteoblast	Osteoid osteoma Benign osteoblastoma	Osteosarcoma
Chondrocyte	Enchondroma Chondroblastoma Osteochondroma (exostosis)	Chondrosarcoma
Fibroblast	Fibrous cortical defect Non-ossifying fibroma	Fibrosarcoma Malignant fibrous histiocytoma
Marrow	Plasmacytoma Eosinophilic granuloma	Multiple myeloma Lymphoma
Vascular	Haemangioma	Haemangioendothelioma Angiosarcoma
Notochord		Chordoma
Unknown	Giant cell tumour (osteoclastoma)	Ewing's tumour Adamantinoma

Cartilaginous Tumours

Osteochondromas (Exostoses)

Osteochondromas—or exostoses as they are often known—may be single or multiple. Multiple osteochondromas are inherited as a Mendelian dominant condition. The tumour is essentially a defect of bone development, and consists of a bony lump with a cap of cartilage. The lump protrudes from the bone surface and continues to grow until skeletal maturity, at which point the cartilage cap becomes completely ossified and only the bony mass remains. Surgery is necessary for cosmetic reasons or for symptoms caused by local pressure effects. Because of a small risk of malignant change, excision is also recommended if an osteochondroma recommences growth or becomes painful in adult life.

Enchondromas

Enchondromas are composed entirely of cartilage. They are most frequent in the small bones of the hands and feet (Figure 1.10). They also may be single or multiple, but, unlike multiple exostoses, multiple enchondromas are not inherited. The condition of multiple enchondromas, or enchondromatosis, is known as Ollier's disease or, when combined with soft tissue haemangiomas, as Maffucci's syndrome.

Chondrosarcomas

Malignant transformation of an enchondroma into a chondrosarcoma happens more frequently than in cases of exostosis, but is still rare. Not surprisingly, malignant change is more common in patients with Ollier's disease (see above) because of the increased number of tumours at risk, but it is still unusual. However, in Maffucci's syndrome, malignant disease occurs in about one third of patients, either as chondrosarcomatous change in a chondroma or as tumours arising in other organs.

Chondrosarcomas may arise in any part of the skeleton and at any age, but are most frequent in the middle-aged and elderly. They usually arise *de novo*, but, as indicated above, may be secondary to pre-existing lesions. Radiologically, they

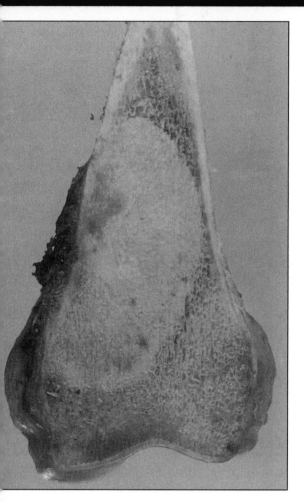

Figure 1.9 Slice through the lower end of the femur of a young adult. The dense white area in the metaphysis corresponds to bone formed by an osteosarcoma. This would have appeared as a sclerotic area on X-ray film.

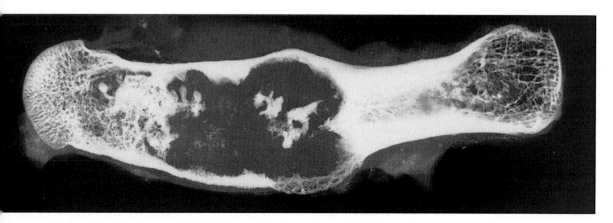

Figure 1.10 X-ray film of a slice of metacarpal containing a cartilaginous tumour. The tumour is both destroying and expanding the bone, and contains areas of calcification.

appear as expanding osteolytic lesions with areas of calcification. They are usually slowly growing tumours, and metastasis occurs late if at all. Because of this, a cure is possible if a correct diagnosis is made at first presentation and the tumour is excised completely; otherwise, recurrent tumours may be difficult to remove in their entirety and death may result from local invasion or late metastasis.

Fibrous Tumours
Fibrous Cortical Defect
Fibrous cortical defect is very common as an incidental X-ray finding in children and resolves spontaneously.

Non-ossifying Fibroma
Non-ossifying fibroma is a very similar but larger lesion than fibrous cortical defect, that fails to resolve and continues growing. It may be the cause of pathological fracture. Cure is effected by simple curettage and, if necessary, bone grafting.

Malignant Fibrous Histiocytoma
Malignant fibrous histiocytoma is a recently described tumour occurring most often in elderly people. It is composed of a mixture of cells with fibroblastic and histiocytic (macrophagic) characteristics. It is usually of high-grade malignancy and metastasises early. Some tumours respond to chemotherapy.

Fibrosarcoma
Fibrosarcoma is closely related to malignant fibrous histiocytoma but lacks a histiocytic element. Many tumours are comparatively low grade and the prognosis is correspondingly better.

Tumours of Unknown Origin
Giant Cell Tumour of Bone (Osteoclastoma)
Giant cell tumour of bone contains numerous osteoclastic giant cells and is also known as osteoclastoma. However, the predominant cell type in this tumour is a mononuclear cell of uncertain origin. It never occurs in a bone that is still growing and it always involves the epiphyseal region of the bone. Like osteosarcoma, it is common in the distal femur and proximal tibia. Unlike osteosarcoma, it is benign. It is almost always cured by complete excision, and metastases are extremely rare and may themselves often be cured by surgery alone.

Ewing's Sarcoma
Ewing's sarcoma is also of unknown cell origin. It is commonest in children but can occur in adults. It used to be rapidly fatal, with widespread metastases, but some improvement in survival has been achieved by modern chemotherapy.

Marrow Tumours
Eosinophilic Granuloma (Langerhans' Cell Granulomatosis)
Eosinophilic granuloma is derived from cells related to the macrophage family, known as Langerhans' cells. It is usually a solitary tumour presenting in childhood. Many cases undergo spontaneous resolution and, provided there is no risk of pathological fracture, may be treated conservatively. Otherwise, simple curettage or low-dose radiotherapy may suffice. Unfortunately, some patients have a progressive form of the disease with involvement of multiple bones and these granulomas may require chemotherapy. When this occurs with pulmonary and pituitary involvement it is known as Hand–Schüller–Christian disease. A rare, widely disseminated form of the disease in infancy (Letterer–Siwe disease) is usually rapidly fatal.

The above diseases are sometimes grouped together under the heading of Langerhans' cell granulomatosis.

Multiple Myeloma
Multiple myeloma, a neoplastic proliferation of plasma cells, is the commonest malignant tumour of bone. It is seen on X-ray film as numerous lytic lesions throughout the skeleton. In the skull it produces the characteristic 'pepper-pot' appearance. All the malignant cells secrete the same abnormal immunoglobulin molecule, which is seen as a monoclonal band on serum electrophoresis. Complications include the development of systemic amyloidosis and renal failure. The malignant cells crowd out the normal antibody-producing cells of the marrow and as a result the immunocompromised patient is at a high risk of death from infection.

JOINTS

Disease of joints may be conveniently considered as osteoarthritis, rheumatoid arthritis, infective arthritis and metabolic arthritis.

OSTEOARTHRITIS
Osteoarthritis, sometimes inaccurately known as degenerative arthritis, is the commonest joint disease. Most cases are of unknown aetiology, but some are secondary to other disorders of the joint or neighbouring bone. Osteoarthritis is common in weight-bearing joints, and its prevalence increases steeply in patients after 50 years of age. In some patients there is probably a genetic component to the initiation or progression of the disease process. In most patients, progression is unrelenting once significant damage to the articular cartilage has occurred (Dieppe, 1995).

The first changes seen in osteoarthritis are degeneration and fissuring of the articular cartilage. This progresses to loss of cartilage and exposure of the subchondral bone—recognised by diminution of joint space on X-ray film. The altered stresses on the bone caused by this loss of cartilage lead to disturbance of the normal bone remodelling activity. The exposed bone becomes sclerotic. Localised areas of fibrous replacement of bone are seen as 'cysts' on X-ray film. Elsewhere—usually at the joint margin—excess production of bone forms osteophytes, and the whole contour of the joint surface is distorted (Figure 1.11).

RHEUMATOID ARTHRITIS

Unlike osteoarthritis, where the first signs of the disease process are in the articular cartilage, rheumatoid arthritis starts as an inflammation of the synovial membrane (Palmer, 1995). In the early stages, this inflammation causes thickening of the synovium, which, together with a fluid exudate into the joint cavity, is evident as painful swelling of the joints on clinical examination and an increase of the joint space on X-ray film. Later, this inflamed synovial tissue erodes the cartilage and bone at the joint margin. This is recognised on X-ray film by the presence of marginal erosions, one of the diagnostic hallmarks of rheumatoid arthritis. The inflamed tissue, now referred to as pannus, then spreads over the joint surface, progressively destroying the articular cartilage. If untreated, and particularly if immobilisation of the joint is allowed to occur, the layers of pannus on opposing joint surfaces fuse to form a fibrous ankylosis of the joint.

In addition to these changes, the intra-articular ligaments, joint capsule and tendons may all be involved in the inflammatory process, leading to weakening, rupture or fibrosis of these structures. It is the combination of these articular and para-articular changes that leads to the characteristic deformities seen in advanced rheumatoid arthritis.

Although its most obvious manifestation is damage to joints, rheumatoid arthritis may also be regarded as a systemic disease. In approximately 20% of patients, rheumatoid nodules develop in the subcutaneous tissues. They are usually seen in the subcutaneous tissue of the extensor surfaces of the elbows or hands, but may rarely involve other organs. Patients with nodules tend to have severe disease and some go on to develop potentially fatal vasculitis.

INFECTIVE ARTHRITIS

Acute infective arthritis is a rare complication of infection elsewhere in the body. Unless diagnosis and treatment are rapid, the disease may progress within a few days to extensive destruction of the articular cartilage and subchondral bone. This is followed inevitably by the development of secondary osteoarthritis.

Chronic infective arthritis may result from infection by organisms of low virulence or be tuberculous in origin.

METABOLIC ARTHRITIS

The principal metabolic cause of joint disease is gout. Gout is a disorder of purine metabolism, and most patients have a raised serum urate concentration. Periodically, precipitation of urate crystals in the synovial fluid causes an acute inflammatory reaction with swelling and severe pain. The diagnosis can be confirmed by identification of urate crystals in the joint fluid by microscopical examination using polarised light.

A second type of crystal, calcium pyrophosphate dihydrate, may be distinguished by its different pattern of polarisation. In many patients it seems to have little effect but in others it may cause a painful pseudogout, and in yet others it is associated with a severe form of osteoarthritis.

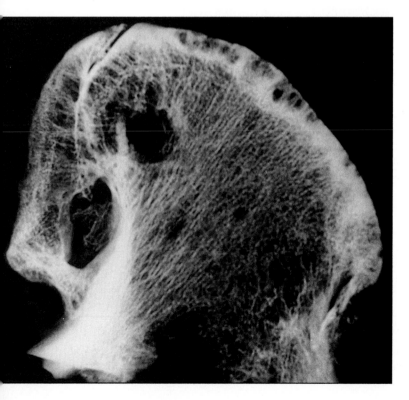

Figure 1.11 X-ray film of a slice through an osteoarthritic femoral head. The articular surface is misshapen and there is a large osteophyte on the left. The subchondral bone is sclerotic and contains several small cystic areas.

Arthritis may also be found in association with the inherited metabolic diseases ochronosis and haemochromatosis.

JOINT REPLACEMENT

Prosthetic replacements of the hip and knee joints are now routine operations, due to the pioneering work of the British surgeon, Sir John Charnley. Unfortunately, some of these prostheses eventually become loose and replacement of the artificial joint is needed by revision surgery. In a small proportion of patients this loosening is due to infection (see Figure 1.2) but in most it is the long-term result of wear of the prosthesis and of the cement holding the prosthesis in position. Initially, cement was thought to be the main culprit and a variety of uncemented prostheses were designed. However, these also become loose. It is now apparent that any sort of wear particle, be it cement, polyethylene, metal etc. can initiate an inflammatory reaction that stimulates resorption of the surrounding bone. Current research is targeted at preventing this resorption of bone and at delaying wear by improving the design of prostheses.

REFERENCES

Beighton P, Giedion ZA, Gorlin R et al. International classification of osteochondrodysplasias. Am J Med Genet 1992, **44**:223-229.

Cormack DH. Bone. In: Ham's histology. Philadelphia: JB Lippincott; 1987:273-323.

Dieppe P. Osteoarthritis and molecular markers—a rheumatologist's perspective. Acta Orthop Scand 1995, **266**:1-5.

Eriksen EF, Langdahl B. Bone changes in metabolic bone disease. Acta Orthop Scand 1995, **266**:195-201.

Lanyon LE. Control of bone architecture by functional load bearing. J Bone Miner Res 1992, **7**(Suppl. 2):S369-375.

MacDonald BR, Gowen M. The cell biology of bone. Baillières Clin Rheumatol 1993, **7**:421-443.

Palmer DG. The anatomy of the rheumatoid lesion. Br Med Bull 1995, **51**:286-295.

Sevitt S. Bone repair and fracture healing in man. Edinburgh: Churchill Livingstone; 1981.

GENERAL READING

Bullough PG. Orthopaedic pathology, 3rd ed. London: Mosby-Wolfe; 1996.

Creamer P, Hochberg M.C. Ostcoarthritis. Lancet 1997, **350**:503-508

Kraus VB. Pathogenesis and treatment of ostcoarthritis. Medical Clinics of North America 1997, **81**:85-112.

Unni KK. Dahlin's bone tumors, 5th ed. Phildadelphia: Lippincott-Raven; 1986.

Salisbury JR, Woods CG, Byers PD. Diseases of bones and joints. London: Chapman and Hall; 1994.

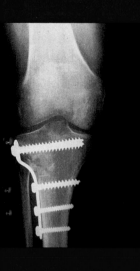

2 P B M Thomas

FRACTURES - CLINICAL

CHAPTER OUTLINE

- **Fractures**
- **Fracture healing**
- **Fracture treatment**
- **Maintenance of reduction**

- **Complications that affect the bone**
- **Complications that affect the limb**
- **Complications that affect the patient**

INTRODUCTION

The word fracture is used to describe any kind of mechanical damage produced in a bone. The damage may range from an undisplaced crack to complete disruption and shattering of a whole bone. While some fractures are so minimal that they cannot even be detected on normal X-ray, others are so gross that their presence is obvious from the deformed appearance of the limb. The force required to produce a fracture varies greatly from one person to another; for example, the femur of a fit athlete may momentarily withstand loads in excess of 100 times the athelete's body weight, while that of an elderly patient who is chairbound may fracture as the person attempts to walk. There are many interrelated factors which determine the strength of bone, and as people age and become inactive their bones become progressively weaker.

SOME USEFUL TERMS

Delayed union: A fracture which has not united in the expected time.

Non-union: A delayed union which appears likely to continue indefinitely.

Atrophic non-union: A non-union in which the bone ends look inert and often tapered.

Hypertrophic non-union: A non-union in which each bone end is surrounded by abundant callus, but the callus has not bridged the gap. It 'wants to unite', whereas the atrophic non-union does not.

Infected non-union: Usually the result of a compound fracture or unsuccessful internal fixation.

Union: The moment when a healing fracture is thought to be strong enough not to refracture.

Malunion: A fracture that has united in the wrong position. There may be rotational malunion, angulatory malunion, shortening or a step in an articular surface.

Fibrous union: A fracture will sometimes heal with fibrous scar tissue bridging the gap. It may be quite solid, but once it is established it will not proceed to bony union.

Pseudarthrosis: Sometimes, gross movement will continue at a fracture site, producing a mobile non-union which is effectively a false joint.

Osteotomy: A planned surgical fracture, usually designed to correct a bony deformity.

Arthrodesis: Bony union which occurs across a joint. It is usually the planned result of surgery, but used to occur in untreated joint infections, particularly tuberculous. It is achieved by the same process as fracture healing.

Callotasis: A technique often used to correct malunions or non-unions. A fresh callus response is started, usually by cutting through the cortex of the bone, and the deformity is then corrected using an external fixator to progressively stretch the callus as it forms.

FRACTURES

MECHANISM OF INJURY

The way in which a bone fractures is often related to the way in which force is applied. The footballer who receives a kick on the shin may well sustain a transverse fracture of the tibia, but the torsional force applied when a skier falls with faulty bindings may result in a long spiral fracture of the tibia and fibula. The cat burglar, unexpectedly disturbed, may fracture both calanei when he jumps from a first-floor window, while the house owner who punches him sustains a fracture of the right fifth metacarpal. Some fractures may even be produced by the violent contraction of a muscle. These avulsion fractures were once seen in patients who received electroconvulsive therapy, and they still occur occasionally in patients with epilepsy and in athletes.

Just as the type of fracture may indicate the mechanism of injury, so the description of a certain type of accident will suggest the possibility of a particular fracture.

DIAGNOSIS

Röentgen's discovery in 1895 revolutionised the treatment of fractures to the extent that almost all fractures are now recognised and treated by reference to X-rays. Before the discovery of X-rays, fractures were diagnosed by examination and categorised by the dissection of amputated limbs and cadavers (Figure 2.1). We sometimes forget the importance of taking a careful history of the accident, but the history will often reveal a mechanism which is known to cause a certain type of fracture. Gentle examination will reveal swelling and tenderness around a fracture and may also reveal deformity or a wound. Most fractures are associated with some degree of damage to other structures, and a careful examination will confirm or exclude abnormalities of the vascular or nerve supply. An examination will also help in deciding which X-ray view to request. X-rays assess the bone from one direction only and a fracture may therefore be missed on a poorly planned X-ray. It is only the fracture lines that run perpendicular to the X-ray plate which show clearly, so most bones are X-rayed in two planes at right angles to each other.

Occasionally, a radioisotope bone scan will reveal a fracture which cannot be seen on X-ray. Scaphoid fractures are sometimes detected in this way. If a fracture has occurred through a carcinomatous deposit, then an isotope scan may reveal other deposits in the skeleton. Tomograms are X-rays taken with a moving tube and plate which blur everything except the structures at the centre of their rotation. This technique produces 'cuts' in different planes through the bone and will sometimes demonstrate a fracture which does not show clearly on a conventional X-ray.

Computerised axial tomography, or CT, uses X-rays which are the basis for computer-reconstructed sections through the body; this is often helpful in delineating complex fractures, and 3-dimensional pictures can be reconstructed by the CT scanner software. The images can be manipulated on the screen, allowing accurate pre-operative planning of the internal fixation of complex fractures, such as those involving the pelvis and acetabulum. It will soon be possible to rehearse the internal fixation of a complex fracture in a virtual reality containing the CT images of the fractured bone as well as those of the screws and plates required to fix it.

When an injured joint is aspirated, liquid marrow fat is sometimes found floating on the surface of the blood and synovial fluid. This indicates that there is a fracture line running into an articular surface.

A fresh fracture is usually exceedingly painful, so examination and X-rays must be performed with great care.

PATHOLOGY OF FRESH FRACTURES

Although most fractures are recognised by the pattern of bony damage seen on X-ray, bone is only one of the many structures which may be disrupted. The amount of damage sustained by soft tissues is roughly proportional to the degree of force. If a force were slowly applied to a bone until it cracked, the surrounding tissue would sustain

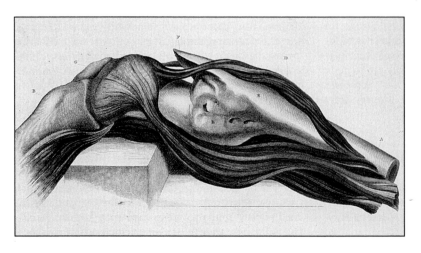

Figure 2.1 Dissection of a femoral fracture. Taken from Sir Astley Cooper's treatise, *Fractures and dislocations* (1824). The healed fracture shows that the patient survived the injury, but the malunion would have shortened the leg and interfered with the quadriceps muscle.

inimal damage. This is mostly because the bone would ot have continued deforming after the fracture had ccurred. Unfortunately, most force which results in a fracture will continue after the bone breaks. The X-ray is thus nly the 'last frame of a movie' in which the bone ends ere displaced during the accident and have returned to a osition of equilibrium. If a motorcyclist hit a car at 80 ıph and sustained a fractured femur, the 'movie' might ave shown that his leg flailed and twisted wildly during ıe accident, although at the end it looked approximately g-shaped again. This violent distortion of tissues causes retching and tearing of all the structures around the bone. he periosteum covering the bone will tear first, and may e stripped back for some distance. Muscle will be retched, bruised or sliced by sharp bone ends, and nerves ıd blood vessels may be contused or torn. An artery which ppears to be in continuity may still not conduct blood ecause of damage to the intimal lining, and nerves not tually divided may cease to function for several months hile an axonotmesis recovers.

Finally, the bone ends may become covered in road dirt grass. All this occurs in the short space of time before astic recoil brings the tissues to rest.

The initial zone of damage may be quite extensive ıd during the first few days after injury the zone of ımage appears to increase. Severely traumatised muse will die immediately, but less severely damaged tisıe will begin to swell as the inflammatory phase of ›aling begins. Skin which was stretched during the .jury may develop 'fracture' blisters after a day or two, ıd skin that looked reasonable to begin with may subquently become black and dead.

Fractures with a wound in the skin are called 'comund', and those without are called 'closed', but a high-veloc- closed fracture may still be surrounded by more tissue mage than a low-velocity compound fracture. As a rough ıide to treatment, compound fractures are graded as:

Grade I, wound <2 cm.
Grade II, wound >2 cm.
Grade III, severe soft tissue damage. Grade III compound ractures are further subdivided according to the degree f tissue loss or contamination.

HYSIOLOGY OF BONE

one is a remarkable tissue. Although it appears inert, its rious components are removed and replaced continuısly, so that the whole skeleton is effectively renewed ery few years.

Bone is designed to withstand stress and, in fact, rives on it; normal or physiological stresses stimulate ne to remain strong. New bone is laid down in response stress and this phenomenon, described as Wolfe's Law, counts in part for the ingenious structure of bones. If the ttern of stress changes, then the bone will slowly remodel accommodate it—the body is very economical. If the ess on a bone is reduced, then it will become weaker as ineral and bone matrix are taken away. This disuse teopenia is seen in astronauts who have spent time in

weightless conditions and, more commonly, in people confined to bed. The bone mineral is sometimes removed so quickly that a patient may develop kidney stones of calcium after a few weeks in bed. Overstressing bone may also cause trouble. Athletes and soldiers on long marches may repeatedly stress bones beyond their physiological limit, causing weakening and an eventual stress fracture. This is unusual, however, and bone, like most tissue, is maintained by use.

FRACTURE HEALING

Fracture healing occurs by two distinct processes which happen sequentially. The first is the callus response and the second is remodelling. In normal physiological bone healing, the callus response occurs in the first few weeks and continues for a few months, while remodelling begins over a few months and continues for several years.

THE CALLUS RESPONSE

Bones are structural and the callus response is nicely designed to re-establish structural strength as quickly as possible. The fresh fracture is initially surrounded by a haematoma and by the remains of damaged tissues, such as periosteum and muscle. Over the first few days this begins to become organised by the influx of specialised cells, and within a week or two, callus begins to appear. On X-ray, the callus is first seen as a faint fluffy opacity surrounding the fracture but lying outside the original boundaries of the bone. As the strength of a tube is proportional to its diameter, by forming outside the bone this shell of callus is well suited to hold the ends of the fracture steady.

Callus is made of immature woven bone and does not have the sophisticated structure of mature bone. As the purpose of callus is to prevent relative movements of the bone ends, it continues to form only until it is strong enough to prevent that movement. The production of callus is therefore initiated and maintained by movement. If there is no movement at all, then no callus will form, but if movement continues, then the blob of callus will carry on growing in an attempt to stop it. If the agitated patient, insensate from a head injury, shakes his or her fractured femur around on traction, a huge ball of callus will form; but if a fracture is held rigidly with a plate or fixator, then callus will not appear at all. This paradox of fracture treatment will be enlarged upon later.

Callus is a 'one-off' response. If it does not occur within a few weeks of injury, it will not occur at all, and movement later on will not induce it to appear (Figure 2.2).

REMODELLING

Once the movement at the fracture ends has been brought to rest by callus, the slower process of remodelling begins. The process is the same as that which reshapes bone to respond to changing patterns of load. Mature bone is made up of lamellae and interlaced by the microscopic tubules of the Haversian system. Osteons are organised groups of cells which move through the bone, constantly removing and replacing it. By the same process, the woven bone formed

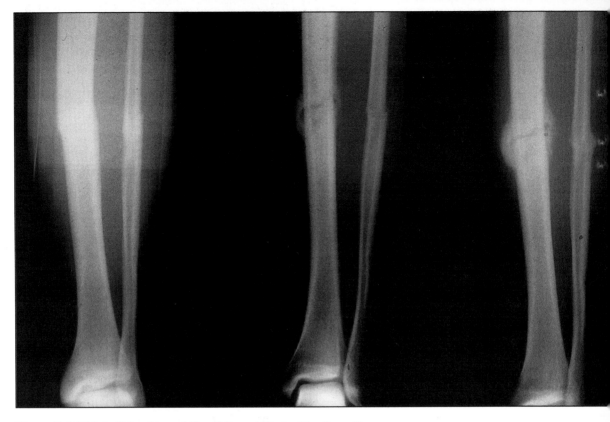

Figure 2.2 Midshaft fracture of the tibia and fibula. The X-ray films were taken on the day of the injury, and at intervals of 4 weeks. An almost spherical blob of callus has formed.

in the callus phase is also slowly replaced by mature bone. The callus response is directed by quite gross movement, which it ultimately controls. The remodelling process is directed by the pattern of stress distribution and ultimately redistributes stress to optimise the strength of the bone. Although the site of a freshly healed fracture is quite obvious on X-ray, the fusiform swelling in the bone steadily remodels so that an X-ray taken several years later may show no obvious abnormality at all.

There is no definite moment of fracture union. The strength of a healing fracture continues to increase to an arbitrary point at which the clinician feels that the risk of refracture is very low. The ability to define a suitable end point is based on experience, using information such as the time from fracture, the X-ray appearance, the clinical feel of the limb and the presence or absence of pain. It is a quality judgement.

Definitions of fracture healing based on stiffness measurements are already used in research and are beginning to be useful clinically. These techniques may eventually improve the informed clinical guess. Plaster, external fixation and traction are usually left on for too long. This is because the surgeon does not want the patient's fracture to deform, and tends to play it safe. Until there are reliable methods of determining when a bone has healed to the point where it will not bend or refracture, fractures wi continue to be treated for too long.

PRIMARY BONE HEALING

This process probably only occurs in undisplaced fracture or in artificial situations created by surgery.

Sir John Charnley discovered that a fresh osteotom through cancellous bone can be made to heal very rapidl by compressing the cut surfaces together with a clamp Unfortunately, this observation was erroneously extrape lated to support the practice of plating the midshaft fra tures of long bones. The Arbeitsgemeinschaft fi Osteosynthesenfragen (AO) group, which was formed i Switzerland by Müller and his colleagues, set out to devel a properly engineered system for the internal fixation of fractures. The plates they designed have holes of a comple shape which allow compression of the fracture surfaces a the screws are tightened. These dynamic compressic plates (DCP) can produce very rigid internal fixation. So el gant was the system, and so persuasive the group's arg ments, that it was quickly taken up throughout the world

There is no doubt that the perfect reduction of certa fractures, such as those involving joints, is beneficial. The is also no doubt that the rigid fixation of fractures allows f early movement of joints, which reduces stiffness ar swelling. Rigid fixation is a necessity to prevent metal fatigue and failure of the plate, but it abolishes the callus response.

The appearance of callus following plating is then taken to indicate movement due to inadequate surgical technique. To the Swiss, callus was anathema. The healing which occurs without callus in a rigidly plated long bone fracture was called primary bone healing. It is probably the same mechanism as remodelling and only progresses slowly across the devitalised bone ends. A plate must therefore last as long as the callus which it prevented, and a plate failure may result in a non-union. Primary bone healing is therefore the second phase of physiological healing, artificially separated from the first phase (Figure 2.3).

FRACTURE TREATMENT

The aim of all orthopaedic treatment is to restore function and to minimise deformity. Immediately before their injury, most patients have full function and no deformity. They have rightly come to expect complete recovery, and the demands of modern fracture treatment are therefore very exacting. The management of fractures consists of pain relief followed by painless reduction, and the maintenance of reduction in a way which does not interfere with bone healing or subsequent function (Figure 2.4).

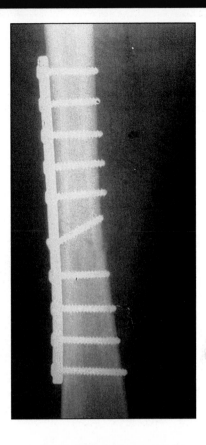

Figure 2.3 Rigidly plated fracture of the femur. After 4 months there is no callus. The plate must now survive for another year to allow healing by remodelling.

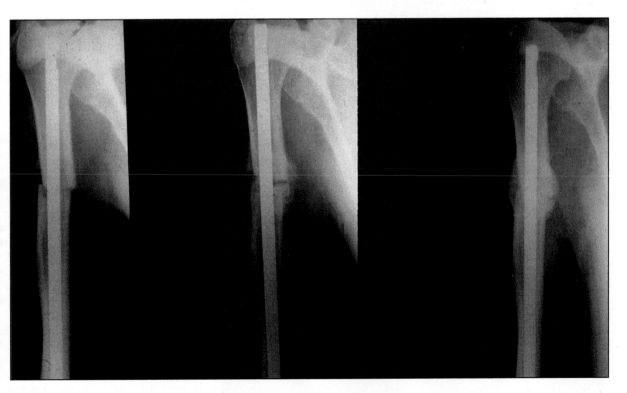

Figure 2.4 Humeral fracture treated with an intramedullary Küntscher nail. The X-ray films were taken after 2 days, 4 weeks and 12 weeks, and show good callus production due to the limited movement permitted by the nail.

REDUCTION

Many fractures are minimally displaced and do not require reduction, but most displaced fractures must either be manipulated or reduced at operation. Accurate manipulation is a subtle skill. Success depends on understanding the mechanism of injury and on taking advantage of the mechanical effect of undamaged soft tissue structures. Undamaged periosteum may act as a 'soft tissue hinge', helping in reducing and holding fractures. This is probably the most useful thing for the manipulator to bear in mind.

OPEN REDUCTION

We know from experience that certain fractures cannot be reduced properly by closed manipulation. We also know that certain fractures will definitely require internal fixation, but some of these are still worth manipulating. If a fractured part is badly deformed, it will not only be extremely painful but will also rapidly develop soft tissue problems. If a badly displaced ankle fracture is left unreduced for a few hours, the skin stretched over the broken fragments may slough, but a timely manipulation will save the skin and will allow an open reduction to be performed later.

There is a wide spectrum of fracture treatment, from the Colles' fracture in an elderly patient, which is almost invariably treated by closed manipulation, to the midshaft fracture of the radius and ulna, which is almost always fixed internally. Each fracture must be judged individually and in its relation to other injuries. Open reduction is almost always combined with some form of internal fixation (Figure 2.5A and B).

Some fractures that are best treated conservatively in isolation are often fixed if they occur in a multiply injured patient. For instance, an isolated fracture of the midshaft of the humerus can usually be treated by a simple hanging cast and a collar and cuff sling. The weight of the arm and cast holds the fracture reduced for the 6 weeks or so that it takes to unite. However, a simple midshaft fracture of the humerus associated with other skeletal injuries will usually be fixed, as in the patient shown in Figure 2.4, who had several other injuries. The fixation of all fractures in multiply injured patients has been shown to reduce mortality if the fixation can be done early. It is easier to nurse the multiply injured patient unencumbered by plaster of Paris or traction, and early fixation of the fractures

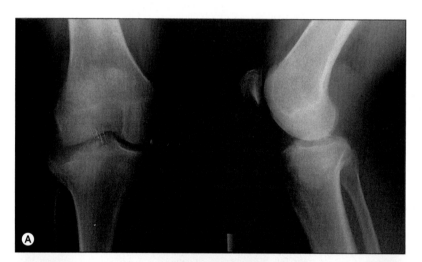

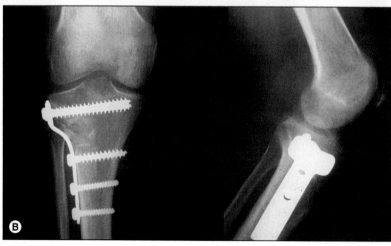

Figure 2.5 (A) Depressed lateral tibial plateau fracture in a pedestrian struck on the lateral side of the knee by a car bumper. (B) The plateau was elevated and held with a cancellous bone graft from the iliac crest; a plate and screws hold the fracture and bone graft in place.

can prevent a malunion occurring unnoticed in an unconscious patient with serious life-threatening problems.

MAINTENANCE OF REDUCTION

When planning treatment it is useful to decide whether a fracture is stable, metastable or unstable. A stable fracture is one that is unlikely to displace, even if left unsplinted. Most undisplaced fractures fall into this category, and they are usually treated with some form of splintage or protection to relieve pain.

Metastable fractures are those which require reduction, but which will then remain stable provided certain movements are limited by external splintage. For instance, in a midshaft tibial fracture, a long leg plaster of Paris cast can control angulation and rotation, but cannot prevent the fracture from shortening. A metastable tibial fracture would be one that cannot shorten under normal weight bearing, provided rotation and angulation are prevented by a plaster.

Unstable fractures are those that cannot be maintained in a reduced position by plaster or splintage. These are usually best treated by external or internal fixation, although some unstable fractures are still treated by traction.

PLASTER OF PARIS

Plaster of Paris has good properties as a splinting material. It is easily applied, remains soft for a few minutes and then suddenly sets hard. When set it is easily cut with a saw and will withstand much patient abuse. It is radiolucent and may be repaired easily by adding extra layers. It also provides a perfect white surface for graffiti! There is danger in a plaster which completely encloses a freshly injured limb, as it will not expand to allow for swelling. The initial plaster is therefore applied as a slab or a cylinder which is split to allow expansion. It may be safely completed to a full plaster after a few days. The position of a fracture may be adjusted after a few weeks by plaster wedging, and windows may be cut out of the plaster for access to wounds. There are several synthetic casting materials, such as Scotchcast and Baycast. These tend to be lighter in weight than plaster of Paris, but are more difficult to apply and more expensive.

Conventional plaster treatment has the disadvantage of immobilising joints. Movement of joints has a beneficial effect on blood and lymph flow, reduces swelling, maintains muscle tone and bone strength, and circulates synovial fluid, which nourishes articular cartilage. Prolonged plaster immobilisation tends to maintain swelling and causes muscle wasting, stiff joints and osteopenia.

TRACTION

The unopposed pull of muscles tends to prevent reduction of long bone fractures. Traction counteracts this pull and straightens out the bone. It is used mostly in fractures of the femur, tibia and cervical spine, but may also be used in supracondylar humeral fractures (Dunlop traction). It allows for early movement of certain joints.

EXTERNAL FIXATION

Threaded pins are screwed into holes drilled into the bone via small incisions in the skin. The pins on each side of the fracture are then joined externally by a bar on which there are mechanisms to allow for adjustment. Once the fracture is reduced, the mechanism is tightened to maintain the reduction (Figure 2.6).

External fixators have the advantage of leaving the skin uncovered. This allows access to areas of tissue loss where further surgery or repeated dressings may be required. Because only the fractured bone is immobilised, the joints may be kept supple and the position of the fracture may be readjusted at any time.

External fixation is useful in multiple fractures, as the fractures may be immobilised, the joints may be kept supple and the position of the fracture may be readjusted at any time. Fractures may be immobilised relatively quickly to allow for soft tissue surgery, e.g. vessel repair. External fixation is easiest to use on subcutaneous bones, such as the tibia. On deep bones, like the femur, the pins must pass through muscle, which sometimes becomes

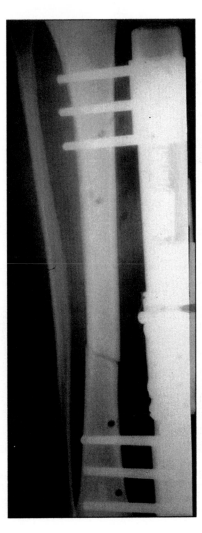

Figure 2.6 Controlled angular motion external fixator maintains reduction in a fracture of the tibia and fibula.

tethered. This can limit joint movement, cause pain and result in infection passing down the pin tracks.

External fixators can be designed to allow a certain amount of movement in a fracture. The ideal external fixator is strong enough to allow full activity without losing reduction of the fracture, and yet allows a small amount of movement in the fracture to maximise the early growth of healing callus. An external fixator may also be used to monitor the movement in a healing fracture. This allows us to determine healing more accurately, and to detect whether a fracture is healing at the desired rate.

INTERNAL FIXATION

The advantage of internal fixation is that even complex fractures may be anatomically reduced and held. The great disadvantage is that periosteum and other tissues are damaged while gaining surgical access to the fracture. Healing may be compromised by rigid fixation, and closed fractures are turned into compound ones.

Although these considerations must be carefully weighed before deciding to operate, there is no doubt that, in expert hands, internal fixation has revolutionised the treatment of many types of fracture. Fractures of the radius and ulna, intertrochanteric fractures of the femur, and femoral shaft fractures are now almost always treated by internal fixation (Figure 2.7A, B and C), and the accurate reduction of intra-articular fractures cannot be achieved by any other means. Probably every type of fracture has been treated somewhere by internal fixation, but as with all surgery the ability to perform an operation is not necessarily its indication (Figure 2.8A and B).

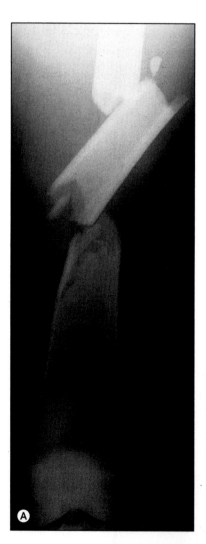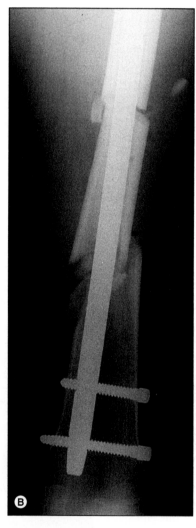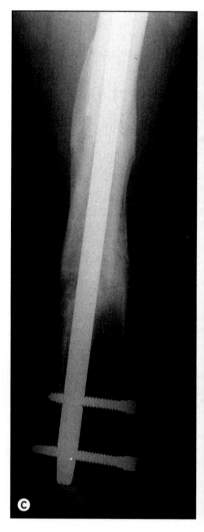

Figure 2.7 (A) Segmental fracture of the femur held with an interlocking intramedullary nail. (B) This second X-ray film was taken immediately after the operation. **(C)** This X-ray film, taken 18 months later, shows that the healed fracture has begun to remodel.

FUNCTIONAL BRACING

This is really just a conceptual shift in plaster of Paris treatment which allows for improved joint mobility.

Sarmiento pointed out that most fractures will not displace any further than the initial displacement caused by the injury. In selected cases, therefore, it is possible to design a cast which allows joints to move but prevents the fracture from displacing too much. Most functional braces employ hinges across joints and rely on the hydraulic effect of soft tissues confined in a cylinder or cone of plaster to control the fracture. Although considered a conservative option, it requires constant vigilance. Like all techniques, when new it was applied to everything, but now it has found its place in tibial fractures and some femoral fractures. A femoral functional brace can be a useful adjunct to internal fixation around the knee, where some protection is required but movement is desirable.

PAIN

Fractures are extremely painful and movement of a fresh fracture may be excruciating. There is hardly ever any reason to manipulate a fracture without proper regional or general anaesthesia. Once a fracture has been reduced and held, the severe pain will be relieved and replaced by a dull ache. Severe pain following reduction is a warning that something is wrong; it is usually caused by ischaemic muscle which has lost its blood supply because of arterial damage, compartment syndrome or a tight plaster. These problems are quite common and must be rectified quickly to prevent disaster. They are discussed in more detail later.

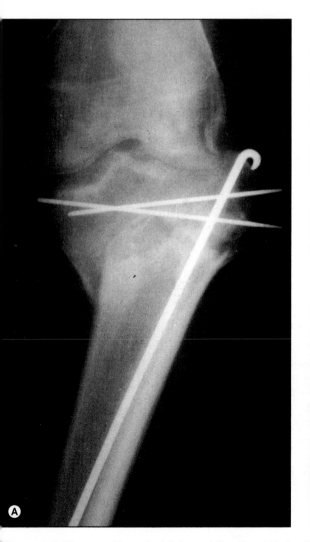

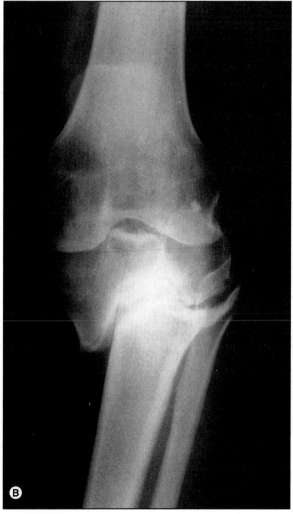

Figure 2.8 Bizarre attempt at internal fixation (A), leading to non-union of a fracture of the proximal end of the tibia (B).

CHILDHOOD FRACTURES

Bones grow in childhood, which gives them some characteristics not found in mature bone. Although an immature bone may break cleanly, it may alternatively undergo a combination of cracking and bending, known as a 'green-stick' fracture. Childhood fractures heal much faster than those in adults, and delayed union or non-union is very rare in children. Malunions, however, are more common. This is because, under certain circumstances, we are prepared to accept a poor reduction knowing that remodelling will come to the rescue. It is safe to rely on remodelling only if its limitations are known. An angulated malunion near a growth plate will remodel better than one at the centre of a long bone, but rotational malunions hardly remodel at all. Remodelling will tend to correct a malunion only while the bone continues to grow, and therefore has less effect in older children.

Fractures involving the growth plate may result in complete cessation of growth. More commonly, only part of the growth plate becomes fused while the rest continues to grow to produce a progressive deformity. This is a difficult situation to treat, but may be remedied by excising the bony tether, by fusing the rest of the growth plate, or by corrective osteotomy or callotasis when growth has ceased. The Salter–Harris classification which is used to describe these injuries is shown in Figure 2.9.

DISLOCATION

When a joint is disrupted in such a way that its articular surfaces are no longer in contact with one another, it is said to be dislocated. The abnormal position is then maintained by muscle spasm, which is extremely painful. Subluxation is the name given to a partial dislocation in which the joint surfaces are partially in contact.

Reduction is usually achieved easily by a suitable manoeuvre once the patient is properly relaxed and anaesthetised, but sometimes it is prevented by the joint capsule or by the presence of a piece of bone or soft tissue jammed in the joint. In this situation, the joint is explored surgically and an open reduction is performed. A dislocation is not cured once it is reduced. The torn capsule and ligaments take several weeks to heal and must be protected by limiting movement during this period. If the patient with a dislocated shoulder is allowed free immediately after reduction, the capsule will heal lax and may allow recurrent dislocations. Dislocations are often associated with fractures and these combined injuries usually require open reduction and internal fixation.

COMPLICATIONS THAT AFFECT THE BONE

INFECTION

Pathogenic organisms may invade a fresh fracture if it is compound or if it is opened surgically. An acute infection may be successfully treated with antibiotics combined, if necessary, by the surgical removal of infected tissue and blood clot.

Figure 2.9 Salter-Harris classification of epiphyseal injuries.

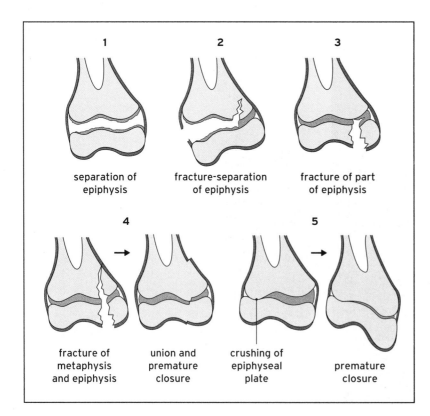

1	2	3
separation of epiphysis	fracture-separation of epiphysis	fracture of part of epiphysis

4	5
fracture of metaphysis and epiphysis	union and premature closure	crushing of epiphyseal plate	premature closure

DELAYED UNION

This is usually due to damage to the blood supply of the bone caused by stripping of the soft tissues in the initial injury. It is therefore more common in high-velocity than in low-velocity injuries.

Delayed union may happen if the callus is abolished by rigid fixation, and it is also more common in certain bones such as the tibia and the scaphoid, which have a precarious blood supply. It is treated by continuing splintage until the fracture eventually unites. The delayed union will be treated as a non-union if it shows no sign of healing after a reasonable length of time. This length of time is arbitrary and will vary from bone to bone and from surgeon to surgeon.

NON-UNION

The treatment of a non-union depends very much on the site, and on whether it is an atrophic, hypertrophic or infected non-union. Atrophic non-unions probably develop because of an inadequate blood supply during the important callus stage of fracture healing. Once the non-union is established, the blood supply to the bone ends may recover, but by this time there is no further callus response and the fracture remains mobile. The aim of treatment is to induce a fresh callus response, and then to hold the fracture ends in such a way that they will join up. The callus response is usually rekindled by 'freshening' the bone ends surgically, and putting in bone graft. The bone may then be held with an external fixator or plaster. The use of a rigid plate would tend to reduce the callus response which the surgeon is trying to produce.

Hypertrophic non-unions probably develop as a result of soft tissue interposed between the fracture ends, or as a result of unphysiological loading of the callus, caused by angulation at the healing fracture site. The bone ends are surrounded by a mass of callus, which is sometimes described as looking like an elephant's foot. Because the bone is still trying to join, and because the callus response is continuing, it is often only necessary to correct the alignment of the bone and hold this with an external fixator. The stresses on the healing callus are brought to within its physiological limits, and it can then bridge the gap.

Infected non-unions present the most difficult problems. Most surgeons now favour the use of callotasis techniques, in which the infected non-union is excised and normal bone is brought in from above or below by bone transport. Plastic surgeons are often involved to bring fresh tissue to the infected area to improve the blood supply and achieve skin cover.

The use of electrical stimulation and magnetic fields is still thought to be helpful by some and is based on the view that if mechanical stimulation produces electricity, which it does, then the application of electricity may stimulate bone to form. Electrical stimulation probably has very little effect when used to treat non-unions, but many surgeons still use it as an adjunct to other forms of treatment.

A longstanding non-union can eventually form a pseudarthrosis or false joint (Figure 2.10A and B).

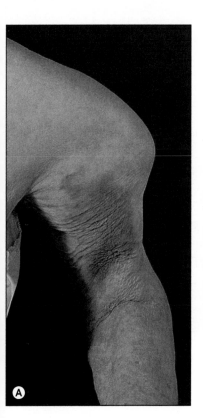
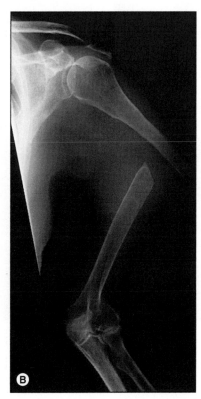

Figure 2.10 (A and B) Established non-union of a midshaft fracture of the humerus, which had occurred 10 years before. Although there was more movement at the non-union than at the elbow, this patient's arm was comfortable, and further treatment was declined.

MALUNION

If the deformity compromises function or is cosmetically distressing, then the bone may be straightened by an osteotomy, or by callotasis (Figure 2.11A and B) using external fixation.

AVASCULAR NECROSIS

In certain bones, such as the scaphoid, the neck of the femur and the talus, a fracture can cause part of the bone to die. This is due to a peculiarity of the blood supply in these bones. The scaphoid, for instance, is supplied with blood only through its distal pole, so that a fracture through the waist will cut off nourishment to the proximal part. If the avascular bone is protected, it will eventually be replaced by creeping substitution of new bone, but frequently the avascular part will simply collapse. Each site requires different treatment, some by bone graft in the early stages and some by excision or prosthetic replacement later on (Figure 2.12).

OSTEOARTHROSIS

If a fracture results in damage to the articular surface of a joint, then the distribution of load over the joint surfaces will change.

This may cause pain and limitation of movement and may eventually lead to the changes of 'wear and tear' arthritis. For this reason, great care is taken to reduce intra-articular fractures as perfectly as possible.

COMPLICATIONS THAT AFFECT THE LIMB

Structures around a fracture are frequently damaged and each poses its own problems.

BLOOD SUPPLY

Arteries may be damaged in any part of a limb, but the commonest and most serious damage is to the popliteal artery in the supracondylar femoral fracture and to the brachial artery in the supracondylar humeral fracture. Sometimes reduction of a fracture will immediately improve the blood supply to a limb, but if there is any doubt then immediate surgical repair of the damaged vessel is mandatory. Dying muscle is extremely painful, and severe pain following a good fracture reduction usually means a problem with the blood supply. If blood flow is not restored quickly, the muscle will die. Muscle which

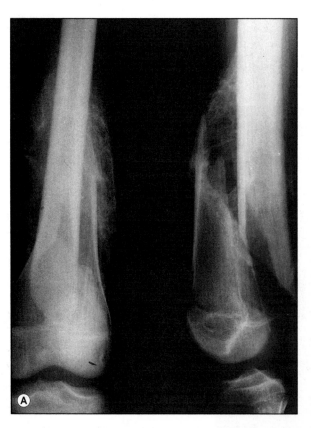
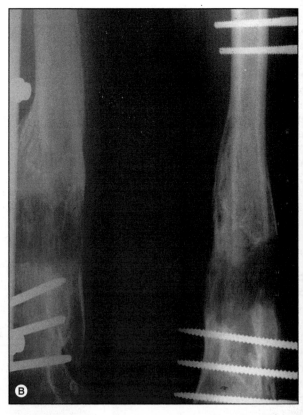

Figure 2.11 (A) Malunion of the distal end of the femur. This patient had a severe head injury and moved his leg a lot in traction, which produced shortening and abundant callus. **(B)** The femur was lengthened again by callotasis using an external fixator. This technique would have helped Sir Astley Cooper's patient in Figure 2.1.

lies immediately will slough and may lead to amputation of the limb. Muscle which dies slowly will contract into a scar and cause clawing of the toes or the tragic Volkmann's contracture of the forearm and hand. This condition should now be preventable, but sadly still occurs occasionally.

A tight plaster may also cause ischaemia and can be very dangerous, especially in children. Again, pain after adequate reduction means that something is wrong.

Ischaemic or dying muscle is even more painful when passively stretched. Gentle passive stretching is a sensitive test for muscle ischaemia, and is particularly useful in children in plaster. If passive stretching of a muscle produces pain, the plaster should immediately be split. If this still does not relieve the problem, then surgical intervention may be required, as described below.

COMPARTMENT SYNDROME

Muscle groups are contained in inexpansile fascial sacs. If the muscle is damaged it swells, and the pressure in the compartment rises. This reduces the entry of blood, damaging the muscle further and causing more swelling. When the compartment pressure exceeds the arterial supply pressure, the muscle will die. The process can be easily reversed by recognising the problem in time and surgically opening the compartments by fasciotomy. A timely fasciotomy will prevent muscle death, but if performed too late it can cause more problems. Patients with a fractured tibia treated in plaster sometimes complain of severe pain for 3 or 4 days, but wake one morning to find that the pain has all gone. The pain stops when the muscle has died. While the muscle is still painful it can be saved by a fasciotomy, but once the pain has gone the muscle is dead. Opening the fascia at this stage can introduce infection into the dead muscle, with serious consequences.

VENOUS THROMBOSIS

Damage to the wall of the vein, sluggish blood flow in an immobilised limb and changes in clotting factor concentrations due to trauma may result in a deep venous thrombosis. This will cause swelling of the limb, which may become chronic, and a clot may travel in the venous circulation, causing a pulmonary embolus. The treatment is anticoagulation.

PERIPHERAL NERVE DAMAGE

Peripheral nerves may be concussed (neurapraxia), or they may be crushed or stretched, resulting in damage to the nerve axons (axonotmesis). Part or all of the nerve may be divided (neurotmesis). A neurapraxia will recover in a few days, but an axonotmesis may take several months, as the axons have to grow back down the nerve, and only progress at about 1 mm per day. Divided nerves must be repaired, and the recovery from a neurotmesis is always poor. It is vital that the patient, with the help of the physiotherapist, maintains a full range of passive movement in the joints of the damaged limb until nerve function returns. A continuing functional deficit may be treated by tendon transfers.

JOINT STIFFNESS

A normal knee may be immobilised for months in plaster and will not become stiff. If an injured knee is immobilised, however, it will become permanently stiff. The stiffness is due to inflamed structures around the joint becoming infiltrated with fibrous exudate and then stuck down by fibrous scar tissue. Ligaments and tendons are thus prevented from sliding normally, reducing the range of motion of the joint. Immobilisation also reduces the nourishment of the articular cartilage by the synovial fluid. Early movements of joints is therefore a good thing, and the modern treatment of fractures aims to allow this to occur as soon as possible.

COMPLICATIONS THAT AFFECT THE PATIENT

BLOOD LOSS

Some fractures result in significant blood loss. A litre of blood will be lost into the thigh of a young adult with a fractured femur and many litres may be lost into a fractured pelvis. Hypovolaemic shock is treated by prompt intravenous fluid replacement, and it is easy to underestimate the blood loss in a patient with multiple fractures.

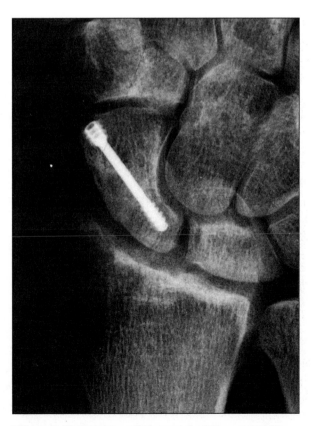

Figure 2.12 Fracture of the waist of the scaphoid was successfully treated with a bone graft and a Herbert screw, which has two threads of different pitches to produce compression. Avascular necrosis has not occurred in the proximal pole.

FAT EMBOLUS

This curious condition is occasionally seen in patients with multiple fractures and at least one closed long bone fracture. Mental confusion is followed by a slight rise in temperature and a petechial rash over the chest. The respiratory rate increases and the patient may become drowsy. Arterial oxygen tension is found to be abnormally low and a chest X-ray shows fluffy opacities over the lung fields.

There is still controversy about the true cause of the syndrome but it is probably a combination of embolising marrow fat (which is liquid at body temperature) and inadequately treated hypovolaemia. Complete recovery usually follows treatment with oxygen, but, in the rare fulminating type, ventilation may be required and the patient may die from disseminated intravascular coagulopathy.

METABOLIC CHANGES

Any injury will produce general changes mediated by an increase in circulating catecholamines and corticosteroids. The patient with multiple fractures will enter a catabolic state for several days following injury, and this often coincides with a period of low nutritional input. Management of this complex changing metabolic situation requires a good understanding of the physiology of trauma, an patients with multiple injuries are often best treated in a Intensive Care Unit for the first few days.

PSYCHOLOGICAL CHANGES

A fracture is a very alarming experience. A patient with fresh fracture or dislocation is often terrified and will happily submit to any treatment which will relieve the pain and deformity. After surgery, the patient awakes in the alie environment of the ward and is immediately assailed b the horrors of injections and hospital food, as well as th indignities of bed pans and communal living. It is hardl surprising that patients feel miserable and withdrawn a they try to imagine their life reorganised around plaster and crutches.

Function is our objective, and a cheerful patient wi regain function much more quickly than a frightened one Much of the problem is fear of the unknown and it is ou job to explain treatment and predict outcome as accuratel as we can. The better we predict each step in a patient' recovery, the better we will be trusted. Once we have th patient's trust, then treatment becomes exciting an rewarding to everyone involved.

GENERAL READING

Basket PJF. Management of hypovocaemic shock. *Brit J of Med* 1990, **300**: 1453-1457.

Bloor RN. Medicolegal reporting in orthopaedic trauma. In: Foy MA *et al*, eds. *Psychological Effect of Trauma*. Edinburgh: Churchill Livingstone; 1990.

Charnley J. *Compression Arthrodesis*. London: E. & S. Livingsone Limited; 1953

Charnley J. *The Closed Treatment of Common Fractures*, 3rd edition.Edinburgh: Churchill Livingstone; 1961.

Cone JB. Vascular injury with fractures. *Clinical Orthopaedic and Related Research* 1989, **243**:30-35.

Crenshaw AH, ed. *Campbell's Operative Orthopaedics*, 7th edition. Washington D.C.: The CV Mosby Company; 1987.

Currey J. *The Mechanical Adaptations of Bone*. Surrey: Princeton University Press; 1984.

Dodson ED. *The Management of Postoperative Pain*. London: Edward Arnold, 1985.

Duis HJT, *et al*. Fat embolism in patients with an isolated fracture of the femoral shaft. *Journal of trauma* 1988, **28**:3, 383-390.

Galasko SCB, ed. *Principles of Fracture Management*, 46-63. Edinburgh: Churchill Livingstone; 1984.

Heppenstall RB. Bone graft surgery for non-union. *Orthopedic Clinics of North America* 1984, **15**:1, 113-123.

Hull RD, *et al*. Prophylaxis of venous thromboembolic disease. *J of Bone and Joint Surg* 1986, **68A**:146-150.

Jensen JE, *et al*. Nutrition in orthopaedic surgery. *J of Bone and Joint Surg* 1982, **64A**:1263.

McKibbin B. The biology of fracture healing in long bones. *J of Bone and Joint Surg* 1978, **60B**:150-162.

Mears DC. *External Skeletal Fixation*. London: Williams and Wilkins; 1983.

Mubarak SJ, *et al*. *Compartment Syndromes and Volkmann's Contracture*. Sanders, 1981.

Muller ME, *et al*. *Manual of Internal Fixation*. New York: Springer-Verlag; 1979.

Omer GE, ed. Peripheral nerve injuries. *Clinical Orthopaedics and Related Resarch* 1982, **163**:1-106.

Rang M. *Children's Fractures*. Toronto: J.B. Lippincott Company; 1974.

Rogers LF. *Radiology of Skeletal Trauma*. Edinburgh: Churchill Livingstone; 1982.

Sarmiento A, Latta LL. *Closed Functional Treatment of Fractures*. New York Springer-Verlag; 1981.

Uhthoff HK, ed. *Current Concepts of Internal Fixation of Fractures*. New York: Springer-Verlag; 1980.

Vaughan J. *The Physiology of Bone*. Oxford: Clarendon Press; 1981.

Watson-Jones R. *Fractures and Joint Injuries*, 280-297. Edinburgh: Churchill Livingstone; 1982.

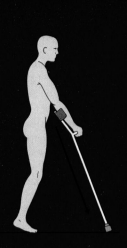

3

J Stallard & R E Major

MECHANICS OF LOWER LIMB ORTHOSES

CHAPTER OUTLINE

- **Force**
- **Moments**
- **Interface pressure**
- **Resolution of forces**
- **Stability**
- **Walking aids**

- **Stabilisation of the foot**
- **Dynamic force**
- **Work done and energy**
- **Inertial forces**
- **Stability, energy and control**

INTRODUCTION

Effective orthotic provision requires the application of mechanics, and it is well known that mechanics are based on Newton's three laws of motion (Williams & Lissner, 1977). It is not suggested that physiotherapists should be able to recite these on demand. However, Newton's third law is not only easy to remember, it is also self-evident and of great benefit to those who wish to have an elementary understanding of orthotics. Newton's law states that 'To every action, there is an equal and opposite reaction'. What this means is that unless there is resistance, there cannot be force. If you pull with a force of 10 newtons, then something must oppose that pull with the same force in order to maintain equilibrium.

FORCE

Force is the physical action which tends to change the position of a body in space. Some confusion exists about the units in which force can be expressed. Many different units have been used over the years, but the one which has been adopted as an international standard is the newton (N). An

appropriate way of remembering the magnitude of 1 N is to think of it as approximately the force that one apple (from which Newton developed his ideas!) exerts at rest under the influence of gravity. Thus, a lightweight man would weigh between 600 and 800 N.

In orthotics, force derives from two main sources: muscles and gravity. These can combine with other mechanical systems to produce force from stored energy, e.g. springs, or from an inertial reaction, which will be discussed in more detail later.

Since force always acts along a straight line it may be represented graphically by a line, the length of which is proportional to the magnitude of force, the direction of which corresponds to that of the force, and the start of which represents the point of application of force. Drawing this line (a vector) is a convenient way of indicating the effect of a force applied to a mechanical system. The application of force by a physiotherapist on the lower limb of a patient (Figure 3.1A) can be represented vectorally (Figure 3.1B), as can the reaction, i.e. the equal and opposite force of the leg on the hand (Figure 3.1C).

The weight of the body acts vertically downwards. There is necessarily an equal and opposite force, and this

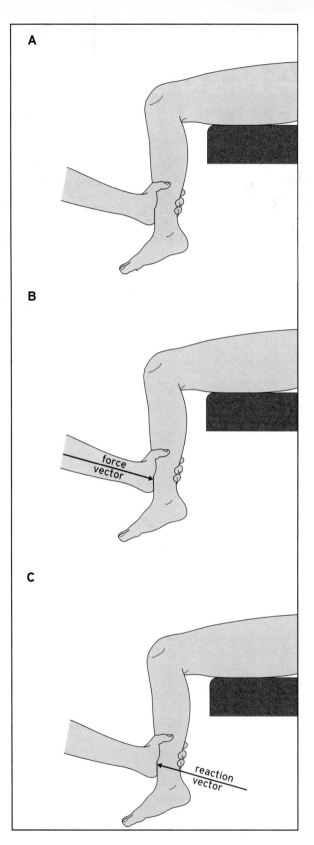

is known as the ground reaction force. Both of these can be represented vectorally (Figure 3.2).

Centre of gravity, or centre of mass, is defined as the point in a rigid body at which the mass may be considered to act. While it may be appropriate to use this concept for individual body segments, it can be misleading when applied to the whole body, which is multisegmental with freely articulated interconnections.

MOMENTS

A force system is rarely simple since it is frequently a combination of forces, and because secondary effects (most commonly moments) also occur. In order to gain some understanding of the problems that result, it is convenient to examine the problem of an unstable knee caused by extensor paralysis. Every physiotherapist knows that with the knee fully extended, the lower limb can support the weight of the body, even when that limb is muscularly deficient (Figure 3.3A). They further know that when this same knee is put into a small degree of flexion (Figure 3.3B), it collapses under the weight which it is carrying. The reason this happens is that the weight

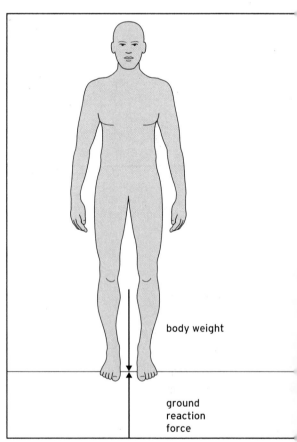

Figure 3.2 Body weight and ground reaction force.

Figure 3.1 Application of force (A) can be represented vectorally (B), as can the reaction (C).

of the body, acting vertically downwards, produces a moment about the knee, the direction of which changes when the knee moves from full extension into flexion. In many instances the effects of moments are much more important than direct forces (a pencil is easily broken in anger through a bending effect but will remain intact if a longitudinal pull is applied).

A moment is the action of a force which tends to cause rotation of a body about a point (known as the fulcrum or moment centre). When giving passive movements to the elbow (Figure 3.4) the physiotherapist applies a force some way from the fulcrum (the elbow joint) in order to cause the forearm to rotate about the elbow. The farther away from the fulcrum the force is applied, the easier it is to produce the turning effect. A moment is the force (F) multiplied by the shortest distance (L) from the line of force to the fulcrum or moment centre. It follows that this distance must be perpendicular to the line of force (see Figure 3.4).

In Figure 3.5A, the moment produced about the knee from the shoe (the weight which acts vertically downwards) is 10 N × 40 cm = 400 Ncm (although metres or millimetres are the preferred SI units of

length, this chapter uses centimetres for distance and Ncm for moments as these are more convenient for normal body dimensions). However, this ignores the weight of the shank of the lower limb, which is itself heavy and very significant. In order to understand the turning effect of the shank, it is necessary to know where its centre of mass is located. Centre of mass is the point at which the mass of a body is considered to be concentrated and is the point of perfect balance (Williams & Lissner, 1977). Figure 3.5B shows the same leg without the shoe, with the centre of mass marked at an 18 cm horizontal distance from the knee centre, and the weight of the shank indicated as 50 N. In the position shown, the shank produces a moment of 900 Ncm, i.e. 50 N × 18 cm. The overall effect when the shoe is worn is shown in Figure 3.5C, and the total moment about the knee is the summation of the two effects, which gives a moment of 1300 Ncm.

To keep the leg stable in that position, it is necessary to provide an equal and opposite moment, and this is achieved by the quadriceps acting through the patellar tendon. From Figure 3.5C it can be seen that the moment arm of the patellar tendon is only 4 cm, and by

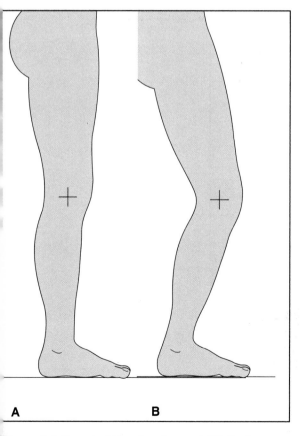

Figure 3.3 Knee in (A) extension and (B) flexion.

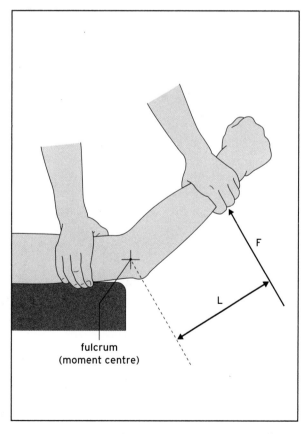

Figure 3.4 Turning moment about the elbow joint.
Moment = F × L. (The distance L must be measured at right angles to the direction of F.)

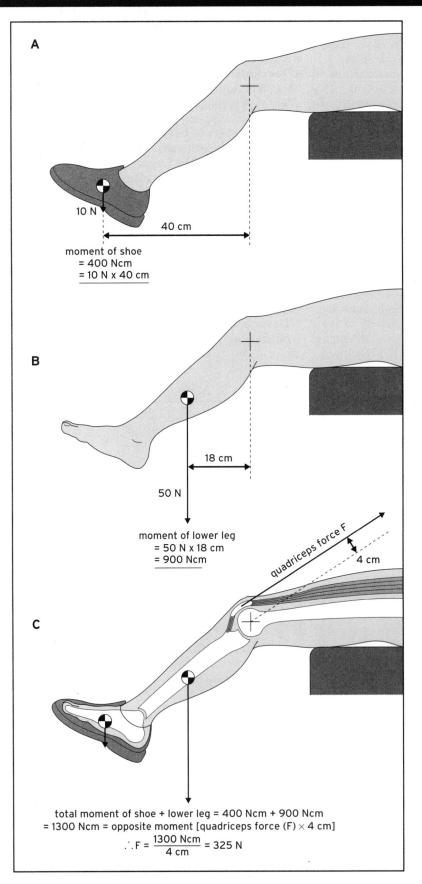

Figure 3.5 Balancing a moment about the knee with the quadriceps muscle. The circles indicate the centre of gravity for **(A)** shoes, **(B)** shank and foot, and **(C)** these combined.

A

10 N

40 cm

moment of shoe
= 400 Ncm
= 10 N x 40 cm

B

18 cm

50 N

moment of lower leg
= 50 N x 18 cm
= 900 Ncm

quadriceps force F

4 cm

C

total moment of shoe + lower leg = 400 Ncm + 900 Ncm
= 1300 Ncm = opposite moment [quadriceps force (F) × 4 cm]
$$\therefore F = \frac{1300 \text{ Ncm}}{4 \text{ cm}} = 325 \text{ N}$$

imple mathematics it can be determined that to produce he balancing moment of 1300 Ncm, the force with which the quadriceps must pull is 325 N, i.e. 1300 Ncm ÷ 4 cm. Notice that the comparatively small moment arm through which the quadriceps acts demands a much greater force than the combined action of the boot and leg weights acting through their respective (much greater) moment arms.

Care must be taken with units when considering moments. Force units (e.g. N), and moment units (e.g. cm), are different and must not be confused.

To return to the unstable knee: it can be seen that ground reaction force passes in front of the knee centre when the knee is fully extended (Figure 3.6A). This produces an extending moment which is resisted by the posterior capsule, thus maintaining the knee in extension. With the knee in flexion, the line of force passes behind the knee centre, thus producing a flexing moment (Figure 3.6B). If the quadriceps are not active, or are insufficiently powerful to balance that flexing moment, then the knee will collapse. The greater the degree of knee flexion, the larger the moment arm and the less likely the quadriceps are to cope.

The orthotic solution to an unstable knee is almost always a long leg caliper (Figure 3.6C). What is perhaps not

well known is the mechanical effect of this device. The term 'three-point fixation' is widely used, but it obscures to many people the real effect. A long leg caliper is simply a manifestation of Newton's third law. When a knee flexion deformity occurs, it is inevitable that a knee-flexing moment will be produced, the magnitude of which will rise as the degree of flexion deformity increases. Without a caliper, a flail knee with flexion deformity has an unbalanced flexing moment applied to it which is equal to body weight (W) multiplied by the perpendicular distance (L) from the knee centre (see Figure 3.6B). When the orthosis is applied, it resists this unbalanced moment by producing an equal and opposite moment through three-point fixation (see Figure 3.6C). Anyone who has ever broken a stick over the knee will understand how this is effective in producing a 'bending' effect (Figure 3.7).

If it can be arranged that the line of force due to W passes directly through the knee joint centre, then clearly no moment would be applied. When a long leg caliper is fitted to an unstable knee with a full range of movement, it is set so that negligible moments are produced about the knee. In this situation the orthosis is merely a stabilising device and only small forces occur between the leg and the orthosis.

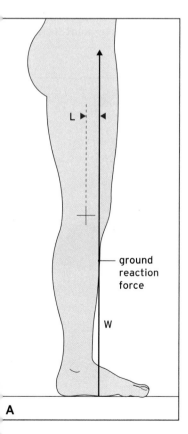
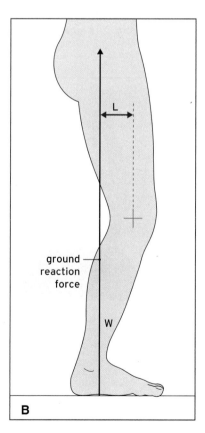
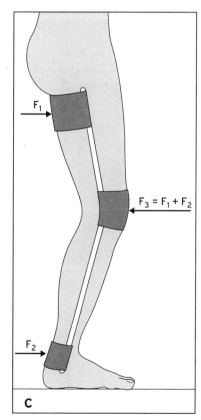

Figure 3.6 Turning effects about the knee joint. (A) Extending, **(B)** flexing and **(C)** flexing effect stabilised by a caliper.

INTERFACE PRESSURE

One difficulty which can occur with a caliper, particularly in the presence of large deformities, is high interface pressure at the knee or, less often, at the thigh band.

Pressure is the intensity of loading applied to a particular area (Figure 3.8). A large load concentrated on a small area will give very high pressure. The only way to reduce this pressure is by increasing the area or decreasing the load. With any type of bracing it is advisable to minimise the applied loads as much as possible, and at the same time spread the loads over the greatest possible area. It is for this reason that, for example, thigh bands on calipers should be made as broad as is practical.

To reduce pressure further, the forces F_1, F_2 and F_3, required to achieve stabilisation of the knee, can be minimised by increasing to a maximum the moment arm through which F_1 and F_2 act (see Figure 3.6C). Moments are a product of both force and moment arm, and increasing or decreasing one has the opposite effect on the magnitude of the other to maintain the same moment. Thus it is in the interest of the patient to position the thigh band as high as possible as this will decrease not only F_1 but also F_3, because (as indicated by Newton's third law) $F_3 = F_1 + F_2$. Figure 3.9 gives a comparison of forces for different application points on a long leg caliper.

Another important fact is that the higher the degree of knee flexion deformity, the larger the forces required to

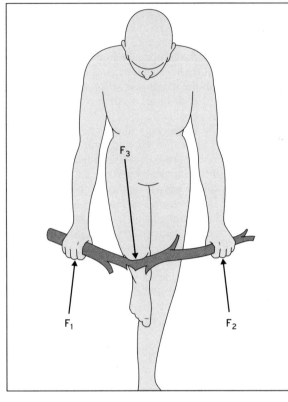

Figure 3.7 Bending effect of three-point fixation.

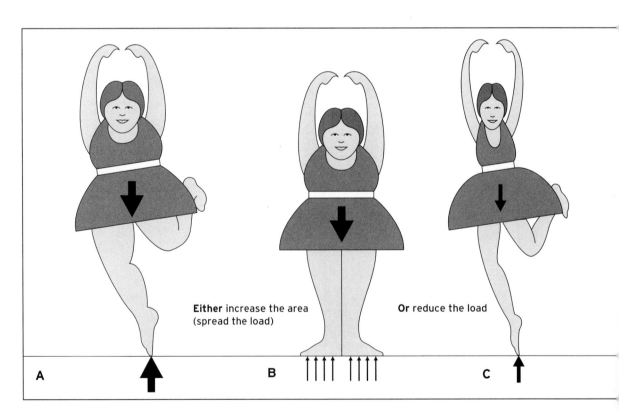

Either increase the area (spread the load)

Or reduce the load

A   B   C

Figure 3.8 Pressure: the distribution of load.

support the leg. Once it is understood how the unbalanced moment about the knee centre is developed, then the reason becomes obvious. As stated earlier, the line of ground reaction force passes behind the flexed knee centre (Figure 3.10A). With larger flexion deformities, the moment arm from knee centre to line of action of force increases (Figure 3.10B and C). Even though nothing else changes (W must stay the same), this increases the flexing moment about the knee in proportion with the increased moment arm, and a consequent increase in stabilising forces occurs.

RESOLUTION OF FORCES

Patients who use calipers, frequently also need to use crutches. Crutches have two primary functions, i.e. to:
• Improve stability by increasing the support area.
• Provide a means of propulsion through ground reaction forces.

In both of these functions it is necessary for the crutch to apply forces to the ground, and this is generally done through the handle along the axis of the crutch. During ambulation the crutches are always sloping, which means that the applied forces are never perpendicular relative to the ground; the implication being that there must be a proportion of the overall force which acts vertically and a further proportion which acts horizontally with the ground

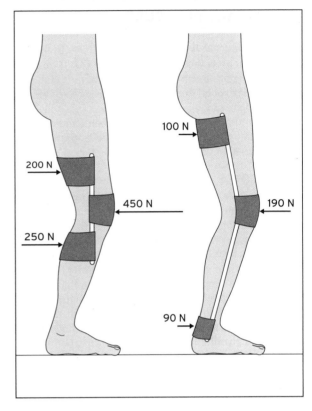

Figure 3.9 Beneficial effect of long moment arms.

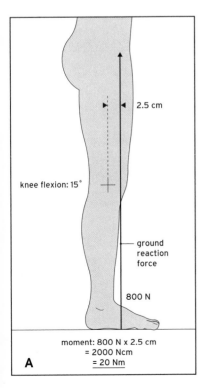

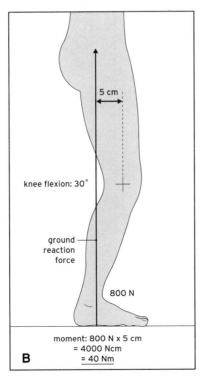

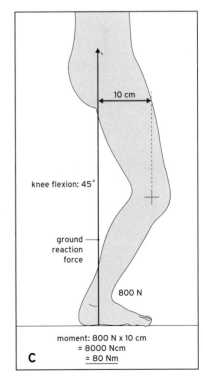

Figure 3.10 (A, B and C) Increase in bending moment with increasing knee flexion (the vertical arrows represent the ground reaction force).

(Figure 3.11). Provided that the magnitude and direction of the force along the crutch axis is known, it is possible to determine these two 'components' of that force by simple manipulation of its vector representation. This is done by dropping a vertical line from the 'top' end of the vector and drawing a horizontal line from the other end (see Figure 3.11). The point of intersection of these two lines will show their magnitude—the direction of force being indicated by following the 'component' vectors around from the top to meet the other end of the overall force vector.

FRICTION

From Newton's third law it can be seen that for a horizontal component of crutch force to exist, there must be an equal and opposite force. This comes from the friction between the crutch tip and the floor surface. Without this frictional opposing force, the crutch would slide on the floor surface and fail to fulfil its function. Coefficient of friction (μ) describes the frictional properties which exist between two surfaces (Figure 3.12). Should the surface be other than horizontal then the weight will need to be resolved into components perpendicular and parallel to the surface. The perpendicular

component will replace the value of W in the formula and the parallel component will either be added to or subtracted from the value of the force F, dependent on whether the motion is up or down the incline. Clearly it is in the patient's interest that crutches should resist slipping, and so the tips are made from a high-friction material such as rubber.

STABILITY

Stability, which crutches can help to provide, is vital for any form of ambulation; an activity which requires both intrinsic and extrinsic stability. Intrinsic stability prevents the human body (a multisegmental structure) from collapsing under itself. Where muscular deficiency exists, e.g. a flail hip or knee, then orthotic assistance in the form of three-point fixation is required. In the static situation, extrinsic stability ensures that an intrinsically stable body does not topple over. This means that the centre of mass, when projected vertically downwards, must be contained within the support area of the body.

An illustration of three forms of extrinsic stability can be shown by a cone (Figure 3.13). On its point, a cone

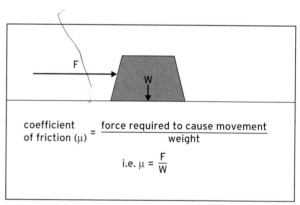

$$\text{coefficient of friction } (\mu) = \frac{\text{force required to cause movement}}{\text{weight}}$$

$$\text{i.e. } \mu = \frac{F}{W}$$

Figure 3.12 Coefficient of friction

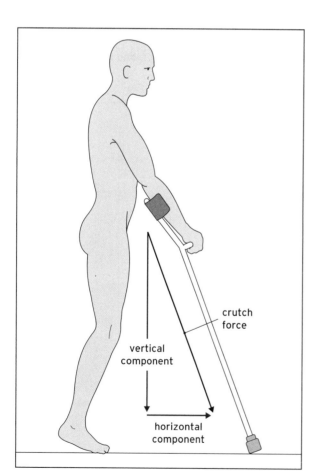

crutch force

vertical component

horizontal component

Figure 3.11 Resolution of crutch force.

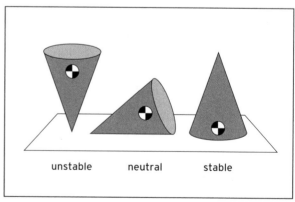

unstable   neutral   stable

Figure 3.13 Stability: conditions of equilibrium.

will require only tiny movements sideways to take the centre of mass outside the support area. This is known as unstable equilibrium. When lying on its side, the cone may be rolled and the centre of mass then follows the support area so that it takes up a new position of equilibrium: this is known as neutral equilibrium. However, when a cone which is standing on its base is tilted, it will drop back to its original position, as long as the centre of mass does not pass outside the support area. This is known as stable equilibrium. Once the centre of mass goes beyond the outside edge of the cone it loses its stable equilibrium and falls onto its side. More interesting is the concept of degrees of stability within the category of stable equilibrium. This can be considered with a truncated cone standing on its large and small ends. When the truncated cone is standing on the small end, it requires a much smaller angular movement before stability is lost (Figure 3.14A) than when the truncated cone is standing on the large end (Figure 3.14B). The more stable situation is better able to resist external disturbances. The implication of this is explored in greater detail on page 42.

WALKING AIDS

Three types of walking aids, providing different functions, are available. These are:
- Sticks, which provide increased extrinsic stability.
- Crutches, which provide a means of exerting propulsive forces.
- Frames, which are part of the intrinsic stabilisation system.

STICKS

Sticks give the lowest level of assistance and in most cases provide a degree of increased extrinsic stability by enlarging the support area. They also enable some injection of propulsive force by reacting against the ground through the arm (or arms). The tripod and quadropod sticks are a specific case (Figure 3.15): because of their multipoint ground contact, they can resist rotation about their vertical axis. Patients who have difficulty with rotational instability around the hips find that these aids can be of great assistance. In addition to their rotational reaction they also have some resistance to forward or side thrust and this enhances the provision of extrinsic stability.

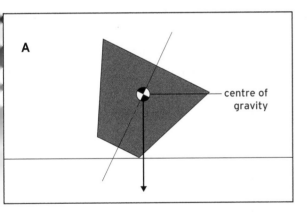

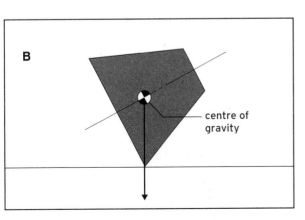

Figure 3.14 (A and B) Degrees of stability of a truncated cone.

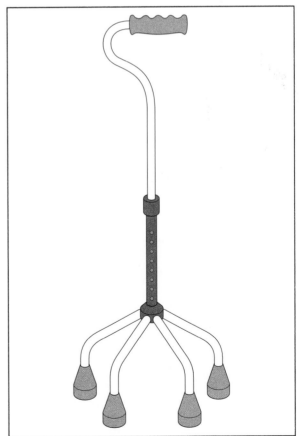

Figure 3.15 Quadropod stick.

CRUTCHES

Crutches provide support across at least one joint in the arm. There are three main types of crutches: axillary, Canadian and elbow (Figure 3.16A,B and C). Axillary and Canadian crutches cross both the wrist and elbow joints and give patients a greater level of stability. In contrast, elbow crutches cross only the wrist joint, and therefore, of the three main types, least enhance patient stability.

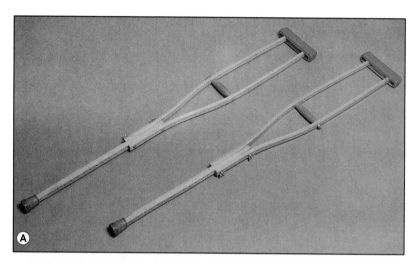

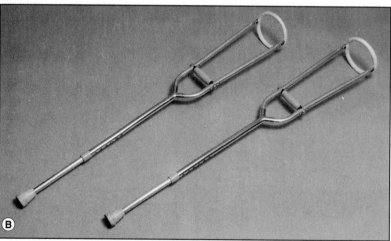

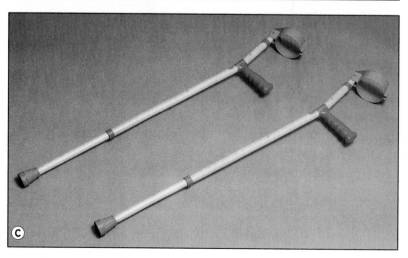

Figure 3.16 Crutch types: (A) axillary, (B) Canadian and (C) elbow.

Crutches are usually grounded at points further from the body than sticks, and because of this give larger support areas. This, coupled with better arm stabilisation, means that they provide a higher level of extrinsic stability (Figure 3.17).

For patients who use long leg calipers and have no hip control, e.g. paraplegics with lesions at lumbar 1 (L1) level and above, crutches form an important part of the intrinsic stabilisation system. By leaning forward to support themselves on the crutches, patients ensure that the applied forces produce an extending moment about the hips (Figure 3.18). This condition must be satisfied at all times for such patients. It is a difficult feat and explains why so few paraplegics are able to ambulate with long leg calipers.

In addition to providing stability, crutches enable patients to exert propulsive forces. The most common means of achieving this is for the arms to pull against the crutches, the equal and opposite reactive forces being the crutch tip/ground interface friction. It is essential for patients to have intact latissimus dorsi muscles if they are

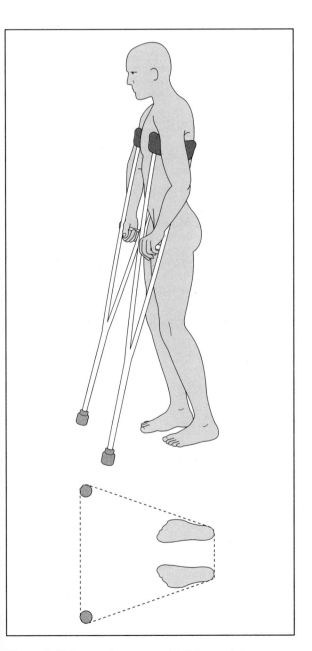

Figure 3.17 Support area provided by crutches. Extrinsic stabilisation is improved with crutches because of the increased support area.

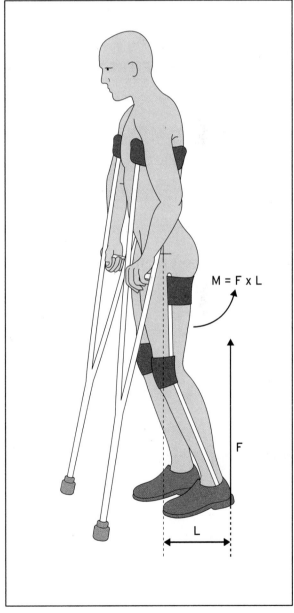

$$M = F \times L$$

Figure 3.18 Stabilising flail hips with crutches. M, moment; F, force; L, length.

to generate these forces, for it is the arms pulling towards the body under their influence which cause the crutch to react against the ground.

FRAMES

Frames come in a variety of forms, e.g. pulpit, rollators. They all provide a large support area for improved extrinsic stability. As many of these frames can also enable patients to partially 'suspend' themselves in the frame using their arms, they can also improve intrinsic stabilisation. All frames have good contact points, making it possible to inject propulsive forces. Some frames, e.g. the Rollator, also have wheels so that frictional resistance is greatly reduced when support points are lifted from the ground. This makes it easier to push the device forward for the next phase of the gait cycle.

STABILISATION OF THE FOOT

The weight-bearing foot has a condition of stable equilibrium. As it supinates (Figure 3.19), the point of application of ground reaction force moves towards the outer border of the calcaneus and fifth toe. Stability will be retained until the point of application reaches the border of the support area. At this point, stability becomes uncertain and collapse may occur because the moment from gravitational forces acting on the body can change from being corrective to one which increases supination.

Limited range in the subtalar joint means that this does not normally occur in pronation. In the rheumatoid foot, however, the centre of mass can move outside the line 3–1(see Figure 3.19) if the disease is in an advanced stage. When this happens, an orthosis of the type shown in Figure 3.20 is necessary if the patient is to walk. As can be seen from the diagrammatic representation, the resolution of forces tends to pull the strap down the outside iron and pull the foot towards the iron. Thus, to make the orthosis work effectively, it is necessary to put a loop on the outside iron to provide the equal and opposite force to the vertical component, and a wedge in the shoe to oppose the horizontal component of the strap force.

DYNAMIC FORCE

One of the aims of a lower limb orthosis is to enable patients to walk. Walking is, in mechanical terms, a dynamic activity

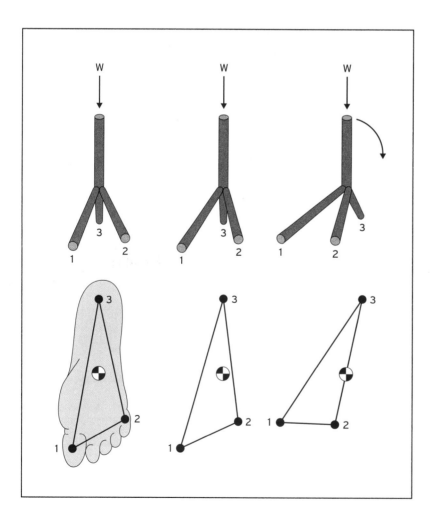

Figure 3.19 Stability of the foot in supination. 1, great toe; 2, fifth toe; 3, calcaneus; W, body weight (the quartered circles show the point of application of the ground reaction force).

in that forces over and above those required to maintain the status quo, i.e. the 'static' situation, are involved. When a change of state occurs, such as starting to walk from standing still or changing speed and direction when walking, extra force is required to bring it about. While it is possible to determine the magnitude of these increased forces, given the variable involved, the mathematics can be complex and it is really only necessary for the physiotherapist to understand the effect of dynamic situations.

During walking, the centre of mass rises and falls and also sways from side to side. This implies that the body is accelerated upwards and downwards and from side to side. The force required to raise the body upwards is over and above that of body weight, and to permit the body to fall back again the force of the body on the ground must be less than body weight. Swaying of the body sideways is brought about by small side-thrust forces on the ground.

Thus it can be seen that the ground forces involved in walking are quite complex. The forces may be monitored by a force platform (force plate). This is a flat rigid plate, set flush into a walkway, which registers components of force applied to the top surface. The use of force platforms during the past 50 years has established the levels and patterns of the various components of ground reaction force for normal walking. For convenience, ground reaction force is split into three components. These are:

- The vertical (F_z).
- Horizontal in line of walking (F_y).
- Horizontal at right angles to line of walking (F_x).

The definitions of F_x, F_y and F_z given here are those adopted by one force-platform manufacturer. Various attempts have been made to define their direction and sign conventions by a number of organisations. It is therefore important to ensure that the same meaning is implied when interpreting force-platform information.

Typical patterns for normal steady pace walking are shown in Figure 3.21.

Notice that the vertical component of force rises to approximately $1.2 \times$ body weight just after heel strike, drops to around $0.8 \times$ body weight at midstance, and rises again

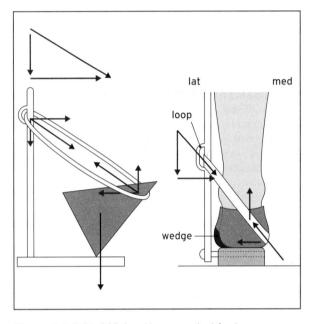

Figure 3.20 Stabilising the pronated foot.

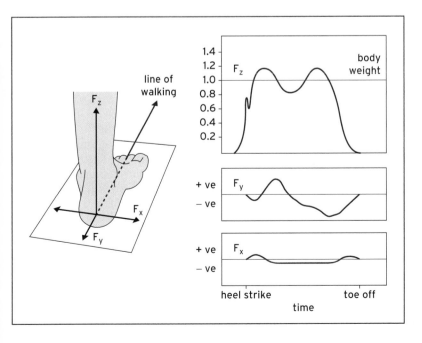

Figure 3.21 Ground reaction forces in walking. F_z, vertical; F_y, horizontal in line of walking; F_x, horizontal at right angles to line of walking.

at the end of single-stance phase—once again to approximately 1.2 × body weight. For running, a different pattern of vertical force emerges, and the force on the lower limb can rise to almost 3 × body weight (Figure 3.22).

In the normal leg, these dynamic forces put greater demands on the bones, tendons and muscles. However, with a braced lower limb, the orthosis also has to bear the increased burden. Many patients perform swing-through gait when wearing calipers and this introduces forces greater than those experienced in reciprocal ambulation (Stallard *et al.*, 1978, 1980). The design of orthotic devices must withstand the extra forces involved in dynamic activities undertaken by patients.

WORK DONE AND ENERGY

One of the reasons for training patients by physical therapy or treating them with orthotics is to enable them to do some work. In mechanics, the term 'work done' has a very specific meaning and it involves moving bodies. Work done is the force applied to a body multiplied by the distance through which the body moves under the influence of, and in the direction of, that force (Figure 3.23). An object can be pushed extremely hard, but unless it moves no 'work' will be 'done'.

Energy, however, is the ability to do 'work' and has the same unit (Nm) as work done. There are many forms of energy. These include:
• Biochemical energy, e.g. muscles.
• Stored energy, e.g. stretched springs.
• Kinetic energy, e.g. motion, momentum.
• Heat.
• Potential energy, e.g. gravity.

Clearly, the act of walking involves doing work and expending the various forms of energy available to the body (biochemical, kinetic and potential energy in particular), and it is the interchange of energy to work done which is at the heart of mechanical dynamic systems. The efficiency with which we move is the ratio of work done to energy expended.

INERTIAL FORCES

Any object tends to retain the mechanical state in which it finds itself. This resistance to change is known as inertia, and dynamic forces are required to overcome this effect. When running to catch a bus, it takes an effort to slow down and stop. That is because of the momentum of the running body and its inertia. To every action, Newton states, there is an equal and opposite reaction, and the reactive effect to forces applied to overcome inertia is known as the inertial reaction. This effect is an integral and important part of walking. At the end of swing phase, for example, the hip extensors apply a decelerative force on the swing leg, and this in turn produces an inertial reaction on the trunk which pulls it forward in space.

Any orthosis applied to the lower limb will alter the dynamics of walking. The increase in weight of the 'lower limb system' will obviously increase its inertia and so affect the inertial reaction. Long leg braces prevent knee flexion, and this limits the ability of the patient to 'smooth out' the rise and fall of the centre of mass during walking. Thus, the amount of energy required to walk will be increased and the overall efficiency of ambulation decreased.

STABILITY, ENERGY AND CONTROL

The definitions of stability discussed so far consider the size of the support area or base and whether the weight of the body falls within the base. This takes into account gravitational effects but gets more complex if inertia is considered. When control is a prime factor, as in the human body, it may be more helpful to further develop the concept of 'degree of stability' (see Figure 3.14) and to relate this to the magnitude of any disturbing force or perturbation (Major & Butler, 1995). The 'degree of stability' has been illustrated by a truncated cone, which can be placed in a position of stable equilibrium on either its narrow or its wide end. In either situation it is, in mechanical terms, stable, but the degree of stability is very different. If placed on its wide end, the cone will return to the original stable equilibrium after the application and removal of a disturbing moment. However, if the same moment is applied to the funnel placed on its narrow end, it is likely to produce sufficient movement that the original condition of stable equilibrium will be lost. It could then be restored only if corrective action is taken by a control system to inject the necessary forces. Different joints within the skeletal structure will exhibit different degrees of stability depending on their construction, position and natural constraints. For example, the ball-and-socket construction of the hip joints

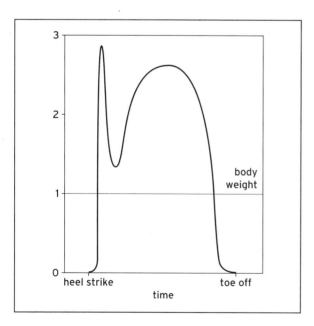

Figure 3.22 Vertical ground reaction force in running.

makes them very unstable, whereas the joints of the spinal column exhibit a small degree of inherent stability, and the knee joints are very stable when in full extension.

Walking requires movement of body segments beyond the limit of inherent stability. The energy required will be related to the degree of inherent stability—the greater the degree of stability, the higher the energy cost to initiate movement. A normal person has a high degree of control and can therefore cope with the low inherent stability necessary to achieve high efficiency of movement. The lack of control which impairment imposes demands assured stability and the greater energy which this requires to produce movement. If stability is mechanically assured, then no muscle activity will be required to maintain segmental stability even though small movements may take place under the influence of perturbing forces. The degree of stability is thus inversely related to the necessity for control, with a greater degree of stability imposing less demand upon the active control system. These three interrelated concepts can be illustrated on a single diagram (Figure 3.24).

The combination of these ideas allows consideration of stability/energy/control situations for both normal and impaired individuals (see Figure 3.24). Viewing proposed treatment strategies in this light can be helpful in estimating the viability of suggested interventions since the interactions between stability, energy and control demands can be readily appreciated. It is important to bear in mind that there is a region at the top of the diagram where energy costs are so high that useful movement may not be practical.

NORMAL

In the normal subject (see Figure 3.24), the skeletal structure has a very low overall inherent stability which will allow low-energy movement provided a high-level control system is functioning. Examples of impaired control follow.

PARAPLEGIA

A suitable example is a paraplegic patient with a mid-thoracic complete lesion who is unable to walk without assistance due to the reduction in control function. Suitable orthotic intervention may introduce sufficient additional passive mechanical control to allow ambulation. Study of Figure 3.24 reveals that the impaired control at this level necessitates a greater than normal level of stability, so a walking aid such as crutches or walking frame will be required. In addition, it would be unrealistic to expect normal energy levels of walking. The provision of an orthotic system, which provides more control than that required to overcome the control deficit, would raise the height of the double horizontal line in Figure 3.24, leading to a yet higher energy cost. Thus, the well-known orthotic maxim, that it is important not to overbrace, is supported by this approach.

CEREBRAL PALSY

A cerebral palsied subject will inevitable have a control deficit. It might be tempting to consider the orthotic options described for paraplegia but in this case it is worth noting that a control system, albeit impaired, is still functioning across all joints of the skeletal structure. If the control function can be improved by therapeutic means, then the horizontal double line in Figure 3.24 will move down, resulting in a lower energy cost of walking, together with a decreased demand on external supports.

CONCLUSION

Lower limb orthoses which adopt the fundamental mechanical principles outlined, do so in an effective and efficient manner and can make an important contribution to the treatment of patients with profound handicaps. The routine provision of hip, knee, ankle, or foot orthoses to

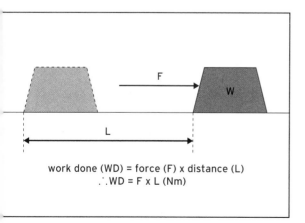

work done (WD) = force (F) x distance (L)
∴ WD = F x L (Nm)

Figure 3.23 Definition of work done.

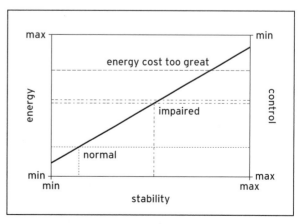

Figure 3.24 Theoretical relation between stability, energy and control. (Reproduced with permission from Orlau Publishing.)

enable paraplegic patients with complete lesions at L1 or above to ambulate, is becoming increasingly common. The objectives are to provide therapeutic benefit and improve independence. Several reports (Rose, 1980; Menelaus, 1987) have shown that ambulation has benefits for paraplegic patients; for example, it improves urinary drainage, bowel function and peripheral circulation, and reduces osteoporosis. This was confirmed in a study of patients with spina bifida (Mazur *et al.*, 1989) which showed that, in comparison with those who use orthoses to walk, nonambulatory patients have five times the number of pressure sores and twice the number of bone fractures. Pressure sores cause much misery and are extremely expensive to treat. On the basis of published figures, the cost of a modern walking orthosis over 10 years can be as small as one third the cost of treating the additional number of pressure sores experienced by non-ambulatory patients over the same period.

In addition to the direct therapeutic benefits of walking, Mazur *et al.* (1989) also showed that children who walk, as opposed to those who do not walk, are more than three times as likely to be independently mobile within the community as teenagers, i.e. using public transport or a car.

The benefits of walking can only be achieved when there is good compliance with the walking programme. This will depend on the effectiveness with which mechanical principles have been applied in individual orthotic designs. Efficiency of ambulation, ease of putting on and taking off the orthosis and the practicality of the walking style will all affect the compliance rate for different groups of patients. Conventional long leg calipers supplied to traumatic paraplegic patients with complete thoracic lesions have had very low compliance rates (one spinal injuries centre reported that less than 10% of patients continue to use them 6 months after supply). However, modern hip, knee, ankle, or foot orthoses (Rose, 1980; Beckman, 1987), which permit reciprocal walking with crutches, greatly increase efficiency. The ORLAU ParaWalker (Butler & Major, 1987) as shown in Figure 3.25 has been widely reported as the most efficient of those currently supplied (Banta *et al.*, 1991; Bowker *et al.*, 1992; Bernardi *et al.*, 1995) (see Figure 3.25). Two compliance studies (Moore & Stallard, 1991; Stellard *et al.*, 1995)

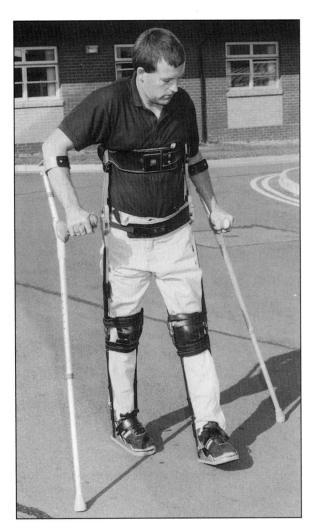

Figure 3.25 ORLAU ParaWalker. (Reproduced with permission from Orlau Publishing.)

showed results ranging from 64% with an average follow-up of 34 months to 58% with an average follow-up exceeding 7 years.

In patients unable to use their upper limbs to inject forces through crutches or walking frames, other aids are available so that they can take advantage of the therapeutic benefits of walking. In particular, swivel walkers (Butler *et al.*, 1982) enable very young patients (from the age of 1 year) or those with hemiplegia, scoliosis, spinal muscular atrophy and muscular dystrophy, for example, to ambulate indoors on flat surfaces.

Attention to detail by physiotherapists can improve the efficiency of their patients. Careful consideration should be given to orthotic devices and walking aids. Even the type of crutch used to perform swing-through gait can affect the efficiency of the patient. Dounis and colleagues (1980) and Sankarankutty and colleagues (1979) showed that Canadian crutches are the most efficient aid for swing-through gait. The need to quantify performance is increasingly a requirement, and new techniques of monitoring ambulation for various levels of ability are becoming available. Functional performance can be established, even in high levels of handicap, using the concept of physiological cost index (Butler *et al.*, 1984), and the effect of ground reaction forces on the joints of the lower limb can be easily monitored using a video vector generator (Stallard, 1987).

REFERENCES

Banta JV, Bell KJ, Muik EA, Fezio J. ParaWalker: energy cost of walking. *Eur J Pediatr Surg* 1991, **1**(Suppl. 1):7-10.

Beckmann J. The Louisiana State University reciprocating gait orthosis. *Physiotherapy* 1987, **73**:393-397.

Bernardi M, Canale I, Castellano V, Di Filippo L, Felici F, Marchetti M. The efficiency of walking of paraplegic patients using a reciprocating gait orthosis. *Paraplegia* 1995, **33**:409-415.

Bowker P, Messenger N, Ogilvie C, Rowley D. The energetics of paraplegic walking. *J Biomed Eng* 1992, **14**:344-350.

Butler PB, Englebrecht M, Major RE, Tait JH, Stallard J, Patrick JH. Physiological cost index of walking for normal children and its use as an indicator of physical handicap. *Develop Med Child Neurol* 1984, **26**:607-612.

Butler PB, Major RE. The ParaWalker: a rational approach to the provision of reciprocal ambulation for paraplegic patients. *Physiotherapy* 1987, **73**:393-397.

Butler PB, Poiner R, Farmer IR, Patrick JH. Use of the ORLAU Swivel Walker for the severely handicapped patient. *Physiotherapy* 1982, **68**:324-326.

Dounis E, Stevenson RD, Wilson RSE. The use of a portable oxygen consumption meter (Oxylog) for assessing the efficiency of crutch walking. *J Med Eng Technol* 1980, **4**:296-298.

Major RE, Butler PB. Discussion of segmental stability with implications for motor learning. *Clin Rehabil* 1995, **9**:167-172.

Mazur JM, Shurtleff D, Menelaus M, Colliver J. Orthopaedic management of high-level spina bifida. *J Bone Joint Surg* 1989, **71A**:56-61.

Menelaus MBD. Progress in the management of the paralytic hip in myelomeningocele. *Orthop Clin North Am* 1987, **11**:17-30.

Moore P, Stallard J. A clinical review of adult paraplegic patients with complete lesions using the ORLAU ParaWalker. *Paraplegia* 1991, **32**:608-615.

Rose GK. Orthoses for the severely handicapped–rational or empirical choice? *Physiotherapy* 1980, **66**:76-81.

Sankarankutty M, Stallard J, Rose GK. The relative efficiency of 'swing through' gait on axillary, elbow and Canadian crutches compared to normal walking. *J Biomed Eng* 1979, **1**:55-57.

Stallard J. Assessment of the mechanical function of orthoses by force vector visualisation. *Physiotherapy* 1987, **73**:398-402.

Stallard J, Sankarankutty M, Rose GK. Lower-limb vertical ground reaction forces during crutch walking. *J Med Eng Technol* 1978, **2**:201-202.

Stallard J, Dounis E, Major RE, Rose GK. One leg swing through gait using two crutches. *Acta Orthop Scand* 1980, **51**:1-7.

Stallard J, Major RE, Patrick JH. The use of the Orthotic Research and Locomotor Assessment Unit (ORLAU) ParaWalker by adult myelomeningocele patients: a seven year retrospective study–preliminary results. *Eur J Pediatr Surg* 1995, **5**(Suppl. I):24-26.

Williams N, Lissner HR. *Biomechanics of human movement*. Philadelphia: WB Saunders; 1977:8,10.

GENERAL READING

Bowker P, Condie DN, Bader DL, Pratt DJ, Wallace WA. *Biomechanical basis of orthotic management*. Oxford: Butterworth Heinemann; 1993.

Condie DN (ed). *Report of a consensus conference on the lower limb orthotic management of cerebral palsy*. Copenhagen: The International Society for Prosthetists and Orthotists; 1995.

D'Astrous JD (ed). *Orthotics and prosthetics digest*. Ottawa: Edahl Productions; 1981.

Department of Health and Social Security. *Classification of orthoses*. London: HMSO; 1980.

Gordon JE. *The new science of strong materials*. London: Penguin; 1991.

Gordon JE. *Structures*. London: Penguin; 1991.

Nordin M, Frankel VH. *Basic biomechanics of the musculoskeletal system*. Pennsylvania: Lea and Febiger; 1987.

Rose GK. *Orthotics: principles and practice*. London: William Heinemann Medical; 1986.

SECTION 2

ORTHOPAEDIC DISORDERS

rthopaedics (orthopædix). That part of urgery which deals with the normnalities, diseases and injuries of e locomotor system.

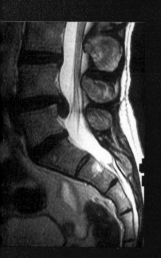

4 S Eisenstein

SURGERY FOR SPINAL DISORDERS – CLINICAL

CHAPTER OUTLINE

- **Spinal disorders and their operations**
- **Indications for spinal surgery**

- **Selecting the patient for surgery**
- **The operations**
- **The Oswestry Disability Index**

INTRODUCTION

There are only two types of surgery for spinal disorders: stiffening of the spine (arthrodesis) and clearing out of the spinal canal to make more room for the contained neural tissue (decompression). Not all spinal disorders require surgery, and not all surgical patients require both types of operation. Within these two categories of operation there is an infinite variation of technique and technology, depending largely on the preference of the surgeon. Traditionally, but quite incorrectly, the various types of stiffening or arthrodesis operations are called 'spinal fusions'. In these 'fusion' operations, surgeons place bone graft on the spine, but it is a natural biological process which achieves the fusion. A newer technique does not even involve a bone transplant but merely a stiffening up of the spinal segments by implanting artificial ligaments (Grevitt et al., 1995). Equally incorrectly, the clearing or decompression operations have been called 'laminectomies'. There is usually much more involved in spinal canal decompression operations than mere laminectomy. Custom and usage have, however, conferred a form of validity on these terms, and we all continue to use them.

In surgery for deformity of the spine, especially for the curvature called scoliosis, various techniques are used to straighten the spine, in combination with the spinal arthrodesis which must always be done. The operations for deformity are described in more detail in Chapter 13.

The role of the physiotherapist in the surgery for spinal disorders may be negligible or critical, depending on the type of surgery and the particular circumstances surrounding the surgery (see Chapter 13). Where spinal surgery is performed frequently, a physiotherapist should be allocated to join the surgical team, performing the vital tasks of pre-operative assessment, preparation for surgery, and postoperative rehabilitation. The major contribution of enthusiastic physiotherapy to the success of surgical treatment is too often taken for granted.

SPINAL DISORDERS AND THEIR OPERATIONS

Some of the more common spinal disorders are described below, in descending order of approximate frequency; the operations which may need to be performed for them are given in brackets.

MECHANICAL PAIN (ARTHRODESIS; UNGRAFTED STABILISATION)

Spinal pain may develop with age-related degeneration of the discs (spondylosis), or as a result of sprain/strain injuries of the spine. The most common spinal disorder of this mechanical type is low back pain. Pain in the neck (cervical spine) of similar origin is the next most common disorder.

In the majority of cases there is no obvious cause for the mechanical pain either in the history or on the plain X-ray films. Occasionally, an X-ray film may show an un-united fracture of part of the lamina of a lower lumbar vertebra (spondylolysis) (Roche, 1949; Eisenstein, 1978). This is a fracture which will have occurred in childhood, usually forgotten or not even known to have occurred, but which presents with pain in adult life. It is never a congenital defect. If the fracture gap has opened significantly, the whole spine above the gap will have shifted forward on the vertebra below (spondylolisthesis; Figure 4.1) (Wiltse, 1962).

DISC PROLAPSE (DISCECTOMY, DECOMPRESSION)

A bulge or actual rupture of a disc annulus posteriorly, is quite common at the lower two lumbar segments, in physically active young or middle-aged adults. The condition comes to light only because the bulging disc mass irritates a root of the sciatic nerve, causing intense pain and paraesthesiae ('sciatica') down one lower limb (Figure 4.2). The irritation of the root is the result of a combination of direct pressure and chemical action of substances leaking from the disc. If non-surgical treatment in the form of rest and analgesics has been entirely unsuccessful for about 10 days, surgical decompression of the nerve becomes necessary to relieve the severe pain. When a large midline bulge of the disc causes paralysis of the bladder (part of the cauda equina syndrome), then this must be considered a surgical emergency.

Disc prolapse also occurs in the cervical spine, causing intense pain and paraesthesiae down one arm, but this is comparatively rare.

DEFORMITY (ARTHRODESIS)

Scoliosis is a side-to-side curvature of the spine with a twist (Figure 4.3), while kyphosis is a forward tilt. These

spinal deformities may be progressive in a young patient, and unresponsive to brace treatment. It is then necessary to perform a spinal arthrodesis with various forms of metal internal fixation to prevent further deformity and to improve the appearance of an unsightly rib hump (see Chapter 13). Physiotherapy has no role in the prevention of these deformities in young people except in the management of a programme of bracing treatment.

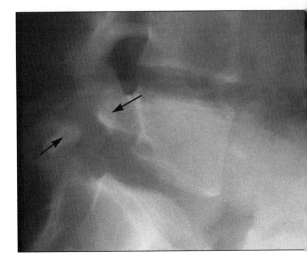

Figure 4.1 Spondylolysis (arrows) with spondylolisthesis, causing backache.

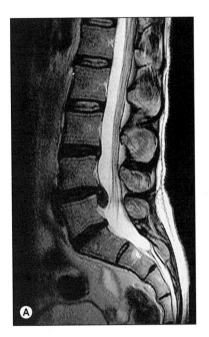

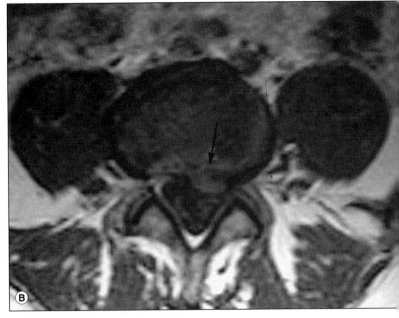

Figure 4.2 Magnetic resonance image of disc prolapse causing sciatica. (A) Sagittal section shows a black bulge at the penultimate disc. **(B)** Transverse section shows a prolapse (arrowed).

SPINAL STENOSIS (DECOMPRESSION, SOMETIMES WITH ARTHRODESIS)

Spinal stenosis is a generalised narrowing of the spinal canal, usually circumferential, at one or several segmental levels (Figure 4.4A and B). Elderly people are most commonly affected. It is the result of bony overgrowth and the buckling of thickened ligaments crowding into the canal. Patients complain of weakness, numbness, tingling and pain in the lower limbs, all of which are aggravated by walking, in spite of good blood circulation (Verbiest, 1954). The symptoms are thought to be caused by the blockage of blood flow in the veins around the nerves in the canal rather than by actual nerve

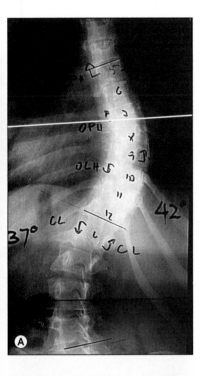

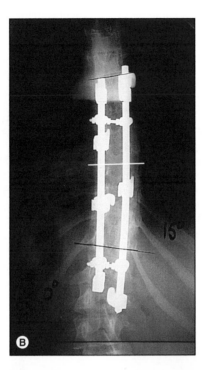

Figure 4.3 Scoliosis deformity (A) before and (B) after fixation and fusion surgery.

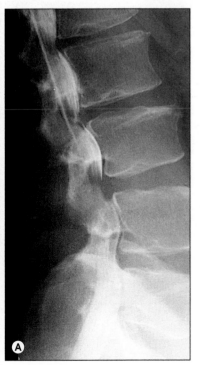

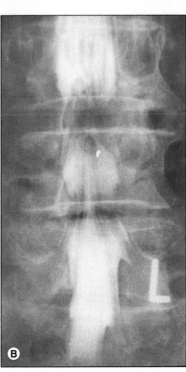

Figure 4.4 Spinal stenosis.
Myelography remains an important imaging technique in this condition. **(A)** Lateral view and **(B)** anteroposterior view show the 'beading' appearance of the contrast, typical of stenosis.

compression. When these symptoms force a patient to stop walking after a certain distance, the condition is called spinal claudication.

Not surprisingly, some of these elderly or late-middle-aged patients have severe low back pain as well. In these circumstances arthrodesis may be offered as part of the surgical treatment.

Spinal stenosis is also associated with achondroplastic dwarfism or may be developmental in origin, but these are rare causes.

Again, physiotherapy has no role in prevention or treatment except in conjunction with rehabilitation and walking education after surgery.

SPINAL INJURY (DECOMPRESSION AND ARTHRODESIS)

Where major trauma has caused a spinal fracture (Figure 4.5A,B and C), with or without dislocation, this frequently results in paralysis of the lower limbs and loss of bladder and bowel control (paraplegia). The management philosophy differs markedly between hospitals and nations. In many institutions it is considered important to operate on these patients to decompress the injured spinal cord and nerves in the hope of restoring some neural function, and to arthrodese the spine for early rehabilitation to mobility.

Where the injury is to the cervical spine, the patient may be paralysed in all four limbs and in some of the muscles of respiration (quadriplegia or tetraplegia). The physiotherapy for spinal cord injury is very intensive and specialised, and is not for discussion here.

INFECTION (DECOMPRESSION WITH OR WITHOUT ARTHRODESIS)

Almost every infecting bacterium and fungus has at some time infected the spine, causing varying degrees of destruction of vertebral bodies and discs (Digby & Kersley, 1979; Charles *et al.*, 1988, 1989; Govender *et al.*, 1991; Osman & Govender, 1995) (Figure 4.6). Paralysis is a possible outcome if the resulting kyphosis deformity and abscess formation produce pressure on the spinal cord and nerves. The two most common infecting organisms are pyogenic (*Staphylococcus*) and mycobacterial (tuberculosis). Decompression may be sufficient in early cases, but it is more usual to have to add a supporting bone graft.

INFLAMMATORY DISEASES (ARTHRODESIS: OCCASIONAL DECOMPRESSION, OR OSTEOTOMY)

Rheumatoid arthritis occasionally causes such destruction of discs and vertebrae that a kyphosis deformity will endanger the spinal cord. More common is the destruction of ligaments which secure the odontoid peg in the upper cervical spine, creating a threat of tetraplegia or sudden death.

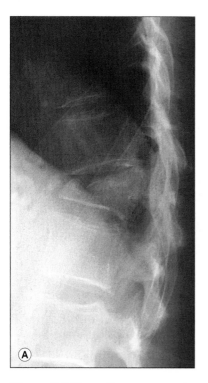
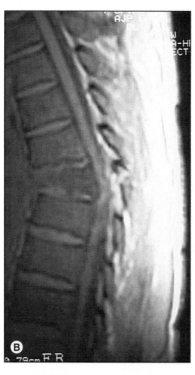
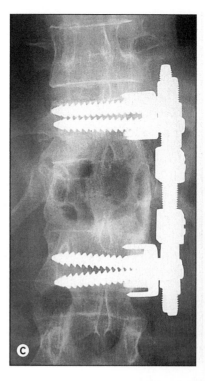

Figure 4.5 Magnetic resonance image of spinal injury. (A) A crush and burst fracture. **(B)** Compression of the spinal cord. **(C)** Anteroposterior view after fixation and fusion surgery.

Ankylosing spondylitis, on the other hand, can produce a spontaneous fusion of the spine of varying extent (Figure 4.7), but often with a kyphosis deformity of the whole spine. These patients are young adults or middle aged, usually male, and are so bent over that they cannot see more than a few feet of ground ahead. In this situation, the vertebral column must be cut across (osteotomy) in the midlumbar area or at the cervicothoracic junction, or at both levels, to improve the deformity and the forward gaze (Simmons, 1977; Thiranont & Netrawichien, 1993). An arthrodesis must be added to secure the correction. These patients have poor respiration, because of the ankylosis of the whole of the ribcage to the spine. This in turn presents a danger for the patient recovering from major surgery.

CANCER (DECOMPRESSION AND ARTHRODESIS)

Cancer originating in the spine is rare, but the spine is a favoured destination for the spread of cancer (metastasis) from breast, kidney, thyroid, lung, bowel and prostate (Figure 4.8A and B). The patient may present with great pain in the spine and established or developing paralysis following the collapse of vertebrae destroyed by the cancer. Decompression and arthrodesis can prevent paralysis (and occasionally improve it), and reduce the pain sufficiently to provide an acceptable quality of life.

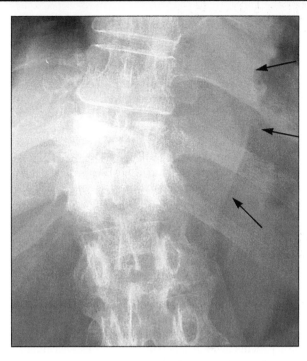

Figure 4.6 Tuberculosis infection. Anteroposterior view shows partial destruction of T11 and T12 vertebrae and the intervertebral disc. Note the outline of the abscess (arrowed).

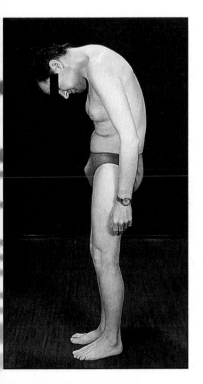

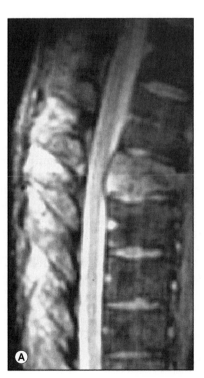

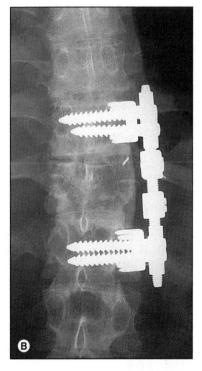

Figure 4.7 Fixed kyphosis deformity of ankylosing spondylitis.

Figure 4.8 Metastatic spread to T11 vertebra. (A) Destruction of vertebral body with pressure on spinal cord, and **(B)** after excision, grafting and fixation.

THE 'SALVAGE' SITUATION (DECOMPRESSION AND ARTHRODESIS)

The best efforts of spinal surgeons occasionally result in failure through a combination of circumstances or for reasons which simply cannot be defined. It is then too easy to point a finger and pontificate that the patient should not have had the surgery in the first place. Spinal surgeons are all too aware that many consider their practice esoteric and of doubtful need, so that decisions for surgical treatment are seldom lightly made. A decompression may need to be repeated, for instance, where a further fragment of disc tissue has emerged to press on a spinal nerve. A spinal arthrodesis may have failed to produce a complete fusion and additional bone grafting will be necessary. Internal fixation may have to be removed or replaced because of displacement or breakage. Infection is an ever-present danger. 'Salvage' or 'revision' surgery is never easy and never as successful as primary surgery, and is plagued by a high complication rate.

INDICATIONS FOR SPINAL SURGERY

Much of this subject has been covered above, from which it may seem that there is no controversy about deciding in favour of surgical treatment. It is widely accepted that the pain of nerve compression in, for example, lumbar disc prolapse becomes more difficult to treat successfully the longer the delay in providing surgical decompression; loss of bladder control is a surgical emergency; certain spine deformities, e.g. congenital scoliosis, are known to be quite unresponsive to non-surgical methods; a spinal abscess needs urgent surgical drainage; spinal cancer may threaten the stability of the spinal column such that only a spinal arthrodesis will suffice; and a few spinal injury patients may be more easily rehabilitated after arthrodesis.

The great dilemma is deciding surgical treatment for the most common spinal disorder: chronic mechanical low back pain. Spinal arthrodesis (or stabilisation) is the only surgical treatment known to have any chance of providing some degree of pain relief when all else (including physiotherapy) has failed. The fact is that the results of surgery are notoriously unpredictable from patient to patient, and symptoms are sometimes claimed to be worse after surgery even when it is clear that the surgery has been technically successful. The condition does not present a threat to life or limb. Most spinal surgeons will act on the basis that 'nobody has to have this operation'. It is therefore inevitable that recommendations for surgery will be made with some reluctance and with many warnings against unrealistic expectations. As far as the physiotherapist is concerned, there is a danger that every patient finally selected for surgery may represent a personal failure. It is closer to reality to regard physiotherapy as a critical stage in the selection process leading to surgery.

SELECTING THE PATIENT FOR SURGERY

There is no difficulty in selecting patients for spinal surgery when they are afflicted with serious spinal disease, deformity or injury: relatively simple rules govern the situation as it presents itself. However, the vast majority of patients attending a spinal clinic have no serious spinal disease: they have 'mechanical' pain, which may have originated from a back sprain or strain, or some degenerative process common to all humans. This mechanical pain will not affect life expectancy nor will it produce paralysis, but it may cause such a disruption of the normal conduct of daily life as to constitute a disability nearly equivalent to paralysis. These patients present the greatest challenge in the matter of selection for surgery, and therefore deserve a little more discussion.

It is important to remember that the vast majority of back pain patients are satisfactorily treated without surgery. The discussion that follows applies to those few patients whose symptoms are refractory to all non-surgical treatments.

DISABILITY

Disability is the cornerstone of patient selection for spinal arthrodesis or stabilisation in mechanical back pain. Pain at any level produces some degree of disability, most of which can be coped with sufficiently well by the majority of patients to continue their daily lives more or less uninterrupted. Pain is a matter of perception, and perception, like beauty, is 'in the eye of the beholder'. It follows that the disability which emanates from the pain is also a matter of perception and will differ markedly between patients. This difference has nothing to do with pain threshold but may have a great deal to do with differing life experience, culture and expectations. Even so, we must all complete certain tasks in our daily living to be able to continue a reasonable existence. When pain, however perceived by the individual, makes this impossible, then disability can be said to be of sufficient degree to justify an attempt at surgical treatment. It is possible to measure disability for a particular patient by means of a questionnaire which covers all aspects of the activities of daily living. The resulting index or score is valid for that patient and is a useful means of measuring progress over time, but it has no validity when making comparisons with other patients. The Oswestry Disability Index (ODI) (Fairbank *et al.*, 1980; see page 60) is usefully comprehensive without being burdensome. The ODI has been validated elsewhere and is now used widely internationally.

PERSONALITY

Apart from being dependent on neurological physiology, pain perception is a function of conditioned mental attitude or personality. Experience of spinal surgeons over the years has produced a wariness of the back pain patient without major pathology, who does not respond at all to conservative treatments and who insists that 'something more' be done. Spinal arthrodesis or stabilisation is the only option remaining. Doctors generally are very conscious of their duty to relieve suffering, but all too often the spinal operation offered in good faith has ended in bitterness. Too often patients have declared that they are much worse even when it can be shown that the operation has been technically successful. Surgeons then begin to question, in retrospect the patient's motivation and sincerity, and the result may be a cynicism which will incline the surgeon to withhold the surgical option from all back pain patients. In seeking to resolve this situation, surgeons have employed a variety of questionnaires designed to assess patients' personalities, in the hope of eliminating those who are likely to perceive a bad result irrespective of technical success. The better known of these tests are the Minnesota Multiphasic Personality Inventory (MMPI), and the Modified Somatic Perception Questionaire (MSPQ) (Beck *et al.*, 1961; Eysenck & Eysenck, 1964; Million *et al.*, 1982; Main, 1983; Main *et al.*, 1992). There are many more. Unfortunately, none of these tests is wholly reliable, nor should one expect them to be, but failed expectations have produced some disillusionment with the concept of personality testing for spinal pain surgery.

In the end, the surgeon's own judgement of the patient's personality may remain the best guide to patient selection, accepting that this judgement will be fallible in an acceptably small number of instances.

SPECIAL INVESTIGATIONS

In the context of spinal pain, special investigations are mainly radiological, i.e. X-ray films of the spine. Most modern imaging no longer uses X-ray technology but we all refer loosely to 'the X-rays'. In time, we will correctly refer to 'the imaging'. Blood tests are useful to eliminate the possibility of infection, inflammation or cancer causing the pain, but it is the imaging which is most likely to give us a working diagnosis and the probable segmental level of the pathology (McCall & Butt, 1987). Plain X-ray films show only the bones of the spine and none of the soft tissues, but

the vertebrae are rarely a source of pain. The discs and ligaments are the major soft tissue stabilisers of the spine and the most frequent source of pain. Discography involves injecting contrast medium into a series of discs to show up internal abnormalities on X-ray film (Figure 4.9A and B), and noting the type and distribution of any pain experienced. Facet arthrography is a similar technique for proving or eliminating the facet joints as a source of pain (Figure 4.10).

If it is uncertain whether lower limb pain is caused by a disc prolapsing onto a spinal nerve, then myelography, also called radiculography (Figure 4.11), will help. Contrast medium is injected into the dural sheath in the spinal canal: no contrast medium will be seen where a disc presses on a nerve. Computerised tomography (CT) scanning produces excellent cross-section views of the spine, (Figure 4.12) usually without the need for an injection. CT scanning is even more accurate when combined with myelography.

Magnetic resonance imaging (MRI) does not use X-rays, but records tissue images as a result of very high magnetic forces being sent through the body to stimulate the tissue ions (Figure 4.13). These images are useful for detecting the extent of various diseases in both the bones and soft tissues of the spine, but are of little use in finding the source of mechanical back pain. Radioisotope bone scans record the concentration of radioactivity in bone after the injection of radioactive technetium[99] (Figure 4.14). Radioisotope scanning is useful for locating cancer, infection and inflammation, but is not helpful in mechanical back pain.

Whenever there is suspicion of a destructive disease—usually cancer or infection—a biopsy of bone or disc tissue will help to make a certain diagnosis. During biopsy, a special wide-bore needle is directed to the diseased area and fragments of tissue are extracted for microscopy and bacterial culture.

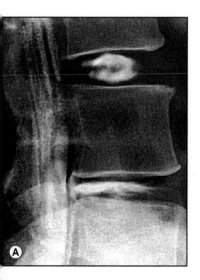
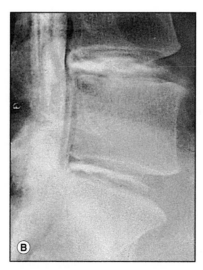
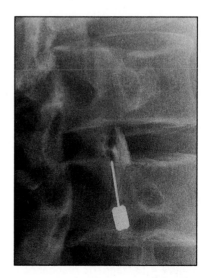

Figure 4.9 Lateral view of lumbar discography. The upper disc **(A)** shows the nucleus only; this disc was painless. The lower discs **(B)** show an abnormal spread of contrast, and the injection reproduced the typical pain.

Figure 4.10 Facet arthrography. Oblique view of lumbar spine showing needle in facet joint and contrast medium in joint.

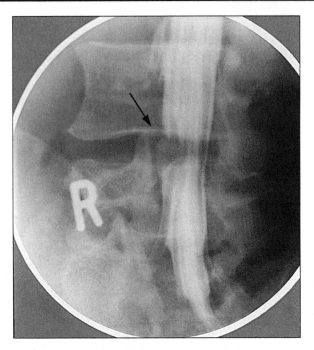

4

Figure 4.11 Myelography (also called radiculography) used typically to show a compressed nerve root, i.e. an absence of contrast medium (arrowed).

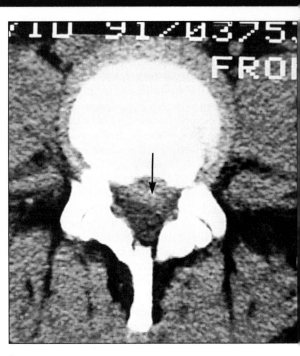

Figure 4.12 Computerised tomogram of a penultimate disc segment of the lumbar spine, showing disc prolapse (arrowed) into the spinal canal.

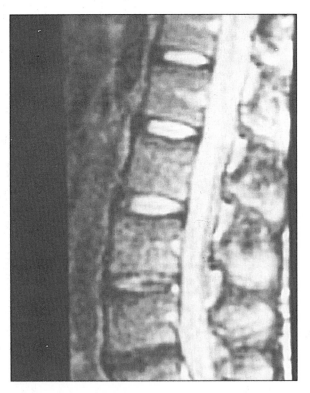

Figure 4.13 Magnetic resonance image showing sagittal section of lumbar spine. Magnetic resonance imaging can show abnormal or age-related changes in disc biochemistry as seen in the lowest disc.

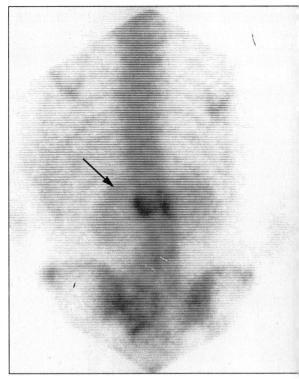

Figure 4.14 Radioisotope bone scan using technetium[99] in a patient suspected of metastatic spread of breast cancer in the spine (arrowed). Dark areas in pelvis are probably normal.

There is still no satisfactory method of imaging or locating common sources of pain which must have arisen in the mass of muscle and ligamentous tissue extending from the back of the vertebral column to subcutaneous fat and from the ribs to the pelvis. This is the single greatest challenge in back pain research today.

THE OPERATIONS

ARTHRODESIS

Arthrodesis, or 'fusion', is a bone transplant operation which can be performed at either the anterior or posterior aspect of the spine, depending largely on the preference of the surgeon and the need for associated decompression surgery.

A posterior fusion anywhere in the spine involves splitting the soft tissues that cover it, usually from a midline incision, and shifting the tissues laterally to expose the bone surfaces of the laminae right out to the tips of the transverse processes. The smooth surface (cortex) of the bone is scraped until it bleeds. Slices of bone graft are taken from the patient's pelvis (autograft) and placed over the scraped surfaces—bone from animals (xenograft) or from other humans (allograft) may be used when there is insufficient of the patient's own bone. Internal

fixation procedures, to keep the spine still and stable while the bone graft consolidates, are now performed routinely, using metal frames of various designs, very like scaffolding. The strongest fixation in the lumbar area is achieved by inserting screws into the pedicles of the vertebrae, and connecting them to a rod or plate on each side of the midline (Figure 4.15A and B). Instead of pedicle screws, it is possible to pass wire loops around the laminae at every segmental level and twist the loops over the rods, known as the Luque system (Luque, 1982).

An anterior fusion can also be performed at any level of the spine, although complex anatomy at the cervicothoracic and thoracolumbar junctions makes for complex surgery at these levels. Once the spine is exposed—via the neck, chest or abdomen—the relevant disc segments are excised, the adjacent vertebral body surfaces scraped till cancellous bone is exposed, and pelvic bone graft blocks pushed into position in the disc space. Where the vertebrae have been crushed by injury or disease, extra stability can be provided by inserting metal internal fixation, anchored to healthy vertebrae above and below. After surgery, the grafted area should be protected by a brace—a firm collar will suffice for the cervical spine for 6–8 weeks, whereas a custom-fitted polyethylene brace is needed for 3–6 months for the thoracic and lumbar spine.

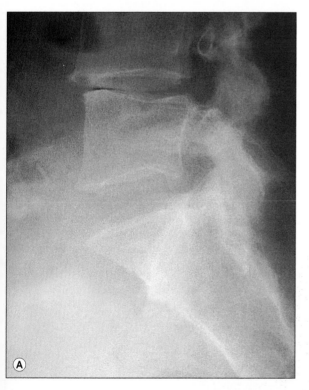

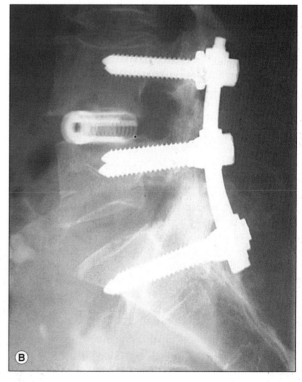

Figure 4.15 Use of pedical screw fixation to assist spinal fusion in painful disc degeneration. Lateral plain X-ray film before **(A)** and after **(B)** surgery. Note the addition of the interbody cage to restore L4/5 disc height.

STABILISATION WITHOUT FUSION

Because of the unpredictability of the results of arthrodesis of the lumbar spine for low back pain, there is increasing interest in less drastic operations. These newer operations may produce pain relief at least as frequently as arthrodesis but with much less scarring of tissues and without the need for bone removal for grafting. These operations depend on affected spine segments being bound by artificial ligaments looped over pedicle screws. The best known of these operations is that developed by Dr Henri Graf of Lyon (Grevitt et al., 1995).

DECOMPRESSION

Lumbar disc prolapse with nerve root compression or irritation is the most frequent requirement for decompression surgery in Western society, whereas in developing countries some entirely different pathology, e.g. infection, may take priority. It is usually possible to perform a discectomy through a fenestration approach, i.e. by cutting a window in the ligamentum flavum on the affected side. When this approach does not give sufficient access to the disc, bone must be chipped away from the adjacent edges of the laminae—a laminotomy. Rarely, an even wider exposure is necessary and a whole lamina is removed—a laminectomy.

In the past, all decompression operations were incorrectly called laminectomies. Such terminology is particularly inappropriate in this era of minimal exposure for many types of surgery. Chemonucleolysis, now less favoured, requires an injection of chymopapain enzyme into the disc (Nordby & Fraser, 1996). Nucleotomy involves removal of a disc through an automated biopsy needle connected to a suction device. Percutaneous discectomy is simply the removal of disc material via a narrow tube inserted from the side of the body through the skin and tissues, much like the technique for arthroscopy of the knee, and using long fine nibblers. A further refinement employs laser technology to vaporise the disc, and video technology to improve visibility for both lumbar and thoracic disc surgery (Figure 4.16).

These minimal approaches are all indirect, i.e. they remove disc material from the disc space but not necessarily that portion which is producing the nerve compression. Microdiscectomy allows a direct approach to the prolapsed portion of disc, as for a conventional fenestration, but through a small incision (2–3 cm) (McCulloch, 1989). An operating microscope affords the surgeon excellent visualisation of the surgical field (Figure 4.17).

The advantages of all these minimal approaches are increased patient comfort and early mobilisation, as well as less time spent in hospital. The task of the physiotherapist postoperatively is much easier, and the mechanical stability of the spine is better preserved. The main disadvantage is the high cost of the equipment required for each of these techniques.

In degenerative lumbar spinal stenosis, it is sometimes necessary to perform a multilevel laminectomy and an undercutting facetectomy, i.e. excision of the whole lamina on both sides and at several levels and widening of the nerve root canals.

In major spinal diseases such as cancer and tuberculosis, and in burst fractures, it may be necessary to decompress the spinal cord from the front, by vertebrectomy, i.e. removal of one or more whole vertebrae. A bone graft is ideal for filling the resulting gap, and anterior internal fixation may be used for extra stability. If this operation has to be performed in the thoracic spine, as is so often the case with tuberculosis, then access through the chest wall is by thoracotomy, and involves the removal of a rib.

The rehabilitation of the patient after major spinal surgery, from recumbency to independent walking, requires dedication and persistence on the part of the physiotherapist. Where a thoracotomy has been performed, the physiotherapist is crucial in helping the patient regain full respiratory function despite pain and the inconvenience of a chest drain.

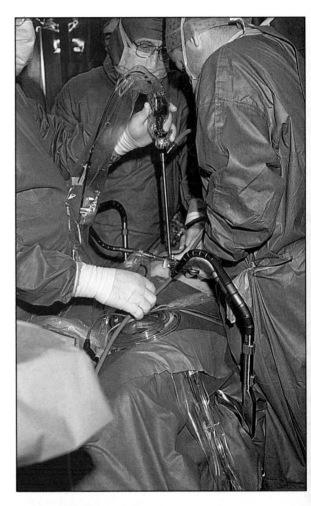

Figure 4.16 Video-assisted endoscopic surgery for a prolapsed thoracic disc.

THE OSWESTRY DISABILITY INDEX

The ODI was developed in 1976 by Judith Couper, Stephen Eisenstein and John O'Brien, and has provided a useful measure of self-reported disability for the activities of daily living, caused by spinal pain (Fairbank *et al.*, 1980). It has been validated by a number of separate studies conducted independently and is in daily use in many countries. An example of this form is shown on page 60.

Each section is scored from 0 to 5, and there are six levels of disability in each section. The scores for all sections are added together and multiplied by 2 to give a score out of 100. Where a whole section is irrelevant for a particular patient, the score is calculated from the reduced possible total. This final score does not in any sense represent a percentage disability in the way that social services may calculate disability for the purposes of compensation. It is merely a score against which to measure progress on subsequent occasions for that particular patient: it is never intended to be compared with the scores of other patients.

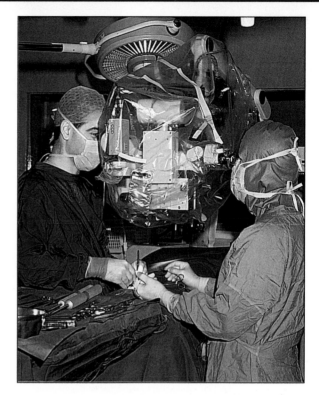

Figure 4.17 Lumbar discectomy. Microscope enables better vision through a small incision.

REFERENCES

eck AT, Ward CH, Mendelson M, Mock JE, Erbaugh JK. An inventory for measuring depression. *Arch Gen Psychol* 1961, **4**:561-571.

harles RW, Govender S, Naidoo KS. Echinococcal infection of the spine with neural involvement. *Spine* 1988, **13**:47-49.

harles RW, Mody GM, Govender S. Pyogenic infection of the lumbar vertebral spine due to gas-forming organisms. A case report. *Spine* 1989, **14**:541-543.

igby JM, Kersley JB. Pyogenic non-tuberculous spinal infection: an analysis of thirty cases. *J Bone Joint Surg* 1979, **61B**:47-55.

isenstein S. Spondylolysis. A skeletal investigation of two population groups. *J Bone Joint Surg* 1978, **60B**:488-494.

ysenck HK, Eysenck SBG. *Manual of the Eysenck personality inventory*. London: University of London Press; 1964.

airbank JC, Couper J, Davies JB, O'Brien JP. The Oswestry low back pain disability questionnaire. *Physiotherapy* 1980, **66**:271-273.

ovender S, Rajoo R, Goga IE, Charles RW. Aspergillus osteomyelitis of the spine. *Spine* 1991, **16**:746-749.

revitt MP, Gardner AD, Spilsbury J, *et al*. The Graf stabilisation system: early results in 50 patients. *Eur Spine J* 1995, **4**:169-175.

uque ER. Segmental spinal instrumentation for correction of scoliosis. *Clin Orthop* 1982, **163**:192-198.

ain CJ, Wood PLR, Hollis S, Spanswick C, Waddell GC. Distress and risk assessment method: a simple patient classification to identify distress and evaluate the risk of poor outcome. *Spine* 1992, **17**:42-52.

Main CJ. The modified somatic perception questionnaire (MSPQ). *J Psychosomatic Res* 1983, **27**:503-514.

McCall IW, Butt WP. The radiological diagnosis of low back pain. *Curr Orthop* 1987, **1**:375-382.

McCulloch JA. *Principles of microsurgery for lumbar disc disease*. New York: Raven Press; 1989.

Million R, Hall W, Haavick-Nilsen K, Baker RD, Jayson MIV. Assessment of the progress of the back pain patient. *Spine* 1982, **7**:204-212.

Nordby EJ, Fraser RD, Javid MJ. Chemonucleolysis. *Spine* 1996, **21**:1102-1105.

Osman AA, Govender S. Septic sacroiliitis. *Clin Orthop* 1995, **313**:214-219.

Roche MB. The pathology of neural arch defects. *J Bone Joint Surg* 1949, **31A**:529-537.

Simmons EH. Kyphotic deformity of the spine in ankylosing spondylitis. *Clin Orthop* 1977, **128**:65-77.

Thiranont N, Netrawichien P. Transpedicular decancellation closed wedge vertebral osteotomy for treatment of fixed flexion deformity of spine in ankylosing spondylitis. *Spine* 1993, **18**:2517-2522.

Verbiest H. A radicular syndrome from developmental narrowing of the lumbar vertebral canal. *J Bone Joint Surg* 1954, **36B**:230-237.

Wiltse LL. The etiology of spondylolisthesis. *J Bone Joint Surg* 1962, **44A**:539-560.

Confidential

THE OSWESTRY DISABILITY INDEX FOR LOW BACK PAIN

The Robert Jones and Agnes Hunt Orthopaedic and District Hospital, NHS Trust, Oswestry, Shropshire, Department for Spinal Disorders

Name .... Date of Birth ....

Address .... Date ....

.... Age ....

Occupation

How long have you had back pain? .... Years .... Months .... Weeks

How long have you had leg pain? .... Years .... Months .... Weeks

Please read: This questionnaire has been designed to give the doctor information as to how your back pain has affected your ability to manage in everyday life. Please answer every section, and mark in each section only ONE BOX which applies to you. We realise you may consider that two of the statements in any one section relate to you, but please just mark the box which most closely describes your problem.

SECTION 1 - PAIN INTENSITY
1 ☐ My pain is mild to moderate: I do not need pain killers
2 ☐ The pain is bad, but I manage without taking pain killers
3 ☐ Pain killers give complete relief from pain
4 ☐ Pain killers give moderate relief from pain
5 ☐ Pain killers give very little relief from pain
6 ☐ Pain killers have no effect on the pain

SECTION 2 - PERSONAL CARE (Washing, Dressing, etc)
1 ☐ I can look after myself normally withought causing extra pain
2 ☐ I can look after myself normally but it causes extra pain
3 ☐ It is painful to look after myself and I am slow and careful
4 ☐ I need some help but manage most of my personal care
5 ☐ I need help every day in most aspects of self care
6 ☐ I do not get dressed; wash with difficult; and stay in bed

SECTION 3 - LIFTING
1 ☐ I can lift heavy weights without extra pain
2 ☐ I can lift heavy weights but it gives extra pain
3 ☐ Pain prevents me from lifting heavy weights off the floor, but I can manage if they are conveniently positioned, eg on a table
4 ☐ Pain prevents me from lifting heavy weights but I can manage light weighs if they are conveniently positioned
5 ☐ I can lift only very light weights
6 ☐ I cannot lift of carry anything at all

SECTION 4 - WALKING
1 ☐ I can walk as far as I wish
2 ☐ Pain prevents me walking more than 1 mile
3 ☐ Pain prevents me walking more than 1/2 mile
4 ☐ Pain prevents me walking more than 1/4 mile
5 ☐ I can walk only if I use a stick or crutches
6 ☐ I am in bet or in a chair for most of every day

SECTION 5 - SITTING
1 ☐ I can sit in any chair as long as I like
2 ☐ I can sit in my favourite chair only, but for as long as I like
3 ☐ Pain prevents me from sitting more than 1 hour
4 ☐ Pain prevents me from sitting more than 1/2 hour
5 ☐ Pain prevents me from sitting more than 10 minutes
6 ☐ Pain prevents me from sitting at all

SECTION 6 - STANDING
1 ☐ I can stand as long as I want without extra pain
2 ☐ I can stand as long as I want, but it gives me extra pain
3 ☐ Pain prevents me from standing for more thatn 1 hour
4 ☐ Pain prevents me from standing for more than 30 minutes
5 ☐ Pain prevents me from standing for more than 10 minutes
6 ☐ Pain prevents me from standing at all

SECTION 7 - SLEEPING
1 ☐ Pain does not prevent me from sleeping well
2 ☐ I sleep well, but only by using tablets
3 ☐ Even when I take tablets I have less than 6 hours sleep
4 ☐ Even when I take tablets I have less than 4 hours sleep
5 ☐ Even when I take tablets I have less than 2 hours sleep
6 ☐ Pain prevents me from sleeping at all

SECTION 8 - SEX LIFE
1 ☐ My sex life is normal and causes no extra pain
2 ☐ My sex life is normal but causes some extra pain
3 ☐ My sex life is nearly normal but is very painful
4 ☐ My sex life is severly restricted by pain
5 ☐ My sex life is nearly absent because of pain
6 ☐ Pain prevents any sex life at all

SECTION 9 - SOCIAL LIFE
1 ☐ My social life is normal and causes me no extra pain
2 ☐ My socil life is normal but increases the degree of pain
3 ☐ Pain affects my social life by limiting only my more energetic interests (dancing, etc)
4 ☐ Pain has restricted my social life and I do not go out as often
5 ☐ Pain has restricted my social life to my home
6 ☐ I have no social life because of pain

SECTION 10 - TRAVELLING
1 ☐ I can travel anywhere without extra pain
2 ☐ I can travel anywhere but it gives me extra pain
3 ☐ Pain is bad, but I manage journeys over 2 hours
4 ☐ Pain restricts me to journeys of less than 1 hour
5 ☐ Pain restricts me to short necessary journeys under 30 minutes
6 ☐ Pain prevents me travelling except to the Doctor or Hospital

INSTRUCTION TO CLINICIAN: CALCULATING THE SCORE

Each Section has six questions. The first question carries a value of O and the sixth question carries a value of 5. The values of the marked questions in the completed Questionnaire, are added together and multiplied by 2 to give a score out of 100. This is not in any way to be seen as a "percentage" disability which could be compared to the score of other patients: the result is merely a figure for the convenience of comparing scores in the same patient on different occasions. When, for one reason or another, a patient cannot or will not complete a Section, then the value of that whole Section, ie. 5, is subtracted from the initial possible total of 50, when calculating the score for that patient.

COMMENTS: ....

Couper, Eisenstein and O'Brien:1976
(Fairbank *et al.*, 1980)

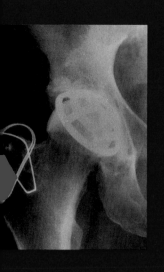

5 M D Northmore-Ball

SURGERY FOR LOWER LIMB ARTHRITIS IN THE ADULT

CHAPTER OUTLINE

INTRODUCTION

Surgery for arthritis in the lower limb may involve one or more of a wide variety of procedures, the main ones being arthroscopy, osteotomy, arthrodesis and the different types of arthroplasty. The first section of this chapter will concentrate on the main characteristics of each of these, followed by their application to the different joints in the lower limb.

TYPES OF SURGERY

ARTHROSCOPY

Arthroscopy is endoscopy of a joint. The first arthroscopy was performed in Tokyo in 1918 by Takaji, although endoscopy had been carried out as long ago as 1806 by Bozzini in Vienna. For a long time arthroscopy was only used for diagnostic purposes, but after the first arthroscopic surgery (an arthroscopic meniscectomy) in 1962 by Watanabe, also in Tokyo, arthroscopic surgery has become a major subspeciality.

OSTEOTOMY

An osteotomy is simply division of a bone, and is frequently part of a surgical approach. If an important ligament or muscle needs to be detached to provide necessary exposure, this can be done by osteotomising the piece of

bone where the ligament or muscle is inserted. At the end of the procedure, the bone is fixed back. The Charnley technique of total hip replacement (THR) provides a well-known example of osteotomy, where the greater trochanter is osteotomised to allow mobilisation of the glutei.

An osteotomy as an operation in itself is usually indicated to correct a bone deformity where there is significant pain or loss of function. An osteotomy is also very frequently performed to deliberately produce an abnormal shape in a previously normal bone, for example, to alter the mechanics to treat a nearby condition such as an un-united fracture or arthritis in a neighbouring joint.

The general principles of the osteotomy technique are: first, to expose the bone surgically (the bone may be easily accessible, e.g. the tibia, or require specially developed methods of exposure, e.g. around parts of the acetabulum); then to divide the bone with an osteotome, a saw or special power tools; frequently, then to change the shape of the osteotomy surfaces; then to displace the bone ends to produce the desired change in shape, usually at the same time bringing the newly shaped bone ends into proximity; and, finally, to hold the skeleton in this new position by internal or external means.

ARTHRODESIS

Arthrodesis, or surgical fusion of a joint, is indicated where significant pain, deformity or instability arises in an abnormal joint, and where it is felt that the resulting complete loss of joint movement is acceptable. With the advent of replacement arthroplasty (see below), these indications are seen much less frequently.

The technique of arthrodesis is: first, to surgically expose the joint, then almost always to dislocate it so as to expose the damaged joint surfaces, which are then suitably treated; then to bring these surfaces together in a position for best overall function, bearing in mind that the joint will no longer move; and, finally, to hold the joint in this position by internal or external means. A fundamental requirement for arthrodesis is that most, if not all, other lower limb joints should be normally mobile.

ARTHROPLASTY

This is a non-specific term covering any surgical refashioning of a joint, with or without the use of artificial materials. An arthroplasty is indicated for pain, deformity or instability in a joint where loss of motion is considered unacceptable, and sometimes for the deliberate mobilisation of a previously fixed joint where this fixity by itself is the cause of significant symptoms, as, for example, in the mobilisation of a previously fused hip for intractable back pain.

There are three main types of arthroplasty: excision, interposition and replacement.

Excision Arthroplasty

Here, one or both of the bone ends forming a joint are excised. The most common example is a Keller's arthroplasty, where the proximal end of the proximal phalanx of the big toe is excised to treat a painful hallux valgus. The resulting weakness and instability of the toe are not felt to be significant. A well-known example of excision arthroplasty in a large joint is the Girdlestone arthroplasty of the hip—now seldom seen except as an end stage following failed hip replacement. After excision of the bone ends, the hope is that a flexible scar will form between them, and therefore an attempt may be made to preserve the gap between the bone ends during the early stages of healing. This is achieved with traction in the case of a Girdlestone arthroplasty or with a Kirschner wire in the case of a Keller's arthroplasty.

Interposition Arthroplasty

This is largely of historical interest. The joint is opened and material is placed between the bone ends. This material may be natural or artificial or a prosthesis and the bone ends may or may not be reshaped. Fascia lata and silastic have been used. An example of interposition arthroplasty is mould arthroplasty of the hip. This procedure was widely used and quite successful, and involved a Vitallium shell being interposed between the reshaped head of the femur and the reamed acetabulum. This type of arthroplasty usually requires a prolonged period of vigorous postoperative rehabilitation, and the results are often unpredictable.

Replacement Arthroplasty

This has almost completely superseded the other types of arthroplasty, and has greatly reduced the indications for osteotomy and arthrodesis in the treatment of symptomatic arthritis. Major joint replacement in the lower limb offer tremendous opportunities for radically decreasing patients disabilities and improving function. In the hip and knee several techniques exist, which, if carefully applied, can be expected to give good results. Limitations of the procedures do, however, still exist and certain quite fundamental questions remain unanswered.

THE HIP

ARTHROSCOPY

Arthroscopy of the hip has recently become possible although its place has yet to be clearly established. It is of benefit in young adults with unexplained hip pain. Specific surgical procedures, such as labral resection and chondral abrasion, are possible, and the concomitant irrigation of the joint may be helpful in treating early arthritis. To perform arthroscopy of the hip, distraction of the hip by traction using special apparatus or a fracture table, and X-ray guidance are needed. Current problems with the procedure include an inability to move the hip into different positions during the arthroscopy, and the need for special instrumentation because of the joint's deep-seated location and spherical shape.

OSTEOTOMY

Before the development of hip replacement, an intertrochanteric osteotomy was very commonly performed for osteoarthritis. In this procedure—the McMurray osteotomy—an osteotome was used to divide the femur and the bone ends were then allowed to fall into a natural position before the hip was immobilised in a plaster spica. Although largely uncontrolled, the McMurray osteotomy gave a good result remarkably frequently—patients are still seen who were treated by this procedure many years ago and they continue to have good function. However, hip replacement has made the McMurray osteotomy virtually obsolete.

In young people, joint replacement has its own problems: a failed joint replacement in a young person, which may be followed later, perhaps, by unsatisfactory revision surgery, can produce gross loss of the skeleton. This has brought about a renewed interest in osteotomy. On mainland Europe, osteotomy has continued to be practised notably by exponents of the priniciples of Pauwels, who analysed the effects of alterations of hip joint alignment on the mechanics of the hip. If osteotomy is carried out using Pauwels' principles and combined with modern technique of internal fixation, e.g. ASIF screws and/or plates, it can produce surprisingly good and predictable results. Under these circumstances osteotomy can be a valid alternative treatment to joint replacement in carefully selected young patients.

In a young adult with developing arthritis or established arthritis of the hip, osteotomy can be used to reduce the load per unit area on the abnormal hip surfaces in two ways: by increasing the effective weight-bearing area an by reducing the total load taken through the surfaces by improving the mechanical advantage of the muscles around the hip (notably the abductors). Occasionally, the latter is supplemented by defunctioning some of the motor muscles, e.g. the psoas.

A careful assessment of the patient and his or her hip X-ray films is needed pre-operatively. This assessment may include special X-ray film views, such as the 'faux profile', an image produced by the patient weight bearing in the oblique lateral plane. This view helps to evaluate the lack of chondral coverage of the anterior head. Computerised tomography (CT) scanning, and sometimes also hip examination under a general anaesthetic with screening using an X-ray image intensifier, may be required.

Osteotomies of the acetabular or femoral sides of the hip, or sometimes both, may be indicated. A common indication for pelvic osteotomy is acetabular dysplasia with deficiency of the acetabular roof anteriorly and superiorly. The osteotomy may then either redirect or enlarge the acetabulum. Redirection in the child is fairly straightforward because of pelvic flexibility, and is achieved simply by opening a transverse osteotomy (Salter) just above the acetabulum. Redirection in the adult, however, requires a considerably more complex operation involving division of all the bony connections of the acetabulum. Several methods for this restorative procedure have been described, for example, the Ganz peri-acetabular osteotomy (Figure 5.1A and B), whereby the ilium is divided coronally to just in front of the sciatic notch, in

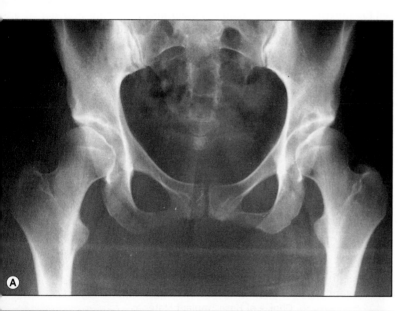

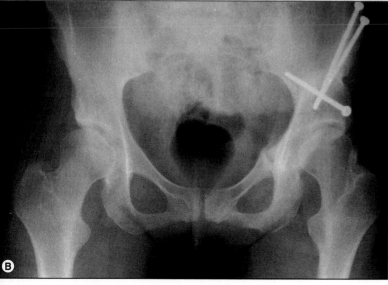

Figure 5.1 (A) Pelvic X-ray film of a 32-year-old woman with bilateral hip dysplasia. The condition is worse on the left, where there is a substantial superior subchondral cyst indicating developing degenerative change. **(B)** Appearances 2 years after a Ganz peri-acetabular osteotomy adducting the acetabulum 15° and extending it 20°. Bony remodelling is still taking place, the pubis not being fully consolidated. There is a little heterotopic ossification of no consequence. The subchondral cyst has completely disappeared and the patient is symptom free.

continuity with a division of the ischium in the frontal plane, and division of the superior pubic ramus. All this is achieved through one anterior approach. Another procedure, the Wagner technique, uses special osteotomes to divide the peri-acetabular bone spherically just deep to the cartilage.

Enlargement of the acetabulum is usually indicated where hip subluxation is too severe for acetabular reorientation. It may be achieved in several ways, notably by the Chiari osteotomy. Here, the ilium is again divided above the acetabulum, but completely into the sciatic notch—the anterior end of the cut may be curved distally over the front of the hip. The osteotomy is then displaced transversely and the hip placed medially some distance in relation to the ilium above it, thus providing a solid load-bearing buttress above the subluxing femoral head. Femoral osteotomy is usually carried out in the intertrochanteric region, as exemplified by Bombelli. A varus femoral osteotomy may be performed for superolateral arthritis, where the acetabulum is normal and the femoral head still spherical but the femoral neck shaft angle is increased. The varus will then increase the force tending to make the femoral head move medially. This procedure is, however, now only rarely indicated in the adult as shortening of the leg, for example, may result. A valgus femoral osteotomy may be performed in quite advanced osteoarthritis but only when the femoral head has become flattened with medial osteophyte formation. Here, the change to a valgus alignment alters the load-bearing fulcrum within the hip joint, moving it medially and thus reducing the load on the hip. Correctly indicated, this procedure can be remarkably effective. Varus and valgus osteotomies are usually combined with extension, i.e. the hip is able to move into a slightly flexed position with the leg in normal position, and often need to be combined with rotation or with medial or lateral displacement. The overall alignment and length of the leg should be considered when planning osteotomies of this kind.

Postoperative Management

This has to be individualised. From about 2 days postoperatively the patient usually undertakes assisted active exercises of the hip and shadow walking for some weeks. A sequence of special exercises is sometimes desirable. A prolonged period of partial weight bearing is then indicated until the osteotomy has united. In the treatment of established osteoarthritis, this will also give the best chance for regeneration of the damaged hip surfaces. This process which has been demonstrated histologically by the growth of islands of fibrocartilage in a previously denuded bony surface, is often confirmed by serial X-ray films showing a gradual increase in thickness of the cartilaginous layer of the hip.

ARTHRODESIS

This has one main residual indication only—the patient is invariably male, extremely young and active, and has an arthritic hip (typically the result of a fracture or fracture dislocation of the hip in an accident) which is painful and stiff. Such a patient should be able to cope with the limitations of a hip arthrodesis and require an absolutely durable surgical procedure. This indication is, however, rarely seen, as most patients have either suitable localised conditions within the hip for an osteotomy, or have too great a residual motion in the joint for them to be prepared to sacrifice this to arthrodesis, preferring instead the relative uncertainties of a future with some other form of operation. An arthrodesis is now usually performed using established ASIF techniques, for example, a long plate running from the ilium above the hip down the lateral or the anterior sides of the femur. A concomitant pelvic osteotomy may sometimes be needed to provide adequate bony contact for fusion to occur. This form of fixation allows very accurate positioning of the hip—about 20° of flexion and neutral or slight external rotation—and does not require plaster immobilisation. A major advantage of this procedure is that, if needed, it is usually possible to convert the arthrodesis to a THR; an arthrodesis should be planned with this in mind.

ARTHROPLASTY

As a procedure for the treatment of arthritis, arthroplasty of the hip is nowadays confined to replacement arthroplasty. The most commonly performed replacement arthroplasty is THR.

TOTAL HIP REPLACEMENT

THR is also known as low-friction arthroplasty (LFA) or, in the USA, total hip arthroplasty (THA).

Implant Design

This may be subdivided into: choice of base implant material; geometry; method of fixation; and materials used for the bearing surfaces.

Choice of Base Implant Material

Nowadays, the base material of the hip replacement stem usually comprises a metal such as stainless steel, cobalt-chrome or titanium alloy. The manufacturer bases his choice of material on strength, resistance to fatigue fracture, flexibility and biocompatibility. The first three depend also on the geometry of the stem: for example, a weak material might be adequate if the stem is thick enough; similarly, the flexibility of an implant, possibly desirable in allowing more uniform loading of the underlying bone, will be as dependent on the thickness of the material as on its intrinsic flexibility. Materials may be good in some respects yet poor in others: titanium, for example, is readily accepted by the body but rather soft, so that it is easily abraded where motion occurs in contact with the skeleton, and produces undesirable debris. Metallic stems are not universal; polymers, sometimes strengthened with a metal core, have been used. The acetabular component is usually made of a high-density polyethylene (HDP). The plastic cups are sometimes composite, with the base material

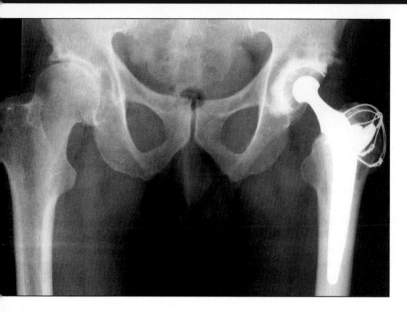

Figure 5.2 Pelvic X-ray film showing a left total hip replacement performed by the classic Charnley technique. A trochanteric osteotomy has been used, with reattachment by cruciate wiring and a Charnley staple clamp. A Wroblewski bone plug has been used to block the femoral canal distal to the cement.

eing exposed as one bearing surface and another materi-
l on the outside (Figure 5.3B). Polyethylene has the advan-
ge of being readily available, a tradition of long use, and
ase of manufacture. It is, however, not without disadvan-
iges (Figure 5.3B). Some cups are made of ceramic, e.g.
lumina, aluminium oxide. Correctly used, ceramic cups
nay have a very low wear rate. Unlike plastic, however,
eramic is subject to fracture.

eometry
he geometry of the femoral stem varies widely between
nplants. The femoral head is made in several sizes rang-
ig from 22 to 32 mm (22.25 mm was the original size cho-
n for the Charnley THR). The size of the head influences
ie rate of wear of the bearing and, in conjunction with the
ze of the prosthetic neck, also influences the range of
iovement allowed by the components before the head lifts
ut of the socket, causing dislocation. For given bearing
iaterials, small heads tend to burrow further into the sock-
: as wear proceeds. Wide variations also exist in the shape
f the section of the stem within the remnant of the
moral neck. The femoral neck is commonly removed to
greater or lesser extent at surgery, and the stem may have
collar which sits on the stump of the neck. The value of
collar remains contentious, some surgeons, e.g. Harris,
insidering it essential, while in the designs of others, e.g.
ing, it is completely absent. The underlying differences
late to where the load transfer is intended to be taken. In
ie Freeman implant, the femoral neck is retained as it has
een shown to have an important influence on torsional
ability of the stem in the femur, for example, when the
itient rises quickly from a chair. The surface finish and
recise shape of the stem within the femoral canal is also
ibject to important variations, for example, in its thick-
ess and taper. In cementless designs, the shape is to some
xtent determined by the internal shape of the femoral
inal, though this shape may be reamed to a desired form

with special instrumentation. If fixed by cement, the
acetabular component is almost always hemispherical. The
Charnley cup has a flange. This flange is cut to fit the prepared skeleton and assists in cement pressurisation.
Several implants have various parts trimmed away to facilitate prosthetic movement. Uncemented cups have a wide
variety of shapes, but are usually either hemispherical,
partly conical, cylindrical and/or threaded. Threaded cups,
however, have not proved successful in the long term.
There are widevariations in opinion as to the correct shape;
these opinions are only gradually being backed up by experimental and/or clinical data.

Method of Fixation
The striking success of the early Charnley THR was
achieved by fixation of the implants with acrylic cement
(Figure 5.2). Sir John Charnley persuaded patients with
successful hip replacements to bequeath their hips back
to him for histological analysis. This analysis showed that
in the majority of cases, the femoral cement was
extremely well accepted by the body in the long term, i.e.
for periods of up to 20 years, though less satisfactory
acceptance was seen in the acetabulum, for reasons
which are still unclear. Cement can, however, break up,
especially when a poorly inserted implant is overloaded.
Broken cement is a cause (see page 66) of osteolysis, a
potentially serious problem resulting in leaching of the
skeleton. So much attention has been focused on this
effect that many view cement as an undesirable material for implant fixation. This has heralded an increase in
systems involving cementless implant fixation. These
systems rely on a 'press-fit', i.e. when the component is
driven into a suitably prepared bed, it fits solidly. The
press-fit can then be supplemented by various forms of
rough or porous surface, for example, beads or mesh,
and, much more promisingly, by a hydroxyapatite (HA)
coating. Bone has been shown, both experimentally and

clinically, to grow up to and bond with HA, and this choice of material is becoming increasingly popular. Its longer-term properties are, however, uncertain; for example, it is thought to slowly resorb, so that late loss of fixation could occur. Further intriguing possibilities include new types of cold curing and bioactive cements.

Materials

The chief requirements of bearing surfaces are that both friction and wear should be as low as possible. The very common combination of metal against plastic is time hallowed and effective, but has finite limitations. However smooth the head, the plastic wears, producing particles, and it has gradually become obvious that these particles are harmful. Particles are a potential cause of major implant loosening from osteolysis, the phenomenon once attributed solely to cement. Although ceramic heads, notably zirconia, produce lower wear, they still occasionally break. This is a problem yet to be fully solved. Recently, the combination of metal against metal has been revived, with considerable promise. There are also experimental materials, e.g. polyurethane rubber, which may reduce wear further or almost abolish it. Particles caused by wear and corrosion products may also arise from the microscopic movement between parts of modular implants and from other surfaces of the implant. As these materials are often metallic, there is the disturbing possibility, especially with cementless implants with porous surfaces, that carcinogenesis could occur in the long term.

Clinical

The main symptoms and indications for THR are pain, loss of hip movement, loss of function—principally the ability to walk adequate distances—or a combination of these. The magnitude of symptoms giving a valid indication for THR depends on the patient. In general, more minor symptoms may be accepted as an indication in the older patient. The pre-operative symptoms should always be tabulated, and several systems for doing this exist. This author uses the Charnley modification of the D'Aubigne and Postel hip chart. In this system, six points each are given for pain, walking ability and range of motion, normality being indicated by the number 6. Patients are also classified into three different grades: A, a patient with one arthritic hip; B, a patient with two arthritic hips; and C, a patient who has some other limitation, e.g. angina, rheumatoid arthritis, such that even with perfect hips there would always be a significant functional deficit. The system allows for an easy comparison between pre- and postoperative function. Secondary symptoms, such as analgesic requirements, the ability to put on socks or stockings, the use of walking aids, and the patient's gait without walking aids, should also be recorded.

Once it has been established that the patient has an indication for operation, a thorough pre-operative screening is needed. This includes a complete medical assessment, a search for potential anaesthetic difficulties, and

elimination of potential sources of sepsis. Attempts to eliminate potential sources of sepsis should include attention to teeth, skin lesions and other possible remote sources. The condition of the peripheral circulation, and a history of prostatism in a male patient, should also be evaluated—further specialist advice and treatment, for example, from a urological surgeon, is frequently required. It is also good practice to arrange for a series of routine blood tests when the patient is an out-patient; these can then be grouped with an antibody screen and a urine clinitest.

As with pre-operative screening, certain aspects of the operation are designed to minimise the possibility of complications. These complications include infection, dislocation and loosening.

Infection

A large international multicentre study sponsored by the Medical Research Council showed that if joint replacement was carried out in the ultraclean air of an operating theatre using laminar flow, the risk of developing a deep infection was reduced to half that of a similar operation carried out in an ordinary operating theatre; this figure was reduced to one quarter if all the surgical team were wearing clothing of a special material or wearing total body exhaust suits. If facilities are available to perform joint replacement operations under these conditions, they should always be used. The reduction in infection is independent of, but equal to, a reduction produced by prophylactic antibiotics. Antibiotics are usually given systemically, peri-operatively, and some surgeons also add antibiotics to the bone cement.

Orientation

The components of an implant are carefully orientated so that the range of motion allowed by their geometry comes within the motion likely to be allowed by the patient. If the orientation is such that the components come to the end of their range of movement while the patient still feels able to move the hip further, e.g. more flexion, then the prosthetic neck may impinge against one edge of the cup, levering out the head, with the threat of dislocation. Dislocation is to some degree also influenced by other factors, such as the surgical approach, and, if the trochanter is detached, on the soundness of its fixation.

Loosening

Loosening of an implant is to a major degree in the hands of the surgeon, and will depend greatly on how strongly the components are fixed. Attention to detail in, for example, cement technique, can markedly reduce the chance of this complication.

It is good practice to use prophylaxis against venous thrombosis, with the potential complication of pulmonary embolism. Prophylaxis includes systemic agents (e.g. anticoagulants, antisludging agents), and mechanical devices allowing regular emptying of the deep veins in the foot and/or lower leg. Some of these devices can be used intraoperatively. Elastic stockings should also be used, though their quality may need to be verified to make sure that they are effective.

Postoperative Management

The patient is usually allowed to stand and walk within the first few days postoperatively, sometimes from the day after surgery. This mobilisation is carried out with careful supervision by a physiotherapist. A frame is usually needed. Walking aids are then progressively reduced, but patients may be recommended to continue on elbow crutches until 6 weeks postoperatively—especially for partial weight bearing in the young patient (see below). Depending on the patient, at some time between 6 weeks and 3 months it should be possible for all restrictions on function to be lifted; improvement usually continues in a subtle way for many months. The result should then be the 'forgotten hip'.

HIP REPLACEMENT IN SPECIAL CIRCUMSTANCES

In young patients, it becomes increasingly likely that while the patient is still otherwise active, a hip replacement will wear out, come loose, or both. One view is that the standard operation should be carried out in such cases, with the full knowledge that revision surgery will be needed later (see below). An alternative view, however, is that some other type of operation should be performed. The non-replacement possibilities have already been described. None may be appropriate; for example, some form of replacement becomes necessary if the hip has morphology unsuitable for osteotomy, the bone is too soft, e.g. inflammatory arthritis, or the joint is too stiff. The types of replacement other than the classical cemented THR include hip resurfacing, replacement of the femoral side only with a bipolar component, and cementless THR. These will now be considered. Unfortunately, there is no uniform agreement about their relative indications.

A fundamental goal for replacement surgery in young patients is that as little bone as possible should be removed, thus preserving it for further surgery. This is the rationale for hip resurfacing (Figure 5.3A and B), in which a hemispherical cup is put onto the surface of the reamed femoral head rather than having a stem down the femoral shaft. This procedure became very popular in the 1970s, but a serious early failure rate became

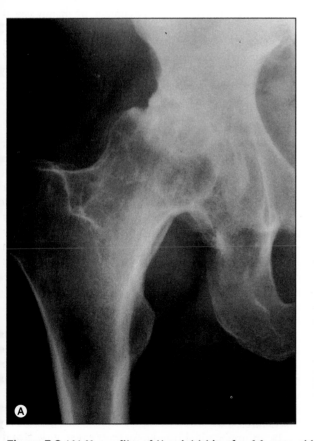
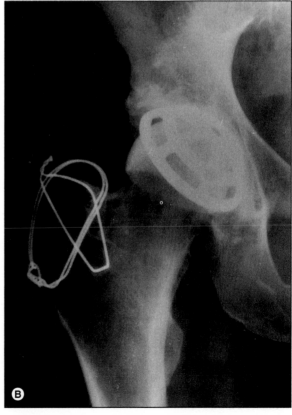

Figure 5.3 (A) X-ray film of the right hip of a 44-year-old woman, showing severe osteoarthritis with collapse of the superior segment of the femoral head. (B) Appearances following Wagner hip resurfacing using a high-density polyethylene acetabular component stiffened with a perforated metal backing and a ceramic femoral cup; both components are cemented.

apparent, and, while to some extent these failures were due to incorrect design features not understood at that time, some of the failures were probably due to intrinsic difficulties in trying to resurface the head of the femur. Thus, the procedure was abandoned by most surgeons, but it has, nevertheless, been continued in a few centres, with gradual improvements in the design. This author has the view that the procedure probably does have a place in the treatment of the young adult, and that the indications may well broaden with improvement in design and materials. Successfully carried out with a good design, the implant can produce a result the same as a THR, with preservation of bone such that subsequent conversion to a THR is not greatly dissimilar from a standard case.

In degenerative hip disease, the clearest indication for a bipolar replacement (stemmed replacement of the femoral head only, in which a separate bearing within the femoral head reduces motion between the outside of the artificial head and the natural acetabulum) is for avascular necrosis of the femoral head, in which the acetabulum is normal. The commonest indication, however, is undoubtedly for fractures of the femoral neck in the elderly. This implant is then used instead of a Thompson or Austin Moore, the additional bearing within the femoral head having been shown to reduce acetabular wear and penetration. Quite commonly, however, no procedure short of a THR will be adequate, the absolute indication for this being absence of the femoral head, for example, when the patient has had a septic arthritis in childhood. At present, there is uncertainty about the type of THR to be used. Many surgeons advocate a cementless THR, but although widely held, this view rests on doubtful evidence (see page 65), and many cementless THR designs have shown very poor results. Whether this situation will be altered by the widely practised current use of HA coatings is still not fully proven.

A small group of patients, for example, those with juvenile rheumatoid arthritis or with an old congenital dislocation, may require special components and/or other measures, such as bone grafting for deficiency of the acetabulum.

The postoperative management of these patients has to be individualised. It has been found that offloading the implant bone interface postoperatively increases the chance of thorough integration of the implant (as with the process of fracture healing). Therefore, young patients should be mobilised later and, wherever possible, kept partial or non-weight bearing for the early postoperative weeks.

THE KNEE

ARTHROSCOPY

Arthroscopic surgery has a major part to play in the treatment of the arthritic knee. Knees with early degenerative change can be debrided arthroscopically. Degenerate meniscal tears can be excised, loose areas of articular cartilage removed, and, particularly with the use of powered tools ('shavers') with special cutting attachments and suction allowing all the debris to be removed, a considerably improved internal appearance of the knee can be produced. Relief of symptoms and the duration of any relief can be good, but are unfortunately unpredictable. The main indications for arthroscopy are the patient who is rather young for major surgery or whose knee X-ray appearances are too good, and the elderly or unfit who have severe osteoarthritis.

OSTEOTOMY

In contrast to the hip, osteotomy is still quite often used as a treatment for arthritis in the knee, provided that this is degenerative rather than inflammatory. Unlike the hip, the knee has three distinct compartments: medial tibiofemoral, lateral tibiofemoral and patellofemoral. The arthritic changes do not usually affect all three compartments equally, and the inference is that the compartment with the greatest arthritic change is being overloaded at the expense of the others. In the case of the two tibiofemoral compartments, it is often obvious which compartment is being overloaded, and a planned realignment of the leg to transfer some of the weight to the less affected compartment can be expected to produce a good result. The underlying biomechanical principles and surgical technique are mainly associated with the work of Maquet. In the typical case, the patient has a varus deformity, probably of long-standing, is aged no more than 60 years—probably much less than this—and has osteoarthritis confined to the medial side of the knee, often associated with arthritis of the patellofemoral joint, but with a normal lateral compartment; a medial meniscectomy will often have been done previously. The patient's symptoms are such that major surgery is necessary, though this will have been preceded by a full course of conservative treatment and possibly also by arthroscopic debridement. Specific pre-operative investigations include a long leg weight-bearing X-ray film. In a normal leg, the hip, knee and ankle lie on a straight line, giving an angle of about 7° between the axes of the tibial shaft and of the femur, due to the medial offset of the femoral head in relation to the femoral shaft. With varus osteoarthritis, this is no longer the case. The actual angle of varus deviation can be accurately measured. A planned correction of this angle (plus 2° or 3° for a slight overcorrection) can be worked out. With a valgus knee, similar calculations can be made, though usually overcorrection is not done.

The osteotomy may then be performed in either the upper tibia or lower femur, or occasionally in both. The choice mainly depends on whether the knee is varus, requiring a tibial osteotomy, or valgus, classically requiring a femoral osteotomy. A developmentally sloping articular surface might require osteotomies of both, but this is rare.

In an upper tibial osteotomy for a varus knee, the osteotomy is usually made at or just above the level of the tibial tubercle, and can be done in several ways: commonly by a wedge removed from the outer side (perhaps with excision of the head of the fibula to gain good surgical access, as in the Coventry osteotomy); by a wedge removed from the outer side and taken to the medial side; or, frequently, using the so-called dome or barrel-vault osteotomy described by Maquet. The advantage of this last form of osteotomy is that the same shape of osteotomy can be used for any planned degree of correction, the bone ends in theory remaining congruent as the osteotomy is displaced. The fibula always has to be divided, otherwise this bone splints the osteotomy and prevents proper displacement. The osteotomy then has to be held in the appropriate position. In the past, plaster was used alone but was often unsuccessful, frequently allowing a shift, with loss of correction and impairment of the result; nowadays some form of fixation is virtually universal. A closing wedge osteotomy may be fixed by staples; barrel-vault osteotomies are commonly fixed with an external fixator, either of the Maquet type or one of the new varieties. When external fixation is used, immobilisation of the knee is not necessary, in principle a considerable advantage. Fixation may be needed for about 8 weeks.

While an upper tibial osteotomy is usually a relatively simple procedure, the occasional complication of non-union may produce serious problems, and the change in shape of the upper tibia may complicate a later total knee replacement, should this become necessary.

Patellofemoral Arthritis

The relation between symptoms and radiographic changes in patellofemoral arthritis is poor. Marked symptoms can be produced from the patellofemoral joint with plain X-ray films showing no abnormality (although in some of these cases more advanced techniques, e.g. arthrography with CT or magnetic resonance (MR) scans, may show abnormalities in the articular cartilage, probably a precursor of radiographic changes); conversely, patients are frequently seen with very severe radiographic changes who state that symptoms are minor or have only recently arisen. The very common clinical problem of anterior knee pain, perhaps associated with patellar malalignment, in the absence of frank osteoarthritic change, cannot be considered here. Symptomatic arthritis of the patellofemoral joint with fairly normal tibiofemoral compartments is not all that common. Simple conservative measures, such as washing out of the microscopic debris in the knee by arthroscopy, other arthroscopic surgical techniques, such as chondroplasty and drilling of subchondral bone in cartilaginous defects, and perhaps realignment procedures, have a very important place and will produce adequate relief in the great majority of cases. Where these fail, relief may sometimes be achieved by a planned alteration of the mechanics by elevating the tibial tubercle. This is intended to increase the lever arm in the extensor apparatus, thus reducing the compressive force between the patella and femur during extension of the knee. This, as noted above, is a fundamental principle in the treatment of arthritis by osteotomy. More than about a 1.5 cm elevation of the tibial tubercle (usually held by a small bone graft) can produce a serious

difficulty with skin healing, and the operation is not without its complications. Its place is, therefore, limited. Patellectomy is considered below.

ARTHRODESIS

Arthrodesis of the knee is a much more satisfactory operation than arthrodesis of the hip, as the loss of movement is much less of a handicap. There is still a clear place for this operation. The appropriate circumstances are where a young patient (often someone with secondary osteoarthritis after injury) develops such severe symptoms of pain, and frequently instability, that radical cure for the condition is required. While many would have the view that such patients should be treated by replacement—reserving arthrodesis for failure of the replacement—this group of patients remains one with a good indication for arthrodesis. Formerly, patients with inflammatory arthritis affecting both knees might have had one treated by replacement and the other by arthrodesis, but, with recent improvements in replacement, this would now seldom be done.

Probably, the commonest indication for arthrodesis of the knee is in the presence of a failed joint replacement, especially where this has been complicated by infection.

Surgical Technique

Where a replacement has not previously been carried out, the ends of the femur and tibia are fashioned into two flat surfaces such that, when apposed, the overall alignment of the leg is correct, with the centres of the hip, knee and ankle on a straight line. A few degrees of flexion is probably desirable. The bone ends are then held together with an external fixator. In such a case, union will usually be quite rapid, there being two large cancellous surfaces in contact.

Where there has been a previous replacement, the nature of the procedure will be governed by the type of replacement removed. If this has been of the resurfacing type, then the procedure as for a primary case will be appropriate. Where, as is commonly the case, a replacement of an earlier type has been used, the cancellous surfaces may have been lost. Many of these earlier implants invade the upper tibia and lower femur, and on removal the bone ends resemble 'ice-cream cones'. Minimal surfaces are then left to bring together and the production of a sound arthrodesis may be very difficult or impossible. While the primary technique may still be appropriate, it will often be necessary to resort to other measures, for example, the use of long locking intramedullary nails, preferably curved, running down the length of the whole leg. While a failed knee arthrodesis may produce an adequate false joint, such that the patient can still get about in a removable brace, this is by no means always the case, and very unsatisfactory instability may result.

ARTHROPLASTY

The patellofemoral joint is perhaps the only major place where excision arthroplasty, i.e. patellectomy, is still occasionally used as a primary procedure. It was formerly thought to be an entirely benign procedure and was carried out readily, but, with the development of more conservative techniques, its indication for arthritis is now restricted. Also, as noted above, symptomatic patellofemoral arthritis is frequently associated with arthritis in the tibiofemoral compartments; if sufficiently advanced, this will usually be treated by knee replacement, and in this procedure the patella may well be resurfaced (see below).

KNEE REPLACEMENT

Implant Design

The underlying principles have much in common with the hip (see page 64). Modern knee replacements (Figure 5.4A and B) are virtually all of a resurfacing kind; hinges, at least

in primary surgery, being outmoded. The generic term 'condylar' is often used, indicating resurfacing of both femoral condyles with one component and resurfacing of the upper tibia. The patella is also commonly resurfaced.

Materials and Fixation

Femoral components are almost invariably made of a metal, the tibial component of HDP on a metal tray, and the patella of HDP. Metal backing of the patella has also been extensively used, but has produced considerable problems.

Geometry and Wear

Although many knee replacements look superficially similar, there are important differences in, for example, the shape of the bearing surfaces. These differences are tied in

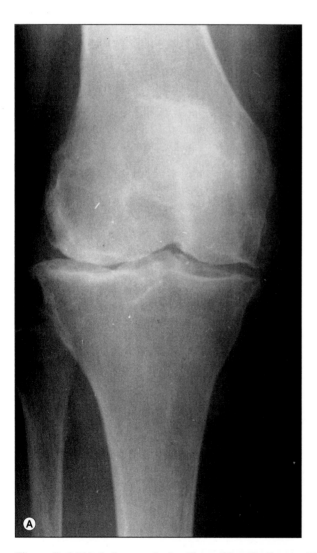
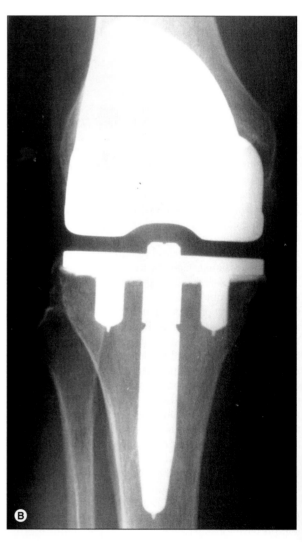

Figure 5.4 (A) Anteroposterior X-ray film of a knee with severe generalised osteoarthritis and an early valgus deformity. (B) Same joint after total knee replacement using Freeman–Samuelson components. The patella has also been replaced, although this cannot be seen in this image.

with retention or otherwise of the cruciate ligaments. If still present, the anterior cruciate ligament is almost always removed; in many designs, the posterior cruciate ligament is intended to be retained. Tension in this ligament influences the relative movement of the tibia and femur in flexion, and this in turn has design implications for the shape of the bearing surfaces. The shape of the bearing surfaces in turn determines the contact areas and hence the pressure applied to the plastic surface of the tibial component. In some designs, the contact areas have been too low and the resulting pressure has produced serious early wear of the HDP. The whole subject remains under active development at present. One group of knee replacements have a third element between the femur and tibia (a 'meniscal bearing') and this principle may represent an important advance, allowing fore-and-aft motion of the tibia while retaining large bearing surfaces. This type of replacement, however, can only be used if the knee is not grossly deformed.

Knee replacements have also gone through a long phase of cementless fixation in the same way as the hip; in fact, cementless fixation of the femoral component has been quite successful. Nevertheless, special X-ray techniques, particularly roentgen stereo photogrammetry (RSA), which is capable of detecting minute movements of an implant in relation to the skeleton, have shown considerably increased movement in the absence of cement, and cement, certainly on the upper surface of the tibia, appears essential.

Where only one side of the knee is affected (most commonly in varus osteoarthritis), it is practicable to carry out a unicompartmental replacement, which allows total replacement later if required. Although theoretically attractive, however, many promising designs have failed and the place of unicompartmental replacement is still uncertain.

Clinical Indications for Total Knee Replacement

In the usual case, the patient has osteoarthritis and is over the age of 55 years, or is a patient of any age with rheumatoid arthritis.

The symptoms are pain, instability (usually due to skeletal collapse) and loss of walking ability. Loss of knee movement is not by itself a good indication for replacement; the more distally one goes in the leg, the more acceptable loss of motion becomes. Simple conservative measures, such as quadriceps exercises and local symptomatic treatment, and simple surgical procedures, such as arthroscopy, dilation and arthroscopic debridement, may well be appropriate before a decision to replace the knee is made.

The symptoms should be documented with some form of chart, allowing a comparison between pre- and postoperative results. This author uses a modified version of the British Orthopaedic Association knee assessment chart.

Pre-operative screening is as for the hip. Pre-operative investigations for knee replacement include a long leg weight-bearing X-ray film and, for some designs, a special X-ray examination of the pelvis with a radio-opaque bar to indicate the position of the hip.

The operation should be carried out with a tourniquet and preferably in an ultraclean air enclosure. At operation, the knee is opened through an anterior or anteromedial incision, and the patella dislocated laterally. The bone ends are prepared using special jigs, unique to any given design, to accept the chosen implants. The upper tibial surface is normally arranged perpendicular to a line drawn from the knee to the ankle, and the femoral component perpendicular to a line drawn from the centre of the knee to the centre of the hip. The latter line is usually at about 7° to the axis of the femoral shaft. As a second, completely separate principle, the soft tissues have to be managed so that when the knee is fully extended the leg is stable to a varus or valgus force and is in correct alignment, i.e. with the hip, knee and ankle in a straight line. This often requires lengthening of contracted ligaments medially or laterally. The knee also has to be stable when an anteroposterior force is put on the tibia with the knee flexed to 90°, and the patella has to track correctly, for which purpose a lateral retinacular release may be required.

Flexion deformities have to be removed at surgery, usually by a combination of posterior capsular release and distal femoral resection.

The development of the soft tissue balancing side of knee replacement has enabled even knees with very severe pre-operative deformities to be replaced using resurfacing types of implant.

Postoperative Management

The knee may be kept still for the first few days, perhaps in a splint or plaster, or placed on a continuous passive motion machine. The latter devices, however, have not completely fulfilled their early promise. While some reports have shown a reduction in analgesic requirements and a more rapid return of knee motion with their use, the difference appears rather marginal, and there may be a tendency for recurrence of any pre-existing flexion deformity. The patient is allowed to undertake partial weight bearing with crutches some time within the first week postoperatively. Physiotherapy is needed while the patient is in hospital but is not usually required after he or she has gone home.

Manipulation Under Anaesthesia

This is now needed infrequently, as return of knee motion is not usually a problem if careful attention has been paid intra-operatively to soft tissue tensions in extension and flexion, and to patella tracking.

THE ANKLE

Symptomatic arthritis in the ankle is usually due either to secondary osteoarthritis following a fracture or to inflammatory arthritis. Except in rare cases where there is a major angular deformity of the ankle following a fracture at or just above it, in which a supramalleolar realignment osteotomy may be appropriate, the treatment, where conservative measures have failed, is by arthrodesis. Loss of motion of the ankle is obviously undesirable, but is not such a great problem as with arthrodesis of the knee. The lower end of the tibia and the lower end of the talus are fashioned into flat surfaces, brought together, and held usually with an external fixator. It is critically necessary to accurately align the foot onto the tibia both in a varus/valgus sense and in a flexion/extension sense. A plantar grade position, or in women a few degrees of flexion, are required. Errors in positioning are a very common source of a poor symptomatic result.

Ankle replacement (usually for rheumatoid arthritis) is technically possible, but in general the results have been poor. Nevertheless, it is possible that improvements in design will give this procedure a wider application.

THE FOOT

Stabilisation of the hind foot by 'triple arthrodesis' of the subtalar and midtarsal joints may be needed in inflammatory arthritis, and arthrodesis of the subtalar joint for badly symptomatic secondary osteoarthritis arising from displaced fractures of the calcaneum. Osteotomy, arthrodesis and arthroplasty all have a major part to play in the treatment of forefoot problems, particularly in painful toe deformities in the adult. Numerous varieties of osteotomy have been described at the distal and proximal ends for hallux valgus, this being sometimes associated with a varus first metatarsal. The Keller's excision arthroplasty of the base of the proximal phalanx for a painful bunion, or for hallux rigidus, is the most common variety of excision arthroplasty. It frequently gives good results provided the patient is not too young. Interposition arthroplasty (see above) of the first metatarsophalangeal joint is often performed using silastic, but when this material is used as an articulating surface, it can wear, leading to undesirable wear debris: this is now lessening its use. Excision arthroplasty following removal of a silastic spacer, however, is usually satisfactory. Osteotomy of the proximal phalanx is sometimes used as a procedure for hallux rigidus in young people. In the treatment of hammer toes, interphalangeal arthrodesis and/or Kellerisation of the metatarsophalangeal joints is often needed. Good results from these procedures are as much dependent on an accurate assessment of the foot as a whole, particularly in relation to where the patient's symptoms lie, as on the details of the surgical techniques used.

REVISION SURGERY FOR FAILED REPLACEMENT

This is a very large and still-expanding subject. Originally, failure of THR was almost always treated by excision (the Girdlestone pseudarthrosis). While many patients do have adequate function with this procedure, it does have severe limitations. If the patient is otherwise fit, the great majority of failures can be treated by insertion of a further joint. The same now applies to the knee.

The chief indications for revision surgery of the hip are mechanical loosening, deep infection or recurrent dislocation; and in the knee, mechanical loosening, deep infection and instability. Combinations of loosening, infection and instability frequently occur. Each case has to be extremely carefully evaluated, and special tests, such as isotope bone scans, CT scanning and preliminary biopsy for bacteriology, are frequently needed. Medical assessment also has to be rigorous, as the operations take much longer than a primary procedure. A very good case can be made for segregation of revision surgery into specialised centres, as the operations are often difficult and require special experience both from the surgeon and the theatre team, special equipment and sometimes special implants. Unless every care is taken, the complication rate is liable to be substantially higher than in primary surgery, and units carrying out this work frequently have patients referred to them who have already had one or more previous revisions. Each revision is, of course, more difficult than the previous one.

Revisions are usually carried out in one operation. The previous components and cement, if present, are first removed, and a thorough debridement undertaken, before inserting the new components, with or without cement. Sometimes in revisions for infection, an interval of some weeks is allowed between these two steps. Even grossly unstable knees can usually be revised using unconstrained implants, provided very special care is taken to restore soft tissue tension by accurate positioning of the components, but sometimes more constrained implants are required. Bone grafting, either with autograft bone or with allograft bone (from a bone bank), is frequently needed, and sometimes striking improvement in the skeleton can be achieved. The postoperative course is always slower than in primary surgery; patients are usually kept in bed for 1 week postoperatively in a straightforward hip revision, and for 3 weeks in a revision for deep sepsis. Longer periods are sometimes required where extensive bone grafting has been performed. In the knee, this author's practice is to keep the knee straight by splintage for 2 weeks postoperatively. On remobilisation, a period of partial weight bearing may then be needed.

Although revision surgery can be taxing for the patient and the surgical team, with suitable attention to detail it can produce improvements in a patient's wellbeing and function comparable to primary surgery. Further discussion of this subject, however, is beyond the scope of this chapter.

GENERAL READING

Black J. *Orthopaedic biomaterials in research and practice*. Edinburgh: Churchill Livingstone; 1988.

Bombelli R. *Structure and function in normal and abnormal hips. How to rescue jeopardized hips*. Berlin: Springer Verlag; 1993.

Charnley J. *Low friction arthroplasty of the hip*. Berlin: Springer Verlag; 1979.

Dandy DJ. *Arthroscopic management of the knee*. Edinburgh: Churchill Livingstone; 1987.

Insall JN. *Surgery of the knee*, 2nd ed. Edinburgh: Churchill Livingstone; 1993.

Liechti R. *Hip arthrodesis and associated problems*. Berlin: Springer Verlag; 1978.

Malchau H, Herberts P, Arnfelt L. Prognosis of total hip replacement in Sweden: follow-up of 92 675 operations performed 1978-1990. *Acta Orthop Scand* 1993, 64:497-506.

Maquet PGJ. *Biomechanics of the knee*. 2nd ed. Berlin: Springer Verlag; 1984.

Pauwels F. *Biomechanics of the normal and diseased hip*. Berlin: Springer Verlag; 1976.

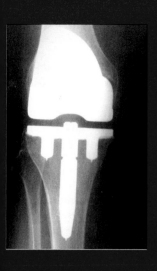

6 A Biggs

PHYSIOTHERAPY AFTER LOWER LIMB SURGERY

CHAPTER OUTLINE

- Aims of surgery
- Pre-operative assessment clinic
- The hip

- The knee
- The ankle

INTRODUCTION

Over the past few years there have been many changes within the management and organisation of the National Health Service. These changes have had an important effect on all staff directly involved with patient care. The impetus for these changes has come from a variety of sources, including the introduction of the Patient's Charter, reforms recommended by the National Health Executive, a general improvement in the health of the population, and significantly increased expectations of the public as a result of healthcare interventions. There have also been initiatives to change the emphasis from procedurally led care to patient-led care, with the development of 'the hospital at home', the identification of pathways of care, and the demand for more accountability regarding clinical effectiveness.

Clinical audit has been introduced to many areas of health care and is now commonly used by the purchasers of healthcare—health authorities, general-practitioner fundholders and extracontractual referrers—to provide evidence of good practice and accurate identification of patient outcome. To facilitate this increased information exchange, greater use is being made of standardised forms. As these forms are still in the developmental stage, the documentation is constantly being evaluated and revised. Examples of summary treatment cards currently in use by this author's unit are on pages 80, 84, 86, and 87.

They are being developed to give comprehensive information about patients' progress in a standardised manner that can be readily interpreted by all interested parties. This facilitates information exchange and provides data in a standard format for use in research and clinical audit. The chart records not only patient performance and response to interventionalist procedures, but also clinical effectiveness of the procedures used and the 'value for money' for purchasers.

This author conducted a clinical audit of patients after hip replacement surgery in her unit between August 1994 and July 1995. The results indicated that there was no evidence or published research to justify patients being prevented from undertaking normal activities at an early stage following arthroplasty surgery. There is, however, still no consensus among surgeons as to the optimum timing for resumption of activities. In the absence of clear instruction from the surgeon, this judgement is often left to the physiotherapist.

Although the rehabilitation process occupies less time than previously and has a different emphasis, it still follows the familiar pattern of:
- Assessment of the patient's condition.
- Treatment planning at all stages of rehabilitation.
- Use of modalities to relieve pain and improve function.
- Education and advice to the patient and family.

There is limited information available to guide patients and their families and general practitioners through the rehabilitation period. To satisfy this perceived need, this author's unit has prepared a booklet containing contributions from all disciplines concerned in patient management.

AIMS OF SURGERY

The aims of lower limb surgery are to relieve pain, improve function and maintain or improve range of movement. Patients admitted to hospital for this type of surgery vary considerably in age and general health; however, all present with similar problems of pain, dysfunction and anxiety about the planned procedures.

PAIN

This is the most usual reason for a patient to seek surgery. The duration, severity and distribution of the pain, considered with the patient's age, will influence the surgeon's choice of procedure.

DYSFUNCTION

Persistent pain will lead to disordered movement with resultant loss of function. As a result of measures taken to avoid unnecessary pain, the patient may develop hypermobility of the affected joint with associated instability in other joints. Alternatively, the joint may become stable but stiff, as a protection against the performance of movements that are painful.

ANXIETY

Many patients are apprehensive about being admitted to hospital. These concerns are focused on:
• The surgical procedure.
• Survival of the anaesthesia.
• Whether there may be a continuance of, or an increase in, the pain postoperatively.
• Whether the outcome of surgery may not be the type expected or desired.

The patient's perception of these factors, and his expectations and motivation, will influence both his postoperative management and his ultimate level of recovery.

PRE-OPERATIVE ASSESSMENT CLINIC

The patient may be admitted to hospital for full pre-operative assessment a few days before surgery. It is becoming increasingly common, however, for patients to attend a pre-operative assessment clinic. This is usually held 1 or 2 weeks before surgery, and provides a forum for detailed assessment of the patient's condition, education about the planned procedure, discussion about the proposed postoperative management, and advice on the patient's role before surgery and during the rehabilitation process.

The following describes a typical pre-operative assessment clinic. Initially, the patient is seen by a clinic-based nurse or a nurse from the ward to which the patient will be admitted. The nurse collects and checks the self-clerking form sent to the patient, takes samples of urine for both simple testing on the ward and laboratory analysis, records current blood pressure, weight and oxygen saturation, arranges for an electrocardiogram (ECG), notes the patient's transport requirements after discharge, and makes arrangements for the patient to be interviewed by the social worker if necessary.

Following the ECG and blood oxygen saturation tests, the patient is seen by a physician. The physician makes a medical assessment and determines whether surgery should proceed. If a major problem is found that could incur significant risk, e.g. a pathological heart condition, surgery is either cancelled or delayed until the results of further investigations and the response to treatment are known. Minor problems that can be treated by the general practitioner may mean surgery is deferred until completion of the appropriate treatment regimen. Alternatively, surgery can proceed as scheduled, with the patient receiving treatment before hospital admission.

If permission to proceed with surgery is given, the patient is assessed by the physiotherapist both subjectively and objectively.

SUBJECTIVE ASSESSMENT

This is concerned with the patient's reason for seeking surgery and the outcome expected from it. It is based on the patient's social history, and information is obtained by asking questions about the patient's occupation, marital status, housing and general lifestyle. The pattern and type of pain experienced by the patient and the use of analgesia are noted. The information will indicate the postoperative rehabilitation requirements appropriate to the patient, ensuring that the maximum benefit is gained from the surgical procedure.

OBJECTIVE ASSESSMENT

In this assessment, the physiotherapist uses physical means to determine the patient's condition. The procedure is logical and follows a pattern to ensure that essential information is not missed. Key instructions are to look, feel, move and test. The main points to consider in this assessment are listed below.

Observation

Observation includes:
• Posture.
• Gait pattern and use of walking aids.
• Localised movement of the joint.
• Condition of the skin, i.e. colour, presence of varicose veins, other lesions, swelling.
• Presence of deformity.

Palpation

Palpation includes the skin's temperature and muscle bulk.

Movement

Measurements to assess movement include the:
- Ranges of active and passive movement in the affected joint.
- Ranges of active and passive movement in adjacent joints, proximal and distal to the affected joint.

Routine Tests

Routine tests include:
- Noting whether there is fixed deformity in the affected joint or adjacent joints.
- Recording abnormal joint movement.
- Determining the integrity of ligaments supporting the joint.
- Determining the power of muscles supporting the affected joint using the Oxford scale.
- Assessing the muscle power of the rest of the body.

In some centres there are specific systems of assessment used by both physiotherapists and surgeons which include many of the points identified above. For hip replacement, for example, there is the Charnley hip assessment, adopted by the British Orthopaedic Association, the Harris hip score and the Merle D'Aubigné. For knee replacement there is the New Jersey Knee score, the Hungerford Knee score and the British Orthopaedic Association Knee score. There are even scores for the ankle, e.g. Tegner.

The patient and spouse or carer are encouraged to express any fears, and the opportunity is presented for them to ask questions. The complete schedule for postoperative rehabilitation is discussed and if possible printed information supplied. The patient may also be offered the opportunity to see the type of prosthesis that is to be used in the planned procedure.

Should the patient require occupational therapy support, a preliminary meeting is arranged. The clinic also provides the opportunity for routine blood tests and X-ray examinations of the affected areas. Finally, the patient is given a dietic form to complete. This completed form may indicate whether the help and advice of the dietician is required.

The last stage of the clinical assessment is part of the routine developed by the pre-operative clinic at the Robert Jones and Agnes Hunt Orthopaedic Hospital following the results of a clinical audit. This format has been developed to save patients having surgery cancelled, and also reduces the need for invasive and expensive investigations not required by the majority of patients.

When a patient is admitted to hospital without having attended a pre-operative assessment clinic, all the investigations outlined above are performed during the few days before surgery. Physiotherapy input is determined by the planned surgical procedure, the surgeon's preferences and the patient's needs.

The remainder of this chapter gives guidance to physiotherapists to enable them to achieve the maximal therapeutic benefit following specific surgical procedures.

THE HIP

Surgery to the hip joint includes arthroscopy with or without debridement, total hip replacement (THR), resurfacing, revision surgery, reconstructive surgery and, more rarely, excision (girdlestone) arthroplasty or arthrodesis.

ARTHROSCOPY

This is performed to assess the state of the joint when clinical findings are not conclusive enough to warrant more extensive surgery.

Pre-operatively, the patient is assessed (see guidelines on page 76) and the postoperative rehabilitation programme discussed. Within a few days after surgery, the patient should be walking unassisted and undergoing an intensive rehabilitation programme in the gymnasium and hydrotherapy pool. The patient's function increases steadily and a return to normal function can be expected within 1–2 weeks if the rehabilitation programme is properly designed. The rehabilitation programme should aim to increase muscle strength, particularly focusing on those muscles that support the hip, e.g. the glutei, hamstrings, quadriceps, and targeting an improvement in the range of movement in all joints of the limb and spine.

TOTAL HIP REPLACEMENT

The majority of hospitals carry out this procedure on a large number of patients each year, and individual surgeons develop their own preferences regarding the type of prosthesis used, the quantity of pre- and postoperative rehabilitation recommended and the expected outcome. Basic physiotherapeutic principles remain paramount, but timescales vary considerably from one institution to another and even from one surgeon to another in the same institution.

It is fair to say that the physiotherapeutic management of each patient will vary slightly from all others. Some of the factors influencing this will include the surgical approach, the surgical procedure, the surgeon's preferences, and the patient's predisposing limitations, past medical history and expectations from the surgery.

The surgical approach used influences postoperative management. For example, the two most commonly used approaches are lateral and posterior. There are merits with each, but the physiotherapist must know which one has been employed, as postoperative management must take into account the incision's location. The lateral approach necessitates an incision over the trochanter of the femur, and a trochanteric osteotomy. The bone is incised below the insertion of the abductor muscles, which allows the surgeon to work within the joint capsule of the hip. The final stage of the operation is to rewire the detached fragment of bone, with its muscle attachment intact, to the proximal end of the femoral shaft. After surgery, it is essential that the hip is maintained in an abducted position. When mobilising the patient, the physiotherapist must ensure that the patient's leg does not fall into adduction, and nurses must also be careful to ensure the abducted position is maintained in bed. The patient is most vulnerable when transferring from a bed to a chair or if rolling to the unaffected side, as the upper leg naturally falls into adduction. These patients should be taught to roll to their operated side if this is required. Care must be taken until the bone and soft tissues around the wound have healed, usually 4–6 weeks.

The posterior approach is also used frequently. During this procedure, the posterior aspect of the capsule is incised to permit surgery to the joint. The capsule is sutured at the end of the operation but remains vulnerable throughout its protracted healing time of 4–6 weeks. During this period, care must be taken to ensure the hip is not flexed beyond 45°. Any flexion beyond this point will force the prosthesis posteriorly and there is a risk of the patient suffering a posterior dislocation of the hip.

The type of procedure used during the operation will also influences postoperative management. For example, many surgeons now implant prostheses without cement. If the patient has undergone a cementless procedure, it is normal for weight bearing to be delayed, and the patient's use of crutches extended, until the surgeon is sure the prosthesis is set firm in the femoral shaft and will not loosen with the movement and leverage of weight-bearing activities.

These restrictions on the patient's level of postoperative activity take account of the factors relative to the surgery, and need to be considered in the rehabilitation programme. All these restrictions are designed to protect the new joint from damage, and the length of protection may vary from a few weeks to months depending on the patient's response and the surgeon's protocol (*Arthroplasty Audit Report, 1995–1996*).

Pre-operative Physiotherapy

If the patient has not already attended an outpatient pre-operative clinic, they are assessed fully and the rehabilitation programme discussed. The pre-operative clinic includes:

- Instruction in the performance of postoperative breathing routines.
- Lessons on how to move about the bed without straining the operation site.
- Instruction on the most efficient and safest way to get in and out of bed.
- Exercises to maintain co-ordination and power of the quadriceps, hip abductors and hamstrings. These are encouraged to ensure the patient is as fit as possible for surgery.
- Exercises to maintain the circulation in the lower limbs. However, where footpumps, anti-embolus stockings and/or anticoagulation drugs are being administered or are anticipated to be required after surgery, circulatory exercises are reduced.

Postoperative Physiotherapy

Once the patient has regained consciousness and is relatively comfortable, general bed activities are encouraged. The physiotherapist must be aware of the surgical approach and procedures and instruct the patient carefully about movements and positions to be avoided during the early postoperative days. As early as 24 hours after the operation, the patient may be allowed to get out of bed, exercise and mobilise under supervision provided the surgeon's protocol is not compromised and there are no complications. This mobilisation normally proceeds without a check X-ray film being taken before the patient gets out of bed for the first time, but it is necessary to check the operation notes to ensure that the surgeon has not specifically requested a check X-ray film before mobilisation commences out of bed.

When getting out of bed for the first time, the patient chooses the side to which they wish to move. Care must be taken to ensure that the operated hip does not fall into adduction or flexion past 90° as these positions apply strain to weakened parts of the joint capsule and may lead to dislocation of the joint. Many patients manage to get out of bed with little or no assistance, although the physiotherapist should be in attendance the first time this is attempted, to advise and provide assistance. On completion of the transfer from lying to sitting on the edge of the bed, patients should be allowed a short time to ensure there is no giddiness and that they are poised for the next step.

When confident, the patient pushes up from the bed into a standing position, supporting their body weight with a walking frame. If the patient's balance is satisfactory and there are no contraindications, e.g. low arterial blood pressure or a feeling of faintness, weight transference exercises can commence, followed by supervised walking. The patient may also be allowed to sit out of bed in a chair at this stage.

Patients gain confidence daily and increase activity levels at their own pace. The physiotherapist supervises the exercise programme, monitors/evaluates progress, deals with patient concerns and progresses the patient's rehabilitation programme.

The rehabilitation programme should include teaching and supervised practice of:

- Safe transfers from a bed or chair to a standing position.
- Walking using appropriate walking aids, e.g. frame, crutches, stick.
- Independent walking, i.e. with or without walking aids.
- Gait re-education, with particular reference to the correct use of walking aids, stride length, timing and rhythm.
- Identification of leg length discrepancy and its correction by the use of shoe raises.

The rehabilitation programme should also include treatment and/or advice on the management of problems associated with the hip disorder, for example, pain in the lumbar region of the back or pain referred to the knee.

Even though the patient may live in a bungalow, there is still a need to be taught the safe negotiation of steps, stairs, slopes and uneven ground. It is essential to remember 'the good leg leads going up steps and follows coming down'; i.e. the good leg is always higher, the bad leg always lower when ascending and descending stairs.

When the patient using crutches climbs stairs, the body weight is supported by both the crutches and the operated leg as the non-operated leg is raised and the foot placed on the step above. By extending the hip and knee of the non-operated leg, the body weight is lifted forward and up, bringing the operated leg and walking aid to join the first leg on the step above. On descending stairs, the opposite occurs. The operated leg and crutches are lowered to the step below, followed by the non-operated leg. This ensures that the strain of lifting the body or controlling its downward movement is taken by the leg that has not been traumatised by surgery.

Occasionally a patient may have a bilateral hip replacement performed on the same day, or some other problem which precludes such clear definition. In this situation, it must be determined which leg is the stronger or most reliable so that the patient can be encouraged to use this leg to lead the climb and follow on the descent of stairs.

Discharge from hospital is determined by the multidisciplinary team after discussion with the patient. Discharge may be as early as 5 days after surgery. Any nursing care required after discharge, e.g. the removal of sutures, is undertaken by the patient's general practitioner, practice nurse or district nurse. Patients are advised to telephone the ward to speak to a nurse or physiotherapist if they have any concerns about their situation or progress following discharge from hospital.

Following discharge, the patient continues to mobilise with the walking aid and will undertake a home exercise programme aimed at strengthening the quadriceps, hamstrings and glutei on the affected side while improving general fitness and mobility of the rest of the body. These exercises are in line with the surgeon's general protocol and adapted to the patient's specific needs. Provided the patient has received and understood the rehabilitation instructions, out-patient treatment should not be necessary. The patient should progress to full independence within approximately 6 weeks, although the timing of resumption of some activities differs from patient to patient according to the surgeon's judgement on the patient's abilities (*Arthoplasty Audit Report, 1995–1996*).

Figures 6.1 and 6.2 show a treatment card for THR. The shaded boxes denote days when activities may commence or continue. The therapist ticks and signs the appropriate box whenever a patient achieves that activity. Not all the boxes will be marked, as obviously patients vary in their abilities, and some activities will be unnecessary or not applicable.

This type of standardised card can be useful for clinical audit. The reverse of the card can be used to record deviations from the expected progress or pattern of care (see Figure 6.2).

COMPLICATIONS OF SURGERY

Deep Vein Thrombosis

Indications

In the affected limb, deep vein thrombosis (DVT) causes pain in the calf, restriction of active and passive dorsiflexion of the ankle and persistent swelling of the limb.

Diagnosis

Diagnosis is by a venogram.

Treatment

Treatment is usually by anticoagulation therapy using either heparin or warfarin. The surgeon will decide if there is to be any restriction on the patient's activity levels during the first few days following a diagnosis of DVT.

Pulmonary Embolism

Indications

Pulmonary embolism causes a severe pain in the chest, particularly on inspiration.

Diagnosis

Diagnosis is by VQ scan or lung perfusion scans.

Treatment

Treatment is by anticoagulation therapy using either heparin or warfarin. The patient's activities may be severely restricted initially and their condition should be monitored carefully once activities resume.

Infection

Indications

Infection causes a raised temperature, a general feeling of malaise and obvious inflammation around the wound.

Treatment

Treatment is with specific or broad-spectrum antibiotics. Movements which aggravate the wound are restricted and the patient may be confined to bed, resting until the infection is under control.

Anaemia

Indications

Anaemia causes tiredness, general malaise and possibly fainting when first getting out of bed.

Diagnosis

Diagnosis is by blood tests to determine the haemoglobin level.

Treatment

Treatment comprises a good, balanced diet and iron supplements. If the haemoglobin level is very low, a blood transfusion may be given. A patient who is anaemic will not progress in the rehabilitation programme as quickly as others with normal blood counts, due to feelings of malaise, general tiredness and lethargy.

RESURFACING OF JOINTS

This operation is usually performed on young patients. The procedure involves the removal of relatively small amounts of bone from the affected joint.

Pre-operative Physiotherapy

This is as for THR (see page 78).

Total hip replacement treatment card													
Date													Initials
Postoperative day	1	2	3	4	5	6	7	8	9	10	11	12	
Circulatory exercises													
Breathing exercises													
Bed exercises													
Bed transfer with help of two													
Bed transfer with help of one													
Stand with frame and help of two													
Stand with frame and help of one													
Gait re-education with frame and help													
Chair transfer with help													
Independent with a frame													
Gait re-education with crutches													
Independent with crutches													
Independent with bed transfer													
Independent with chair transfer													
Stair practice													
Patient education and advice													

Figure 6.1 Total hip replacement treatment card.

Reverse of the hip replacement treatment card		
Record of postoperative problems or delays	Date recorded	Signature
Operation day / / Expected day of discharge / /	/ /	

Figure 6.2 Reverse of the hip replacement treatment card.

Postoperative Physiotherapy

The rehabilitation programme follows the same sequence as that for THR, except the timescale is shorter. Patients are encouraged to resume normal activities within 4–6 weeks provided recovery is uncomplicated.

REVISION PROCEDURES

Pre-operative Physiotherapy

This is as for THR (see page 78).

Postoperative Physiotherapy

The rehabilitation programme is decided by the surgeon. Sometimes the joint condition after revision surgery permits a rehabilitation programme the same as for a primary hip replacement. However, it is more usual for the patient to be confined to bed for a longer period than for a primary hip replacement. In this situation, exercises of all limbs are encouraged to maintain circulatory flow and reduce the tendency for the development of DVT. Patients are also taught tatic muscle contractions of the quadriceps and glutei and active exercises for the non-operated leg and upper limbs. In the upper limbs, exercises concentrate on strengthening the shoulder depressors and elbow extensors to prepare the patient for using walking aids. Wrist extension is also necessary, but if not achievable, the physiotherapist must arrange for a walking aid that does not require support of the body weight on the extended wrist.

Revision surgery is often undertaken in stages, the patient being confined to bed for a number of days if not weeks, so these exercises are important for both their physical and mental wellbeing.

When mobilisation commences, the rehabilitation programme follows the pattern for THR, but is progressed more slowly. The surgeon will decide the length of time walking aids are to be used when weight bearing can commence.

JOINT RECONSTRUCTION

The rehabilitation programme, undertaken in hospital, is similar to but slower than that of a patient undergoing a hip replacement. On discharge, out-patient physiotherapy must be continued to improve the pattern of gait and increase muscle strength, particularly of muscles surrounding the reconstructed joint and the quadriceps on the same side.

EXCISION ARTHROPLASTY: GIRDLESTONE

This operation is rarely seen these days as hip replacement prostheses are now extremely sophisticated and can be replaced more than once if they fail. The girdlestone operation is a salvage procedure involving the removal of the femoral head. It may still be used in the elderly when all other surgical procedures have failed. It may also be used in patients confined to wheelchairs when there are problems with sitting due to associated hip dislocations.

Postoperatively, patients will be confined to bed for up to 6 weeks—often with skeletal traction through the upper end of the tibia. It is desirable to position patients in supine if their condition allows, or, even better, to lie them prone for periods throughout the day to help prevent fixed flexion deformities at the hip. This is particularly important for the patient who is wheelchair bound. Provided the medical condition permits lying, the patient is advised to continue this on discharge.

Once traction is removed, the patient is mobilised. Initially a walking frame is used, with the patient progressing to crutches then a walking stick as experience and confidence are gained.

Young patients are encouraged to delay weight bearing on the operated limb for several weeks to reduce the limb shortening that occurs as a result of surgery. However, some limb shortening will be inevitable and a compensatory shoe raise will be required to keep the pelvis level and enable walking with a minimal limp.

The elderly find non-weight-bearing walking impossible due to poor balance control, reduced co-ordination, generalised muscle weakness and lack of confidence.

These patients will bear weight on the operated limb as soon as mobilisation starts. They will require compensatory shoe raises as soon as mobilisation commences, as limb shortening on the operated side will be very pronounced.

Patients are discharged as soon as they gain independence with their walking aids. Patients may progress from walking with a frame to using crutches or walking sticks, but it is rare for a patient to walk without any aid after surgery.

ARTHRODESIS

Arthrodesis is the surgical fusion of the joint. It is not often required nowadays as improvements in the design of prostheses enabling surgical revision procedures have dramatically reduced the numbers of joints irreparably damaged by previous surgery.

Rarely, arthrodesis is used to relieve pain in the joint. The procedure is performed when only one hip is affected and the adjacent joints are able to compensate for the loss of movement that results.

Pre-operative Physiotherapy
This is as for THR (see page 78).

Postoperative Physiotherapy
Bed rest is maintained until the patient is comfortable, when mobilisation will commence.

The timing of mobilisation and weight bearing is determined by the surgeon. Discharge from hospital is arranged once the patient is independent and mobile using crutches.

Any splintage used to support the fused joint is removed once the arthrodesis site is united. The patient continues guided rehabilitation until full weight bearing on the affected limb is allowed and normal activities can be resumed without the risk of injury.

UPPER FEMORAL OSTEOTOMY
This is performed on the young patient who complains of severe joint pain although there is little evidence of joint destruction. A joint replacement may be required in the future.

The patient is assessed pre-operatively, and postoperative rehabilitation is discussed.

Postoperative rehabilitation is similar to that of a joint replacement, and the surgeon determines any variation on commencement of mobilisation and protected weight bearing. If out-patient physiotherapy is indicated, this will be arranged.

THE KNEE

Surgery to this joint includes arthroscopy with or without other procedures, total knee replacement, unicompartmental knee replacement, arthrodesis, ligament reconstruction, chondral grafting, chondrocyte grafting and meniscal grafting.

ARTHROSCOPY

Arthroscopic procedures are often performed as day surgery, and may or may not require physiotherapeutic intervention. Where physiotherapy is indicated, it is usually postoperatively. This may consist of:

- A functional assessment of gait, and provision of appropriate walking aids to enable comfortable mobilisation. Walking aids are usually only required for a few days.
- Instruction on exercise. For the quadriceps and hamstring, the patient is advised to increase activities slowly back to normal, providing the knee is comfortable and not swollen. Continuation of exercises are encouraged to maintain muscle strength and range of movement. The use of number sets, drills or timings of these exercises may be included, but are not necessary as long as the patient exercises throughout the day. An icepack may be applied for 15 minutes to relieve pain or reduce swelling in the joint. There is no limit to the frequency of application of the icepack, but a check should be made to ensure exercises are being performed accurately. If the knee becomes swollen, the patient is instructed to rest with the leg in elevation. Normal activities are resumed when possible, depending on the patient's feelings and the stresses to which the knee will be subjected.
- Provision of out-patient physiotherapy. This is provided only if necessary or requested.

Other Procedures

These may include partial menisectomy, meniscal repair, osteochondral drilling and lateral release.

Physiotherapy is undertaken as part of the postoperative management only where indicated or considered necessary. Provision of walking aids and careful instruction in their use is often required, particularly after meniscal repairs, where the surgeon may order restricted weight bearing for up to 6 weeks.

The patient is discharged when walking safely with a walking aid, often the day after surgery. Physiotherapy is arranged on an out-patient basis and is directed at maintaining or reducing swelling. This is achieved by resting with the limb in elevation, icepacks, compression, movement, and techniques to maintain or increase muscle strength and range of movement, e.g. free or sliding board exercises, steps, rowing machine, bicycle (in the gymnasium), proprioceptive neuromuscular facilitation.

TOTAL OR UNICOMPARTMENTAL KNEE REPLACEMENT

Pre-operative Physiotherapy

This will consist of an assessment and discussion of the postoperative rehabilitation programme and the patient's reason for surgery. The patient is taught to perform breathing and circulatory exercises, and is encouraged to practise these exercises during the time before surgery.

An assessment of the patient should include a subjective and objective assessment (see page 76), remembering to look, feel, move and test.

Look

The patient should be observed for:

- Gait pattern and any use of walking aids.
- Posture in standing, sitting and during movement.
- Presence of deformity or knee instability in weight-bearing and non-weight-bearing activities.
- Muscle bulk, particularly of the quadriceps, hamstrings and calf muscles.
- Presence of swelling of the calf and foot.
- Colour of the skin.
- Presence of varicose veins.
- Presence of lesions.

Feel

Feel the temperature over the affected joint.

Move

Measure the range of movement of the knee, noting any inhibiting factors.

Test

Determine the muscle power of the quadriceps and hamstrings, ligament laxity and patella mobility.

Postoperative Physiotherapy

Patients may be nursed in bed for approximately 24 hours postoperatively, during which time they are encouraged to perform the breathing and circulatory exercises they were taught pre-operatively. If anticoagulant therapies are in use the need for circulatory exercises is diminished. The patient is also encouraged to practise static quadriceps exercises. A knee immobiliser, e.g. a resting splint or plaster of Paris cast may be in situ, the patient could be on a continuous passive motion (CPM) machine or free in bed. The surgeon will usually determine the length of use of a splintage or CPM.

After 24 hours, active mobilisation usually commences with the patient getting out of bed and standing and supporting themselves with a frame supervised by the therapist. If the patient's balance is good and there are no adverse effects of the surgery (e.g. drops in blood pressure, feeling faint), they are encouraged to practise weight transference exercises, progressing to walking when able.

Rehabilitation progresses within the patient's tolerance and should cover:

- Progression to walking with crutches or sticks.
- Gait re-education to correct stride pattern and rhythm.
- Safe negotiation of steps, stairs, slopes and uneven ground.
- Mobilisation of the knee. This may be started immediately postoperatively or, dependent on the surgeon's protocol, delayed for up to 5 days. Mobilisation may be achieved by the use of CPM, or free and/or facilitatory exercises.

Many papers have been written on the use of CPM. Some papers state that CPM increases the range of flexion in the early stages of rehabilitation, while others state that over about 6 months there is no difference in the achieved range of movement between CPM and free exercises.

The patient's tolerance of CPM has to be taken into account when considering this method of knee mobilisation. The need to remain totally immobile while the machine is being operated reduces the patient's confidence. Also, the effective use of several of the designs requires a greater range of hip movement than many patients possess. Free exercise and the use of the sliding board may be needed to encourage movement. As the patient's range of movement and strength improves they may progress to participating in pool and gymnasium exercises. These exercises increase the physical demands made on both the patients and their knees. Icepacks may be used to reduce or prevent swelling, which allows the knee to move more easily.

The duration of hospital stay will depend on the patient's capabilities, their safety in mobilising, the range of movement achieved at the knee and the absence of any complications. Discharge may be as early as 5 days postoperatively. Many surgeons are happy for their patients to return home providing they can achieve full extension at the knee and a range of active flexion from 60° to 90°.

If knee mobilisation is particularly slow, some surgeons use manipulation under anaesthesia (MUA). The timing of such a procedure depends on the surgeon's preference.

Patients may or may not need to attend the hospital for physiotherapy. Some surgeons would always advise they do, while others make individual judgements based on the patient's progress in hospital, level of independence before discharge, level of motivation and knowlege of the condition.

To allow rehabilitation to progress unhindered, the patient must be given adequate analgesia to control any postoperative pain.

The complications and managment of knee replacement are as for the hip (see page 79).

A possible pattern of the rehabilitation programme for patients after knee replacement surgery is shown in Figure 6.3.

ARTHRODESIS

Arthrodesis is performed infrequently nowadays because of the sophistication and versatility of knee replacement surgery. If arthrodesis is the procedure of choice, however, its pre-operative physiotherapy management is the same as for knee replacement (see page 82).

After surgery, the patient is returned to the ward with the arthrodesed joint immobilised by internal or external fixation or a combination of both—this will be retained until joint fusion is assured. Once the patient is comfortable, mobilisation can begin. The surgeon will indicate the timing of weight-bearing activities, but initially weight bearing will be protective. Once the patient is independent on crutches and able to undertake normal activities of daily living, they are discharged.

The walking aid is discarded once the patient is free of pain and confident in all walking activities. This may occur as early as 6 weeks postoperatively, but some patients never achieve this level of independence.

LIGAMENT RECONSTRUCTION

As a result of research there have been modifications to the treatment regimens after surgical reconstruction of ligaments.

Previously, rehabilitation programmes were based on timed intervals from the operation; however, research has demonstrated that patients recover at such variable rates that a more realistic guide would be the patient's physical status. Rehabilitation programmes are divided into several stages, the patient progressing to each stage as their condition allows.

Stage I: the Pre-operative Period

During this stage, non-surgical measures are used to support the knee and attempts are made to educate the patient, particularly if this stage occurs immediately after injury. A knee brace may be used to stabilise the knee in the initial post-injury period; however, they are unsightly, uncomfortable and cumbersome and not always effective, so are used less frequently these days. Natural splintage from improved muscle power is more effective, if it can be achieved. Physiotherapy aims to restore normal function and includes measures to eradicate swelling of the affected area, and to regain full range of movement in the joints adjacent to the damaged ligaments.

Treatment consists of icepacks applied to the joint, elevation of the limb, protected weight bearing and exercise to the muscles surrounding the joints. The use of ice, elevation and protected weight bearing decreases as the swelling reduces. Active resisted exercises are introduced and the patient progresses to gymnasium work as the joint becomes increasingly free of pain and more mobile. Once the patient has returned to normal levels of activity, it may be decided not to proceed with surgery. However, if the knee still gives way and does so sufficiently frequently to be a problem, surgery will be undertaken.

Stage II: Hospital Stay

During the time the patient is in hospital, the objectives of physiotherapy are to:
• Prevent or minimise swelling.
• Enable full extension of the knee to allow locking.
• Enable flexion to 90° to allow the patient to ascend and descend stairs and sit in comfort on a chair of normal height.

Following surgery, the patient may be required to start mobilising the knee using a CPM machine. Alternatively, knee movement may be encouraged using a sliding board. There is considerable pain after surgery, and sufficient analgesia should be administered before CPM, to ensure pain inhibition does not interfere with the quality of movement. Icepacks applied to the knee joint and elevation of the limb help to prevent or reduce swelling of the knee. Before applying the icepack, the wound dressing should be protected by a waterproof covering to prevent it becoming soggy. Wound dressings are minimal after surgery and, when changed, the knee is flexed maximally before the new dressing is applied.

Early mobilisation is encouraged, with the patient normally using crutches after 24 hours, to reduce pain on weight bearing of the affected limb.

The length of hospital stay varies from overnight to 1 week depending on the surgeon's preferences and the patient's capabilities. If the surgeon requests it, some centres use knee bracing in this early postoperative stage.

The patient is taught to apply icepacks to the knee after discharge from hospital, and is encouraged to mobilise without the use of aids as the pain reduces and confidence returns. Care must be taken to ensure that the pattern of gait is not compromised. If swelling persists, Tubigrip may be applied. This will help alleviate swelling and increase proprioception at the knee.

Treatment card for hospital stay following knee replacement													
Date													Initials
Postoperative day	1	2	3	4	5	6	7	8	9	10	11	12	
Circulatory exercises													
Breathing exercises													
Bed exercises													
Bed transfer with help													
Stand with frame and help													
Gait re-education with frame													
Chair transfer with help													
Independent with frame													
Use of knee immobiliser													
Independent in all transfers													
Use of cryotherapy													
Use of CPM machine													
Static exercises													
Commence knee flexion													
Free exercises													
Hydrotherapy													
Functional re-education exercises													
Gait re-education with crutches													
Independent with crutches													
Progress with sticks													
Stair practice													
Patient education and advice													
Range of movement													
Out-patient physiotherapy													

Figure 6.3 Treatment card for hospital stay following knee replacement.

Stage III: the Immediate Post-discharge Period

Physiotherapy continues following discharge. Muscle strengthening exercises, knee mobilisation and elimination of any swelling continue until the patient returns to full independence with normal muscle power and range of movements in the joint.

The timing of this stage is variable, as patients recover at different rates according to their physical states and motivation.

Physiotherapeutic techniques include:
- Icepacks to reduce or eliminate swelling of the joint.
- Active assisted exercise to encourage the correct use of weak muscles.
- Active resisted exercise as muscle power improves, to strengthen the muscles.
- Hydrotherapy to mobilise the knee and improve muscle power—hydrostatic pressure also helps control swelling.
- Gymnasium activities, e.g. bicycles, steps, running. These improve power, mobility of the knee and co-ordination in complex activities.
- Proprioceptive exercises—wobble board to improve power and control, leg squats for strengthening, mobilisation and co-ordination, and walking on uneven surfaces to encourage co-ordination and control.

Stage IV: Final Rehabilitation

The patient may now resume sporting activities provided the knee is free of swelling, there is full range of movement, muscle power is normal and there is no evidence of ligament laxity. Some patients recover quickly and will progress to stage IV within 4–6 weeks, whereas others will never achieve this and plateau at stage III, making the decision not to return to sport.

CHONDRAL, CHONDROCYTE AND MENISCAL GRAFTING

In the United Kingdom, these procedures are recent additions to the surgical repertoire. Specific postoperative treatment regimes are determined by the surgeon.

Pre-operative assessment follows the same pattern as for all knee surgery (see page 82). Postoperatively the patient is returned to the ward, possibly on a CPM machine. When comfortable—about 24 hours after surgery—the patient will be allowed out of bed and will mobilise using crutches for protected weight bearing.

Exercises to increase the range of knee movement within limits are performed, the range of movement allowed being determined by the surgeon's protocol. A knee brace may be worn and, if used, will be set to allow only the prescribed range of movement.

The length of time the patient remains in hospital depends on their speed of recovery. The patient is discharged when they are comfortable and confident on walking.

On discharge, physiotherapy is continued—initially to supervise the continuation of protected weight bearing and gentle active exercise to the knee. The treatment may last up to 6 weeks. From 6 to 12 weeks, weight bearing is gradually increased, as is the range of movement allowed

at the joint. Resistance to exercise is also increased.

From 3 to 6 months, the patient gradually progresses all rehabilitation activities, and a return to normal levels of functional activity is expected within this time. Resumption of contact sports is delayed for a further 3–6 months.

THE ANKLE

Surgery at this joint consists of arthroscopy, ankle replacement and arthrodesis.

ARTHROSCOPY

The treatment of a patient who has had an ankle arthroscopy is the same as that for the knee (see page 82). As this is often performed as day surgery, physiotherapy may not be required. Where physiotherapy is required, it is usually undertaken postoperatively. The following procedures may be indicated:
- A functional assessment of gait and provision of appropriate walking aids. The patient is normally allowed to bear full weight on the limb following an arthroscopy; however, if the pattern of gait is compromised through pain, walking aids (e.g. crutches, sticks), may be required for a few days.
- Instruction and advice on the use of icepacks and limb elevation to control swelling, rest, exercise to monitor integrity of ankle movements and the resumption of daily activities. Daily activities are gradually resumed as pain and swelling allow.
- Provision of out-patient physiotherapy. The patient may be required to continue the rehabilitation programme under supervision once discharged from hospital.

ARTHRODESIS
Pre-operative Physiotherapy

This involves an assessment of the patient's condition and discussion of the postoperative care. Assessments are subjective and objective, as described for the hip and knee (see pages 76 and 82).

The patient returns to the ward with the fusion held by internal or external fixation or a combination of both. When on bed rest, the patient is instructed to keep the limb elevated.

The patient is mobilised once comfortable, the surgeon determining the timing of weight bearing. Once the patient is independent using a walking aid, discharge and readmission for removal of the fixator may be arranged. The patient is discharged once the fusion is solid. The length of time and the degree of restricted weight bearing are determined by the surgeon. Following discharge, physiotherapy may be arranged on an out-patient basis.

Figure 6.4 shows a typical treatment card for a patient who has had an ankle arthrodesis.

ANKLE REPLACEMENT

The pre-operative physiotherapy is as for surgery of the hip and knee (see pages 76 and 82). Postoperatively, the patient is instructed to rest the limb in elevation to minimise

Ankle arthrodesis treatment card													
Date													Initials
Postoperative day	1	2	3	4	5	6	7	8	9	10	11	12	
Circulatory exercises													
Breathing exercises													
Bed exercises													
Elevation													
Cryotherapy													
Splintage (please state)													
Mobilise NWB with frame													
Mobilise NWB with crutches													
Stair practice													
Patient education and advice													

Figure 6.4 Ankle arthrodesis treatment card.

swelling when not exercising. This may be necessary for 2–3 months.

Following surgery, the patient remains on bed rest for approximately 24 hours with the limb in elevation. The patient then commences mobilisation with a walking frame, progressing to crutches then a stick. The speed of these transitions is dictated by the surgeon and the patient's comfort and ability.

Rehabilitation will include:
• Gait re-education.
• Ankle mobilisation. Both dorsiflexion and plantar flexion may be gained by active exercises, active assisted exercises, hydrotherapy and gymnasium activities. Splintage of the ankle will prevent mobilisation for about 6–8 weeks.
• Proprioceptive exercises, e.g. wobble board, squats, walking on uneven surfaces, to encourage stability, balance and co-ordination.

Once the patient is mobile with a walking aid, they will be discharged and out-patient physiotherapy provided until the patient is fully rehabilitated.

Figure 6.5 shows a typical treatment card for a patient who has had an ankle joint replaced.

The rehabilitation period will depend on the surgeon's preference and the patient's abilities and motivation. It may take from 6 weeks to several months before the patient achieves full independence.

ACKNOWLEDGEMENTS

We thank all the surgeons, physiotherapists and other clinicians, and the Arthroplasty Audit Team (Mr A. Roberts FRCS, Mrs A. Biggs MCSP, Mrs D. Lloyd BOAT and Ms K. Jones RGN), of the Robert Jones and Agnes Hunt Orthopaedic and District Hospital, NHS Trust Oswestry.

Ankle replacement treatment card

Date													Initials
Postoperative day	1	2	3	4	5	6	7	8	9	10	11	12	
Circulatory exercises	▓	▓											
Breathing exercises	▓												
Bed exercises	▓	▓	▓	▓	▓	▓	▓	▓	▓	▓	▓	▓	
Elevation	▓	▓	▓	▓	▓	▓	▓	▓	▓				
Cryotherapy	▓	▓	▓	▓	▓	▓	▓	▓					
Range of movement exercises	▓	▓	▓	▓	▓	▓	▓	▓	▓	▓	▓	▓	
Plaster of paris													
Gait re-education with frame		▓											
Gait re-education with crutches		▓	▓	▓	▓	▓	▓	▓	▓	▓	▓	▓	
Independent		▓	▓	▓	▓	▓	▓	▓	▓	▓	▓	▓	
Stair practice				▓	▓	▓	▓	▓	▓	▓	▓	▓	
Patient education and advice	▓	▓	▓	▓	▓	▓	▓	▓	▓	▓	▓	▓	
Range of movement													
Out-patient physiotherapy													

Figure 6.5 Ankle replacement treatment card.

GENERAL READING

Pynsent, Fairbank, Carr. *Outcome measures in orthopaedics*. Butterworths-Heineman; 1993.

Rehabilitation programme following chondrocyte transplantation. Sweden: Gothenburg Medical Centre, Gruvgatan 6, 30 Vastra Frolunda.

Van Arkle ERA, de Boer HH. Human meniscal transplantation. The Nertherlands: Department of Orthopaedic Surgery, De Wever Hospital, Heerleen.

7 A J Carr
SURGERY TO THE UPPER LIMB

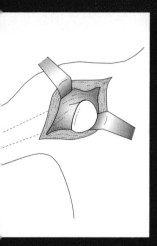

CHAPTER OUTLINE

- Subacromial decompression
- Arthroscopic subacromial decompression
- Rotator cuff repair
- Stabilisation of the acromioclavicular joint

- Shoulder replacement
- Shoulder stabilisation
- Arthroscopy and distension of the shoulder with manipulation under anaesthetic
- Elbow replacement

SUBACROMIAL DECOMPRESSION

INDICATIONS

Subacromial decompression is indicated for impingement syndrome or painful arc. Usually the patient has undergone conservative treatment including rest, avoidance of exacerbating factors, physiotherapy, anti-inflammatory medication and cortisone injections into the bursa.

Anterior acromioplasty may also be undertaken in patients who have irreparable rotator cuff tears.

INVESTIGATIONS

Making a correct diagnosis is essential if treatment is to be successful, and a thorough history-taking and clinical examination are important. Examination should involve impingement tests which assess whether there is pain in the mid-range of abduction of the shoulder. Sometimes this pain is reduced with an injection of local anaesthetic into the bursa.

Plain X-ray films may show some sclerosis on the undersurface of the acromion and the formation of osteophytes on the anterior edge of the acromion. Sclerosis of the greater tuberosity is also a feature. In more advanced impingement, the distance between the acromion and the humeral head may be narrowed to less than 7 mm.

Generally, the standard X-ray views for assessing the shoulder are anteroposterior and axillary. Better information can be obtained from plain X-ray films if a caudal tilt view of 30° is used.

Ultrasonography is increasingly used for assessment of the rotator cuff, but an experienced practitioner is required for the information to be valuable; in these circumstances, the sensitivity and specificity of the test approach those of magnetic resonance imaging (MRI) scanning. The advantages of ultrasonography are that it is relatively inexpensive and quick. Many shoulder clinics employ ultrasonography, which enables advice to be given to the patient about the best treatment at the time of the clinic visit.

Magnetic resonance imaging scanning is the most sensitive and specific investigation for assessing the rotator cuff, and an accuracy level of almost 95% has been reported. Magnetic resonance imaging scanning has the advantage over arthrography of being non-invasive. The disadvantage of MRI scanning is that it requires a visit to hospital, and it is relatively expensive.

TECHNIQUE

The patient is placed in the beach-chair position, enabling the surgeon access to both anterior and posterior parts of the shoulder. A superior strap incision is made over the lateral border of the acromion, exposing the anterior edge of the acromion and the junction of the anterior third and posterior two thirds of the deltoid muscle (Figure 7.1). This muscle is then split in the line of its fibres, detaching the deltoid from the anterior portion of the acromion. This exposes the coracoacromial ligament, which is released from the front edge of the acromion (Figure 7.2). The anterior edge of the acromion is then excised and any osteophytes or 'beaking' of the acromion removed (Figure 7.3). Bigliani has described three shapes of acromion;

types I–III (Figure 7.4). It is probable that the increased 'beaking' of the acromion is acquired rather than congenital. Once the acromioplasty has been undertaken the rotator cuff can be inspected from its superior surface. Often a glenohumeral arthroscopy will have been undertaken, before open acromioplasty, to allow inspection of the bursa from the joint surface. It is possible that a rotator cuff tear may be found at the time of surgery and this may then be repaired. The deltoid is closed with interrupted sutures. The muscle can usually be reattached to the periosteum of the acromion, but sometimes bone sutures are required to allow a stable and secure repair (Figure 7.5). The wound is then closed and often infiltrated with local anaesthetic. A sling is then placed over the arm.

ANAESTHETIC

Many shoulder operations are undertaken under general anaesthetic and relatively few under local anaesthetic. In the case of acromioplasty, this procedure is often performed with a combination of general anaesthesia and regional anaesthesia. The regional anaesthetic most commonly used is an interscalene block. This allows a period of 6–8 hours postoperatively where there is little or no pain. The slight disadvantage is that the arm is paralysed during this period and is susceptible to damage if not protected properly.

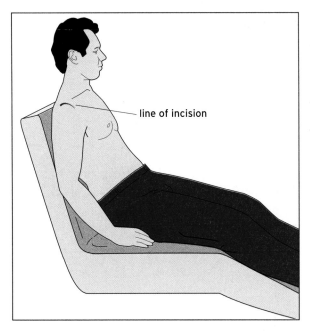

Figure 7.1 Strap incision used for anterior acromioplasty and rotator cuff repair. The patient is in the beach-chair position.

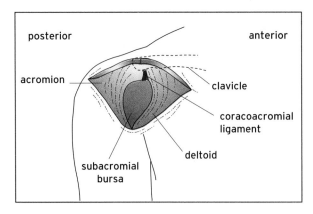

Figure 7.2 Deltoid split along its fibres.

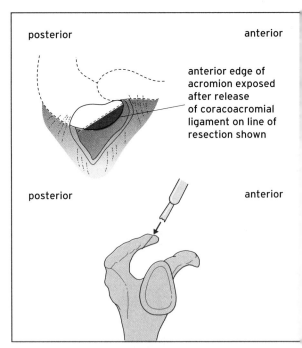

Figure 7.3 The anterior edge of the acromion is exposed by releasing the deltoid from its anterior edge. The coracoacromio-ligament is divided and the anterior edge of the acromion resected using bony burrs.

POSTOPERATIVE MANAGEMENT

Immediately after surgery the patient should be visited and instructed in maintenance exercises to the neck, shoulder, elbow and wrist. Early passive movements of the shoulder are also commenced. Patients are advised to use the sling for the next 24–48 hours, then to remove it for short periods, as comfort permits. Driving is usually not possible for 1–2 weeks and manual work should be avoided for 4 weeks.

COMPLICATIONS

Failure may occur because the operation has been undertaken for incorrect indications. If undertaken for correct indications, then 80–85% of people will have significant resolution of their symptoms by 6 months postoperatively. Infection may occur, and any redness or increase in pain during the first few weeks after surgery should be taken seriously and the patient advised to consult his or her general practitioner or return to hospital. In open anterior acromioplasty, the deltoid may become detached from the anterior acromion, causing a step deformity that is palpable on clinical examination and that produces some weakness of flexion of the shoulder.

Very occasionally, postoperative stiffness may develop. This is similar to capsulitis of the shoulder and is associated with a global restriction of movement. This is a very rare complication but will considerably slow up the postoperative recovery. The stiffness may take up to 12 months to resolve.

ARTHROSCOPIC SUBACROMIAL DECOMPRESSION

The operative technique for this is based on the same principles as for open acromioplasty. However, rather than making an open incision through the deltoid, the coracoacromial ligament is released from within the bursa and the anterior edge of the acromion removed using arthroscopic burrs; the advantage being reduced postoperative morbidity. The wounds are much smaller and heal more quickly (Figures 7.6–7.8). Manual work can usually be resumed after 4–6 weeks and driving between 1 and 2

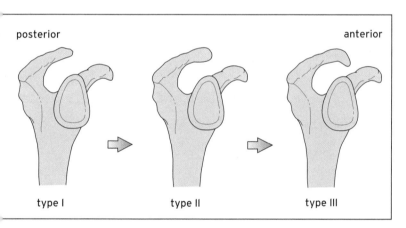

posterior   anterior

type I   type II   type III

Figure 7.4 Impingement and rotator cuff disease are associated with progressive curvature of the acromion. Osteophytes form on the anterior edge of the acromion.

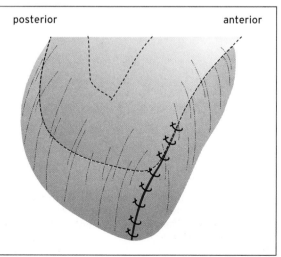

posterior   anterior

Figure 7.5 The deltoid reattached to acromion using sutures passed through bone. It is important to obtain a secure fixation of the deltoid if anterior deltoid weakness is to be prevented.

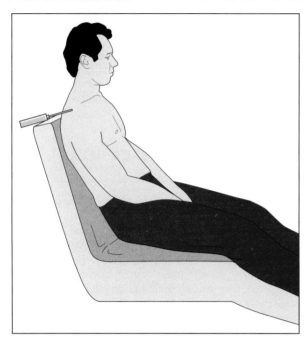

Figure 7.6 Arthroscopic arthroplasty. The patient is in the beach-chair position. Both joint and bursa are viewed from the posterior portal.

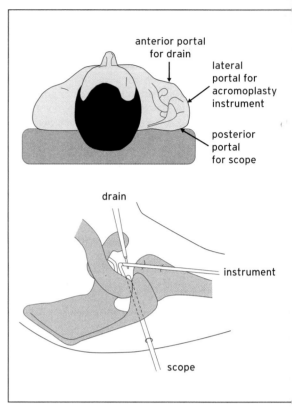

Figure 7.7 Arthroscopic arthroplasty.

weeks. Arthroscopic subacromial decompression does not appear to confer any advantage over open decompression at six months.

ROTATOR CUFF REPAIR

INDICATIONS
The indication for this operation is symptomatic tear of the rotator cuff. Patients will have usually undergone conservative treatment in the form of modification of activity, rest, physiotherapy, analgesics, anti-inflammatory medication and often one or two cortisone injections.

The most common tendon to rupture is the supraspinatus (Figure 7.9A). The rupture occurs almost always through a degenerative process, although traumatic rupture is described. A minor fall may cause an acute tear of a previously degenerate tendon. The patient presents with a combination of pain, weakness and restriction of movement. The pain is characteristically on movement, but may occur at rest and at night with larger tears. Examination may reveal typical painful arc and, in more substantial tears, there may be evidence of weakness of either the supraspinatus or infraspinatus muscles.

If the patient fails to respond to conservative treatment and is medically fit, then surgery is indicated. In the patient with relatively mild symptoms, arthroscopic decompression may be chosen to see if this relieves the pain, therefore precluding the need for more major open surgery. It is advisable for young patients to have a rotator cuff repair even if

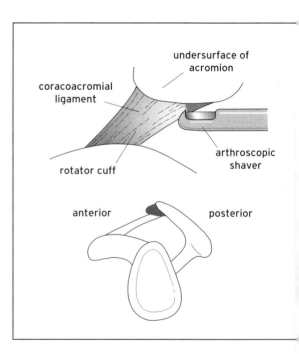

Figure 7.8 Arthroscopic instruments are used to release the coracoacromial ligament and resect the anterior acromion.

their symptoms are not severe, because of the possibility of the tear extending. It must be assumed that large tears were once small. In the frail and elderly, an arthroscopic decompression may be preferred because of the much lower risk to the patient and the faster recovery rate.

INVESTIGATION

History taking and clinical examination are often supplemented by the use of plain X-ray films and some more formal assessment of the state of the rotator cuff. Traditionally this was with an arthrogram, but more recently this investigation has been superseded by ultrasonography and MRI scanning.

Ultrasonography is quick and inexpensive but is very operator dependent. The most sensitive and specific investigation of the cuff at present is MRI scanning.

If a decision has already been made to operate on a patient, then ultrasonography will usually suffice in determining whether or not a rotator cuff tear is present. If greater accuracy is required for establishing a diagnosis or determining the precise size of the tear, then MRI scanning is preferred.

TECHNIQUE

The patient is positioned as for open anterior acromioplasty (see above). The initial steps of the procedure are also the same. A strap incision is made, the deltoid split, the coraco-acromio ligament divided and an anterior acromioplasty performed. The rotator cuff is then exposed and the extent of the tear defined.

Once the tear has been assessed and the bursal tissue overlying it excised and debrided, then the thickness and quality of the residual cuff muscle are evaluated.

Small tears less than 3 cm usually only involve part of the insertion of the supraspinatus and can be relatively easily drawn back down onto the greater tuberosity. These tears are repaired by inserting them in a groove cut in the upper surface of the greater tuberosity, and are attached using bone sutures. The bone sutures draw the rotator cuff edge down into the groove and hold the cuff in that position (Figure 7.9A, B and C).

For medium-sized tears of 3–5 cm, some dissection of the rotator cuff may be necessary to allow them to be drawn back down onto the greater tuberosity. The size of the cuff does not always determine its ease of repair and some medium-sized tears can be very difficult to repair because they have become rigid and inelastic. Nevertheless, it is usually possible to repair a medium-sized tear, and this is undertaken in a similar fashion to smaller tears

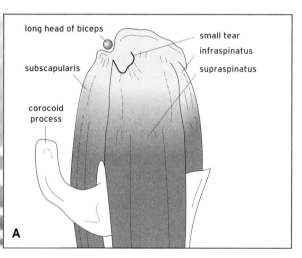

A

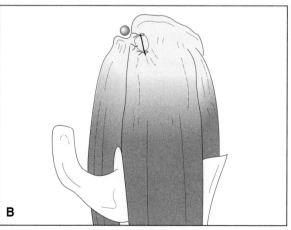

B

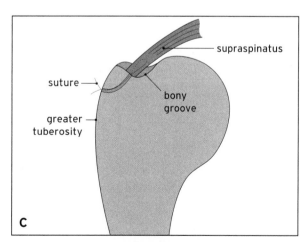

C

Figure 7.9 Rotator cuff repair. **(A)** Tears fo the rotator cuff usually begin at the anterior edge of the supraspinatus next to the long head of biceps. **(B)** In repair of the rotator cuff the tendon is drawn down onto the greater tuberosity and secured with sutures. **(C)** shows acromial section of the humerus demonstrating the reattachment of the supraspinatus to the greater tuberosity with sutures through bone.

using a groove cut in the greater tuberosity and intra-osseous sutures (Figure 7.10A and B).

The medium-sized tear of 3–5 cm may take on either a 'U' or an 'L' shape. In the latter shape, the tear not only involves the whole of the supraspinatus, but also extends along the rotator interval (Figure 7.11A and B). In the former shape, both the subscapularis and, more commonly, the infraspinatus may begin to be involved (Figure 7.12A, B and C). In this type of tear it may be impossible to draw the supraspinatus back down onto the greater tuberosity, and therefore it may be necessary to transfer either the upper part of the supraspinatus or whatever remains of the infraspinatus onto the greater tuberosity (Figure 7.13).

In the L-shaped tear, it may be possible to close side to side the rotator interval and some remaining part of the supraspinatus. Another option is to include the biceps

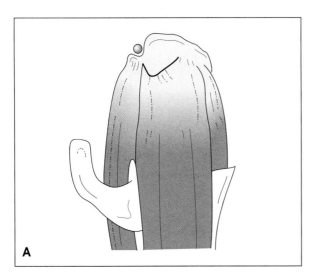
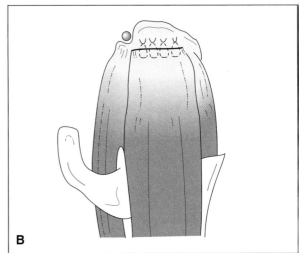

Figure 7.10 (A) The tear (measuring 3–5 cm) usually extends posteriorly towards the infraspinatus. At this stage, the supraspinatus may still be functioning. **(B)** Larger tears are also repaired using osseous sutures, with the tendon being held in a bony groove.

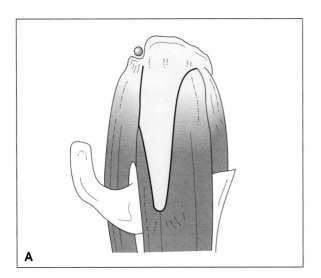
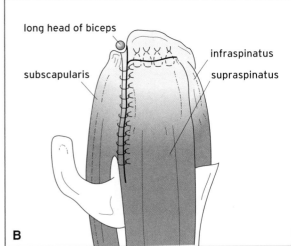

Figure 7.11 (A) The tear (measuring 3-5 cm) may become 'L' shaped rather than 'U' shaped, if it extends along the rotator interval. (B) Repair is often difficult and it may be necessary to repair the supraspinatus to the long head of the biceps anteriorly.

tendon in the repair, performing a tenodesis of this tendon to whatever remains of reparable rotator cuff. Some surgeons will use suture anchors if they find the greater tuberosity too osteoporotic. Once the rotator cuff has been repaired, the bursa is closed, if possible, over it.

The subsequent closure is identical to that of anterior acromioplasty, with interrupted sutures to the deltoid and then closure of the skin.

POSTOPERATIVE MANAGEMENT

It is best to repair the rotator cuff so that the arm can be left by the side without placing undue tension on the repair. In 90% of cases, this is possible, and only rarely does some form of abduction splint have to be used (Figure 7.14). Passive mobilisation should begin immediately and instructions given for mobilisation exercises for the elbow, wrist and neck. During the first 2 weeks

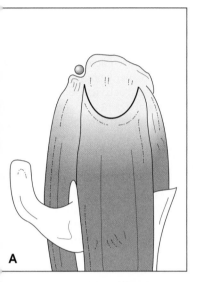
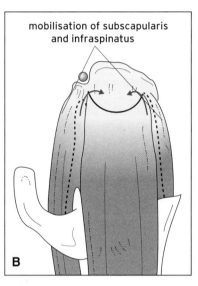
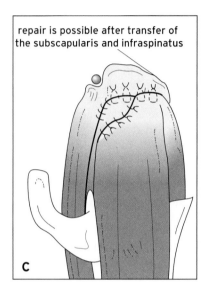

Figure 7.12 (A) As the tear enlarges, the infraspinatus becomes involved. The long head of the biceps becomes flattened and frayed. **(B)** Larger tears may be unrepairable. Mobilisation and transfer of the infraspinatus and subscapularis may be necessary. **(C)** If the muscle is mobile, then a total or partial repair may be achieved. Sometimes the long head of the biceps is incorporated in a tenodesis.

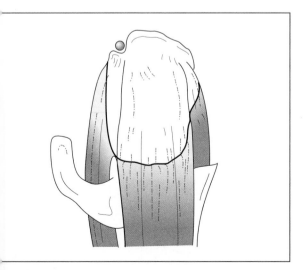

Figure 7.13 In massive tears (measuring >5 cm), the subscapularis and teres minor muscles are also involved. The long head of the biceps is usually ruptured. Repair is usually impossible in this situation.

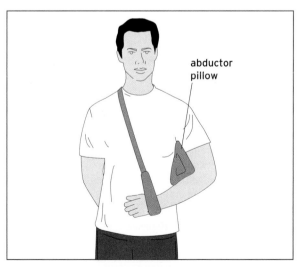

Figure 7.14 Sometimes an abduction pillow made of a wedge of foam may be used to rest the arm in approximately 30° of abduction.

after surgery, no active movement should be allowed, although pendulum movements and passive flexion in extension should be encouraged to prevent any postoperative stiffness.

After 3–4 weeks, further passive movements should be encouraged and some passive assisted exercises commenced. Active work does not usually begin until 6 or 8 weeks. The precise nature of the programme will depend on the size and security of the rotator cuff repair, and to this end it is important to liaise with the surgeon.

COMPLICATIONS

Generally, 80% of patients who have their rotator cuff repaired will have good relief of pain and improvement in strength by 6 months.

There is a tendency for the rotator cuff to re-rupture and this re-rupture rate may be up to 30%. Even if the cuff does re-rupture, the anterior acromioplasty may still afford some relief of pain.

Infection is always a concern with this type of surgery and any increase in pain or abnormal redness in the area should be taken very seriously and the general practitioner consulted.

A further complication of this type of surgery is postoperative stiffness. This is a form of capsulitis of the shoulder and presents with a global restriction of movement. This considerably slows down the recovery from the surgery, and the stiffness may take up to 12 months to resolve. It is unclear whether this significantly adversely affects the outcome of the rotator cuff repair.

STABILISATION OF THE ACROMIOCLAVICULAR JOINT

INDICATIONS

Most patients who sustain an injury to the acromioclavicular joint can be managed conservatively. The mechanism of injury is often a fall onto the point of the shoulder either from a bicycle or a horse, causing disruption of the ligament apparatus around the distal end of the clavicle. The most substantial ligament stabilising the distal end of the clavicle is the ligament between the coracoid process of the scapula and the clavicle. Trauma to this region may be so severe that the clavicle becomes buttonholed through the trapezius or lodges beneath the coracoid process; in these circumstances, an acute repair is required. This is a rare situation and the majority of injuries to the acromioclavicular joint involve subluxation, known as grade I or II injuries, or complete dislocation with a variable amount of disruption, referred to as grade III to VI injuries (Figure 7.15).

If at 6 months symptoms of pain and discomfort continue, due to impaction of the end of the clavicle on the acromion in abduction or flexion, then stabilisation may be indicated. Sometimes patients complain of a feeling of heaviness of the arm. This is because with disruption of the ligament apparatus the scapula and arm fall down from the clavicle. Sometimes surgery is indicated because of a concern about the viability of skin overlying what is often a fairly significant cosmetic deformity at the site of the injury.

INVESTIGATIONS

Usually the abnormality can be detected clinically and on plain anteroposterior X-ray films of the shoulder. Specific views of the acromioclavicular joint including weight-bearing views are sometimes used.

SURGICAL TECHNIQUE

A variety of different surgical techniques have been suggested for stabilisation of the acromioclavicular joint including the use of plates between the clavicle and acromion, the use of percutaneous K-wires, and screw fixation between the clavicle and coracoid process. One method that seems to be particularly popular involves an attempt to reconstruct the coracoclavicular ligament by transferring the coracoacromial ligament to the end of the clavicle and securing it to the bone. This repair is often supplemented either with a screw between the clavicle and the coracoid or with sutures. This procedure has been made popular by Weaver and Dunn.

Through a strap incision overlying the acromioclavicular joint, the origin of the deltoid muscle is detached and reflected laterally and inferiorly, exposing the distal clavicle, the coracoid process, the coracoacromial ligament and the end of the acromion. There is often a significant amount of scar tissue in this region. The very tip of the clavicle is removed with a saw and the end hollowed out. Two holes are drilled in the superior surface of the clavicle to take a suture. The coracoacromial ligament is removed from the acromion with a sliver of bone. A suture is then passed through the ligament in a zigzag fashion, and the end of the ligament, along with the small flake of bone, is drawn into the end of the clavicle with the suture ends having been passed through drill holes prepared in the end of the clavicle (Figure 7.16). The clavicle is pressed downwards at the same time and the ligament is securely fixed into the end of the clavicle. This procedure effectively reconstitutes the coracoclavicular

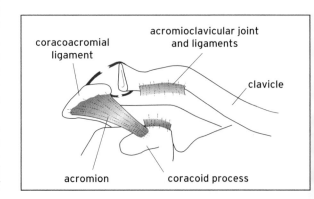

Figure 7.15 Acromioclavicular joint reconstruction.

gament. To supplement and protect this ligament repair during the first few months, sutures are passed either round the clavicle and the coracoid or through drill holes n the clavicle and coracoid. A very strong number 5 uture is used for this augmentation (Figure 7.17). At the nd of the procedure, the deltoid is reattached to the clav- :le and acromion and the wound closed. A sling is placed ver the arm.

POSTOPERATIVE MANAGEMENT

he arm is rested in a sling for 3–4 weeks, during which me maintenance and pendulum exercises begin. ollowing this, passive exercises are increased and early ctive movement commenced. Sports, particularly contact nes, e.g. rugby, should be avoided for a minimum of 3 ionths.

COMPLICATIONS

variety of complications have been described with this urgery, particularly with the use of K-wires and tension and wires. The wires tend to migrate and have been found s far away as the lungs and the superior vena cava. 1ethods that use a screw fixation between the clavicle and ie coracoid process are prone to loosening of the screw, nd this often has to be removed.

Occasionally the new ligament ruptures or there is a fail- re of the augmentation sutures, both leading to a reappear- nce of the cosmetic deformity and recurrence of pain. With xcision of the distal end of the clavicle, some of the pain may e improved, because of reduced impingement between the nd of the clavicle and the acromion in abduction.

SHOULDER REPLACEMENT

INDICATIONS

he commonest indication for shoulder replacement in the Inited Kingdom is rheumatoid arthritis. Other indications iclude primary osteoarthritis and osteoarthritis secondary trauma or rotator cuff rupture.

The principal reason for considering shoulder replacement is uncontrolled pain that is affecting the qual- ity of an individual's life. A secondary reason is loss of movement in the shoulder either through stiffness, mus- cle weakness or pain. Shoulder replacement, like other joint replacements, is effective at relieving pain.

The shoulder has a phenomenal range of movement, and restoring this is difficult following shoulder replace- ment surgery. This is because arthritis of the shoulder usu- ally involves some contracture of the soft tissue around the joint, and because there is often associated damage or loss of the rotator cuff. This loss of the rotator cuff not only removes motor units that control shoulder movement but also causes disruption of the normal positioning of the humeral head relative to the glenoid. This malposition of the two bony elements of the shoulder causes considerable biomechanical disadvantage and is one of the reasons that shoulder movement is often impaired following replace- ment surgery.

Two types of shoulder replacements are possible: a total replacement, where both the humeral and glenoid surfaces are replaced, and a hemiarthroplasty, where the humeral component alone is implanted. If the bone stock is ade- quate and the rotator cuff is intact and functioning, then a total shoulder replacement will probably give the best func- tional results both short and long term.

If, however, the rotator cuff is not functioning properly and is badly torn or the glenoid is significantly eroded, then a hemiarthroplasty is usually chosen. There seems to be a high rate of glenoid component failure if a total shoulder replacement is used in this situation. The hemiarthroplasty functions very well, although there is probably less pain relief than with a total shoulder replacement.

INVESTIGATIONS

Good-quality anteroposterior and axillary X-ray films should be obtained. The axillary view is particularly useful for determining the amount of glenoid erosion. Sometimes additional imaging with computerised tomography (CT) or MRI scanning is needed to assess the state of the bones and surrounding soft tissues.

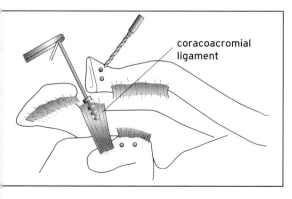

Figure 7.16 Preparation of drill holes in the end of ie clavicle.

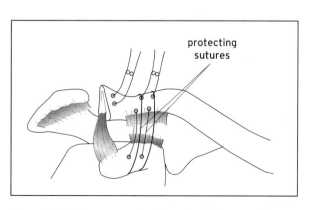

Figure 7.17 Strong number 5 sutures are used to protect the ligament repair in the first few months.

TECHNIQUE

The patient is positioned in a beach chair position with the shoulder over the edge of the table, enabling the joint to be extended during surgery. An anterior delto-pectoral approach is used. The cephalic vein is identified in the space between the deltoid and pectoralis muscles (Figure 7.18). The con-joint tendon muscles are then identified. Some surgeons will remove the coracoid process and then reattach it at the end of the procedure. Often the muscles can be retracted simply by releasing them close to the coracoid. The subscapularis muscle is then divided over stay sutures (Figure 7.19). A retractor is placed round the neck of the humeral head to protect the axillary nerve. Once the capsule and subscapularis muscle have been retracted, the joint is exposed. It is sometimes possible to dissect the capsule and subscapularis separately, but often the osteoarthritic or rheumatoid process has produced so much scarring they have to be divided in continuity. The capsule is released around the inferior aspect of the joint, allowing dislocation of the joint. The humeral head is exposed and an assessment is made of the integrity of the rotator cuff muscles, particularly the supraspinatus (Figure 7.20). An osteotomy is then made in the humeral head, retroverting it 35° relative to the axis of the forearm. With the osteotomy accomplished, the medullary shaft of the humerus is then reamed to take the standard trial instrumentation for the humeral component (Figure 7.21). It is important to sit the component at the correct level. If it sits too low or too high then an abnormal relation will be made between the prosthetic component and the glenoid. Most humeral components are modular these days and different sizes of head can be tried for the best fit.

The glenoid is then exposed by using retractors placed behind and in front of the glenoid (Figure 7.22). Several implantation systems exist for the glenoid, but essentially it is reamed to provide a smooth concave surface. A hole is

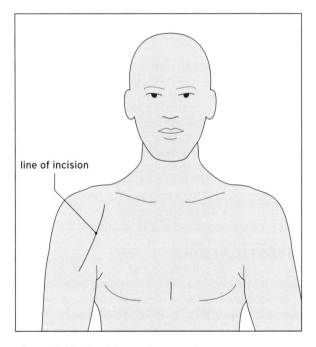

Figure 7.18 Shoulder replacement.

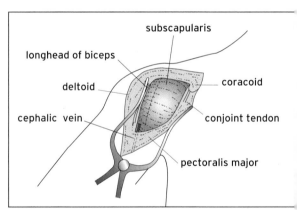

Figure 7.19 Anterior deltopectoral approach.

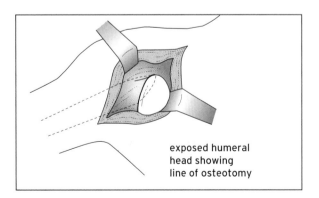

Figure 7.20 Exposed humeral head, showing line of osteotomy.

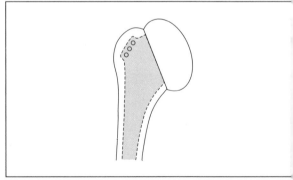

Figure 7.21 Reamed medullary shaft of the humerus.

then made in the base of the glenoid to accommodate the keel or pegs of the glenoid component. Once the trial reduction has been accomplished, definitive components are then cemented into position (Figure 7.23). It is important to be certain during the trial reduction that the joint is not too tight or too loose. This means assessing the relation of the glenoid and humeral components in different positions (Figure 7.24). The subscapularis muscle is then closed, the aim being to repair it in continuity without any shortening (Figure 7.25). Sometimes the muscle can be shifted superiorly if the rotator cuff is absent, to allow some downward pull of the muscle, which may help to reduce the humerus on the glenoid. The coracoid muscle is repaired and the wound closed.

POSTOPERATIVE MANAGEMENT

The management of the patient will depend very much on the circumstances, but can be usefully divided into three phases. During the first phase, passive movements and gentle active assisted movements occur and these can begin the day after surgery, lasting 2–3 weeks. In the second phase, an active assisted programme is commenced, avoiding active internal rotation or undue passive external rotation to protect the subscapularis repair. Strengthening and isometric exercises are included in this second phase. In the third phase, the patient is encouraged to further stretch and strengthen the arm. Most improvement in movement appears to occur within the first 6–12 months.

COMPLICATIONS

Peri-operative complications include fracture, particularly of the proximal humerus, and damage to nerves and vessels. Very rarely, damage can occur to elements of the brachial plexus, usually the musculocutaneous nerve or the axillary nerve.

Dislocations of the joint may occur postoperatively. This is rare, other than in revision surgery or in surgery after fracture. Usually there is sufficient soft tissue envelope to prevent dislocation. Sometimes dislocation may occur because the components are malpositioned. This is especially so if the humeral component is placed too low in the humeral shaft after fracture. In these circumstances, the humerus will be inferiorly subluxed beneath the glenoid.

As with all joint replacements, infection is a potential risk, although the incidence is probably less than 1%. Antibiotic prophylaxis should always be given. Aseptic loosening may also occur, although this seems to be more with the glenoid component than the humeral component, particularly if there is a mismatch due to rotator cuff failure.

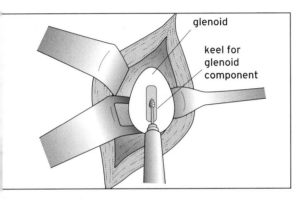

Figure 7.22 Exposed glenoid.

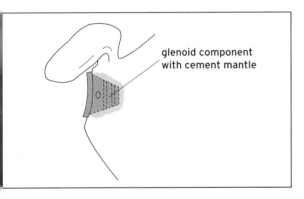

Figure 7.23 Cementation of definitive components.

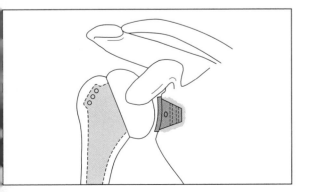

Figure 7.24 Relation of the glenoid and humeral components in different positions.

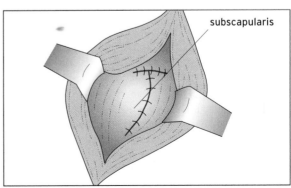

Figure 7.25 Closure of the subscapularis muscle.

Thromboembolic disease is less of a problem in the upper than lower limb.

RESULTS

To date, relatively few large long-term series for shoulder replacement have been published. The indications are that 90% of implants last 5–10 years. Shoulder replacement is therefore similar in this respect to knee and hip replacement.

SHOULDER STABILISATION

INDICATIONS

The shoulder is the most frequently dislocated joint in the body. The majority of shoulder instability occurs following a traumatic event such as a fall. In most of these cases the shoulder dislocates anteriorly or anteroinferiorly. This dislocation usually causes damage to the capsule and its ligaments. A lesion may be created where the capsule is stripped off the front of the glenoid, known as a Bankart lesion. This part of the capsule includes the inferior glenohumeral ligament.

Often the capsule does not reattach, and most people who have a dislocation, particularly if they are young, will have further episodes of either subluxation or dislocation.

If the instability is troublesome and affects the quality of life, then surgery is indicated. Surgery for this type of instability involves tightening or repair of the damaged tissues at the anterior and inferior part of the joint. Such surgery is generally very successful.

Other forms of shoulder instability also occur. Rarely, these are caused by trauma involving a different direction of dislocation, usually posterior but sometimes inferior. Traumatic posterior dislocation often occurs after an exceptional event such as an epileptic fit or electric shock.

Another important group of people who are susceptible to shoulder instability have congenital laxity, sometimes associated with poor muscle co-ordination. These patients often have lax shoulders and a tendency to sublux the joint in a number of directions. There may be a predominant direction and this is usually posteroinferior. The dislocations may be precipitated by a relatively minor event such as throwing or swimming.

The management of this group is much more difficult and is usually with physiotherapy and rehabilitation exercises. Sometimes surgery is undertaken with a capsular shift, but a much higher rate of recurrent dislocation should be anticipated.

INVESTIGATIONS

Usually, instability is clear from the history. It is important that care should be taken with the history and when asking the patient to describe what events precipitate his or her problems. This should be followed up with a careful examination involving testing for apprehension when moving the shoulder into different positions. If dislocation has occurred, this may have been confirmed with X-ray films taken at the time of presentation to a casualty department.

If doubts still remain about whether the shoulder is subluxing, then further investigation may be necessary. Plain X-ray films with an axillary view may demonstrate the presence of a Hill–Sachs defect on the posterior aspect of the humerus. Sometimes a chip fracture of the anterior rim of the glenoid is present where the capsule has stripped away. If no abnormality is noted, then further investigation with CT scanning or MRI scanning may be helpful; these usually have to be supplemented with some form of arthrogram. Unfortunately, instability, particularly that which is difficult to diagnose clinically, may not be associated with gross anatomical abnormalities and therefore the imaging may not be helpful. In these circumstances, an examination under anaesthetic, including an arthroscopy, may be necessary to determine whether the joint is dislocating.

TECHNIQUE
Inferior Capsular Shift

This type of shoulder stabilisation was once used principally for the multidirectional pattern of instability. It is increasingly used for traumatic, anterior and anteroinferior instability because it preserves a greater range of external rotation than some other methods.

The patient is placed in the beach-chair position and an incision made in the line of the delto-pectoral groove as inferiorly as possible to allow a more cosmetic scar (Figure 7.26). The deltopectoral groove is opened and the cephalic vein retracted. The coracoid muscles are then exposed and released close to their origin. A retractor placed over the coracoid muscles allows the incision to be lifted superiorly over the shoulder joint. The top 80% of the subscapularis muscle is identified and the anterior circumflex vessels swept inferiorly (Figure 7.27). A retractor is then placed between the lower 20% of the subscapularis muscle and the capsule.

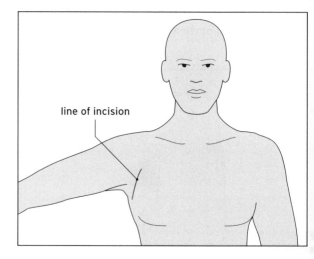

line of incision

Figure 7.26 Anterior stabilisation of the shoulder.

This retractor protects the anterior circumflex vessels and the axillary nerve (Figure 7.28). The subscapularis muscle is then divided approximately 1 cm from its insertion, taking care to preserve the capsule beneath. The interval between the subscapularis and the capsule is opened and the subcapularis retracted with stay sutures. The capsule is then identified beneath the subscapularis and divided 1 cm from its insertion (Figure 7.29). The capsular incision is extended as far as possible posteriorly by externally rotating and abducting the arm. The joint is then inspected and the presence of a Bankart lesion ascertained (Figure 7.30).

The capsule is then divided horizontally to create a 'T' shaped incision with two flaps—one inferior the other superior (Figure 7.31). The capsular shift involves lifting the inferior flap superiorly up to the rotator interval and holding it in place with sutures. The capsular flap is then closed on its lateral margin. This procedure alone stabilises the joint and it is noteable that when the joint is externally rotated and abducted this flap of capsule tightens preventing further subluxation or dislocation (Figures 7.32 and 7.33).

The superior flap is then brought down over the inferior flap and closed with interrupted sutures (Figure 7.34). Throughout the capsular repair, the movement of the joint should be tested so that 30°–40° of external rotation is possible but the joint feels stable and no anterior subluxation is possible. The subscapularis muscle is then closed, without shortening, using interrupted sutures, followed by the coracoid muscle and skin.

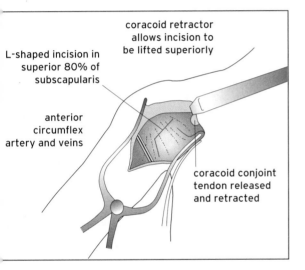

Figure 7.27 Exposure of coracoid muscles, subscapularis muscles and anterior circumflex vessels.

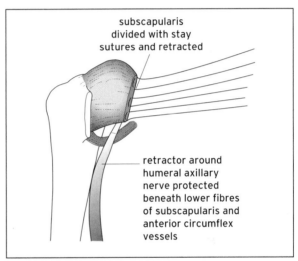

Figure 7.28 Placement of the retractor.

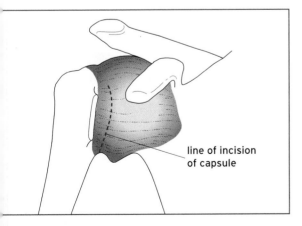

Figure 7.29 Opening of the interval between the subscapularis and capsule.

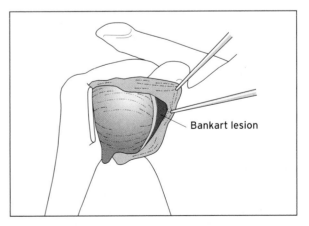

Figure 7.30 Capsule incised from rotator interval to posterior aspect of joint, and retracted with stay sutures.

Putti-Platt Operation

In the Putti-Platt operation the approach is identical to that for the capsular shift except that the T-shaped incision is not made in the capsule. Rather than attempting to provide flaps in the capsule, the capsule is simply overlapped by approximately 1–2 cm. A similar overlapping of the sub-scapularis muscle is undertaken using interrupted sutures. This overlapping of the anterior structures significantly restricts the amount of external rotation and thus stabilises the joint (Figure 7.35).

Bankart Repair

In a Bankart repair, the approach is similar to that of the capsular shift. The T-shaped incision is not made in the capsule but the Bankart lesion is identified at the base of the capsule on the anterior surface of the glenoid. The capsule is then sewn to the roughened anterior surface of the glenoid using either sutures passed across the corner of the glenoid or by inserting suture anchors into the anterior surface of the glenoid. This repair closes the defect causing the instability (see Figure 7.32)

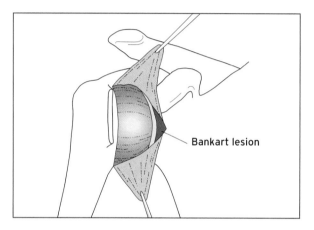

Figure 7.31 T-shaped incision down to Bankart lesion.

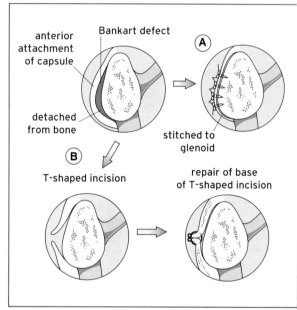

Figure 7.32 Two methods of closing the capsular defect are shown. In **(A)** for a large Bankart defect the capsule is reattached using suture anchors or by conventional Bankart repair. If the Bankart lesion is relatively small thne the T-shaped capsular shift incision can be closed using a suture at the base of the T-incision.

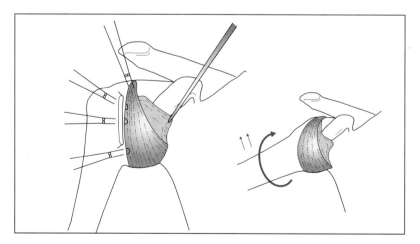

Figure 7.33 Lower flap of capsule is moved superiorly and sutured to the rotator interval. The lateral edge is then closed under the subscapularis using interrupted sutures.

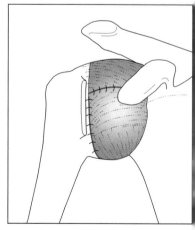

Figure 7.34 Upper flap is then closed over the lower flap to complete the capsular shift.

POSTOPERATIVE MANAGEMENT

The arm is usually managed in a sling for 3 to 6 weeks postoperatively. The precise time will depend upon the individual circumstances. Early passive movements are begun to prevent joint stiffness, but external rotation is limited both actively and passively for at least 3 weeks. Patients with joint laxity and multidirectional instability will usually be immobilised for longer. Thereafter the patient is stretched to regain a full range of passive movement after which strengthening is accomplished. A good range of movement is usually achieved by 3 months.

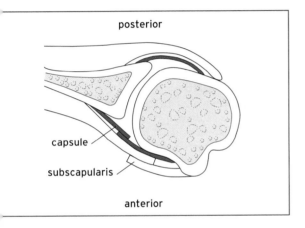

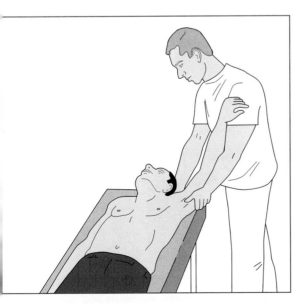

Figure 7.35 In a Putti-Platt repair, the capsule and subscapularis are shortened by overlapping and suturing. External rotation will be restricted.

Figure 7.36 Manipulation under anaesthetic and arthroscopic distension by abduction.

COMPLICATIONS

Rarely, complications may arise due to damage to the musculocutaneous or axillary nerves during surgery.

The main complications are due to overtightening of the tissues, producing excessive stiffness and restriction of movement. This is particularly so with procedures that involve shortening of tendons and muscles. If the dominant arm is affected, then excessive restriction of movement can produce problems with certain activities, e.g. racquet sports and overhead throwing.

Recurrent dislocation may occur and is variously reported in between 2% and 20% of cases. It is much more common in patients with joint laxity than in those with traumatic unidirectional instability.

ARTHROSCOPY AND DISTENSION OF THE SHOULDER WITH MANIPULATION UNDER ANAESTHETIC

INDICATIONS

This procedure is indicated for individuals with frozen shoulder or shoulder capsulitis resistant to non-surgical treatment. The patient may have diabetes or have been involved in trauma. Usually, this procedure will be undertaken after the first painful phase of frozen shoulder is over but where the joint remains stiff despite attempts to stretch it.

Manipulation under anaesthetic involves stretching of the joint in flexion, abduction, adduction and external rotation (Figures 7.36–7.39). In some patients, dramatic improvement in the range of movement can occur with a sudden give or snap of the capsular structures. In other patients, however, the joint remains extremely stiff, and

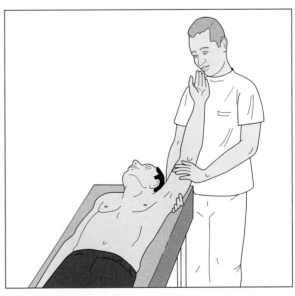

Figure 7.37 Manipulation under anaesthetic and arthroscopic distension by elevation.

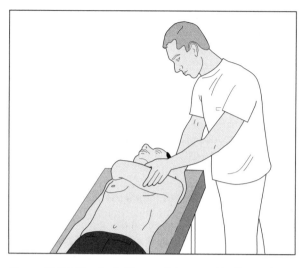

Figure 7.38 Manipulation under anaesthetic and arthroscopic distension by adduction.

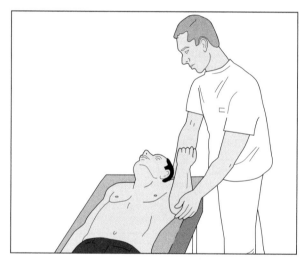

Figure 7.39 Manipulation under anaesthetic and arthroscopic distension by external rotation.

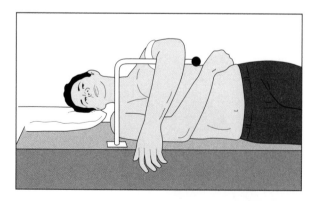

Figure 7.40 Elbow replacement. The patient is positioned on his side with his arm over an armrest. A tourniquet is usually used.

despite forceful manipulation, no additional movement is obtained. It is difficult to predict how much movement will be possible postoperatively, but generally frozen shoulders in patients with insulin-dependent diabetes are much more resistant to manipulation than in people without diabetes.

Several surgeons now perform an arthroscopy and distend the joint using a fluid management pump, once the manipulation has been undertaken. This seems to produce some additional benefit and may help to break the cycle of fibrosis that occurs in capsulitis. Distension is achieved by introducing the shoulder arthroscope through the posterior portal and distending the joint for 5–10 minutes.

COMPLICATIONS

Complications may result from overzealous manipulation including tearing of muscles and possibly fracture of the proximal humerus. Fracture should always be suspected if there is excessive pain after this procedure.

ELBOW REPLACEMENT

INDICATIONS

Elbow replacement is invariably undertaken for rheumatoid arthritis, although it is now being performed for osteoarthritis, particularly post-traumatic osteoarthritis. Rarely, elbow replacement may be performed for an acute fracture in an elderly patient where reconstruction of the fracture is felt to be possible.

INVESTIGATION

Investigations are usually by plain X-ray films; alternative imaging is rarely required.

TECHNIQUE

The patient is positioned in the lateral position with the arm over an armrest and a tourniquet applied to the upper arm (Figure 7.40). A posterior approach is then made to the elbow through a midline incision. The ulnar nerve is identified and released but not transposed (Figure 7.41).

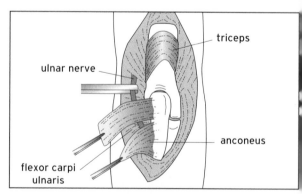

Figure 7.41 The triceps, anconeus and flexor carpi ulnaris muscles are exposed.

The triceps is then split using a lambda-shaped incision. This incision allows good exposure of the joint and a strong reattachment of the triceps at the end of the operation (Figure 7.42). It is essential to preserve the ulnar collateral ligament in elbow replacements that are not of the hinged variety. The incision is carried down the lateral aspect of the joint, lifting the anconeus muscle from the ulna exposing the radial head and neck. The radial head is then removed (Figure 7.43). With the radial head removed and the joint exposed and dislocated, the humeral component is then fitted onto the end of the humerus after preparation of the bone using saws and burrs (Figure 7.44). Once the humeral component is fitted satisfactorily, the ulna is prepared to accept the ulnar component, which is fitted into position as a trial (Figure 7.45). Once a successful trial reduction has been obtained, the definitive components are

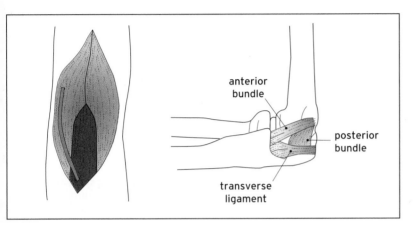

Figure 7.42 The triceps is split in the midline to 2-3 cm from the ocecron, and the incision extended down the lateral side of the ulna. Care is taken to avoid damage to the ligament, particularly the anterior band of the medial ligament.

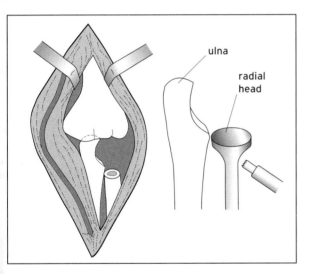

Figure 7.43 The distal humerus is exposed and then the radial head and neck. The radius is then osteotomised, and the radial head removed.

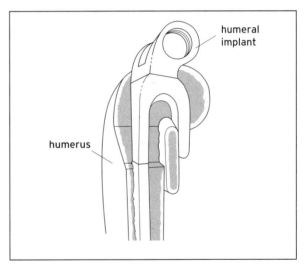

Figure 7.44 The humerus is then cut and reamed so that the implant fits well and can be cemented into position. The precise technique will depend on the implant.

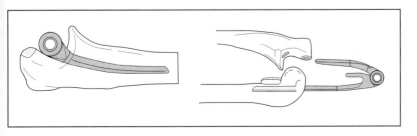

Figure 7.45 The ulna is prepared to take its component.

cemented into position. A check is made for adequate flexion and extension.

Closure is to the ligaments if these have been accidentally damaged, and subsequently to the triceps muscle using interrupted sutures (Figure 7.46).

POSTOPERATIVE MANAGEMENT

The arm is usually managed in a sling for 2–6 weeks postoperatively. If there is difficulty in getting full extension, the arm may be splinted in extension for a few days after surgery. Early passive movements are begun to obtain as much movement as possible. Active extension is avoided for 4–6 weeks because of the repair to the triceps. It is often impossible to correct fixed flexion deformity that was present pre-operatively, and patients should be advised of this. Good return of flexion is often obtained with surgery.

COMPLICATIONS

Complications are common with elbow replacement surgery and these include ulnar neuritis, problems with wound healing and failure of the triceps repair. Both septic and aseptic loosening have been reported, and dislocation can be a problem with unlinked implants.

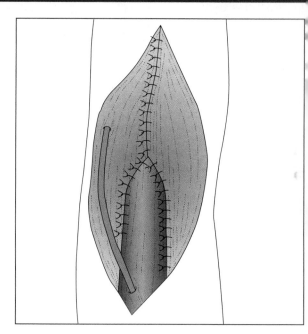

Figure 7.46 The triceps is closed first, reattaching the medial part of the triceps to the ulna. Then the main division in the triceps and the anconeus is closed.

REFERENCES

Bigliani LU, Morrison D, April EW. The morphology of the acromion and its relationship to rotator cuff tears. *Orhop trans* 1986, **10**:228.

Weaver JK, Dunn HK. Treatment of acromioclavicular injuries especially complete acromio-clavicluar separation. *J Bone Joint Surg* 1972. **54(A)6**:1187-1197.

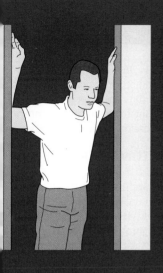

8 K Barker

PHYSIOTHERAPY AFTER UPPER LIMB SURGERY

CHAPTER OUTLINE

- **Total shoulder replacement**
- **Shoulder stabilisation**
- **Subacromial decompression (without rotator cuff repair)**

- **Rotator cuff repair**
- **Total elbow replacement**
- **Outcome measurement after upper limb surgery**

INTRODUCTION

To achieve a satisfactory result after any major surgery to the upper limb, the patient must participate actively and co-operate fully with the rehabilitation process and with the physiotherapist. The patient must also be involved in setting realistic targets and both the physiotherapist and patient must have a clear idea of all the functional improvement that can be expected after the surgery.

A thorough pre-operative assessment should be completed and a clearly documented record made before surgery. Assessment should include both the affected side and the contralateral side, including the function of the adjacent joints. The assessment should also involve:
- Distribution of pain and patterns of pain.
- Posture of the joint.
- Active and passive ranges of movement.
- Muscle power.
- Sensation.
- Impairment of other joints.
- Evaluation of functional activities.

Irrespective of the planned operative procedure, the role of physiotherapy will be to facilitate restoration of the functional use of the involved limb (Harris & Leffert, 1988).

Throughout the rehabilitation programme, soft tissue healing and postoperative precautions will need to be considered and the postoperative protocol tailored according

to these. Harris & Leffert (1988) cite the following guidelines as common to all rehabilitation programmes:
- The exercise programme should not cause pain.
- The scapular musculature should be included.
- Restoration of normal functional movement patterns should be the ultimate goal.
- Realistic goals should be set, based on clinical status and surgery.
- The quantity and quality of exercise should be carefully selected and patients should accept responsibility for their own care.

Several surgical procedures are covered in this chapter, although not those involving the wrist and hand. However, the assessment and principles of rehabilitation described would be applicable to most operative procedures of the upper limb.

The exercise regimens described are intended as a guide only and may be altered in accordance with the surgeon's preferences or with the specific rehabilitative goals of the physiotherapist.

TOTAL SHOULDER REPLACEMENT

ARTHROPLASTY

Upper limb arthroplasty is most commonly performed on the patient with rheumatoid arthritis but can also be used for those with osteoarthritis and after fractures involving the humeral head. The objective when undertaking the procedure is primarily to relieve pain and secondarily to improve range of movement and improve function.

The outcome of the rehabilitation programme after total shoulder replacement will vary according to the amount and degree of damage to the joint, soft tissue and tendon of the upper limbs as well as the patient's underlying condition.

Most patients undergo total replacement, i.e. both replacement of the humeral head and provision of an articulating component in the glenoid. However, some patients, particularly where there is insufficient bone stock to allow good fixation of the glenoid component, will only have the humeral head replaced. This is referred to as a hemi-arthroplasty of the shoulder. There are also variations as to whether the total shoulder arthroplasty is cemented or cementless; the latter relying on a press-fitting of the humeral components. Some authors suggest that cemented total arthroplasties are less prone to complications and loosening (Cofield, 1994).

Irrespective of the underlying reason for the replacement surgery, or the surgical procedure that has taken place, most patients will follow a postoperative rehabilitation programme based on Neer's original protocol (Neer, 1990). The time scale for commencement of mobilisation will vary according to whether the rotator cuff muscles are intact, or if they have been repaired, when extra protection may be required. It will also vary with the surgeon's preference, mobilisation usually starting early, on day 1 postoperatively, although in some centres this may not occur until day 5 postoperatively.

The postoperative treatment programme follows a logical sequence allowing for tissue healing, joint mobilisation and muscle strengthening (Brems, 1994). The programme will start with the pre-operative assessment. This is performed by the physiotherapist, and the postoperative programme should be explained and discussed so that realistic goals and expectations can be set. The patient should be reassured that it is normal for the shoulder to feel stiff and painful after surgery and he or she should be encouraged to take analgesics on a regular basis.

Day 1 Postoperatively
Immediately postoperatively, most patients will have their arm supported in a body sling or firm bandage holding it across the trunk. They will usually have a drip, drain and an intravenous line for patient-controlled analgesia (PCA).

Patients should have analgesia 30 minutes before physiotherapy and be encouraged to perform the full range of active movements of their hand, wrist, forearm and cervical spine. The physiotherapist will support their upper arm to allow active elbow movement through the full range. These exercises will prevent stiffness.

Day 2 Postoperatively
The drain is removed and the Neer regimen started, initially concentrating on increasing the range of movement, while protecting the healing tissues. All exercises occur after the

provision of adequate analgesia and, if required, icepacks or moist heat (hot pack); ice and hot packs may make it easier for the patient to comply with the exercise programme. Each exercise should be carried out for about 60 seconds and repeated 2–3 times in short sessions about four times a day.

EARLY MOBILISATION EXERCISES
Pendular Swinging Exercises
The patient leans forward, inclining the trunk, with the affected arm hanging so that the shoulder musculature is in a position of minimal gravity and gentle traction is exerted on the glenohumeral joint by the weight of the arm (Figure 8.1). The arm is gently exercised by forwards, backwards and circular movements, each occurring for 60 seconds. These are sometimes referred to as Codman's exercises (Codman, 1934).

Assisted Passive Elevation
The patient lies supine without a pillow so that the shoulder and scapula rest on the bed. The physiotherapist elevates the arm while applying slight traction to the humerus until the patient feels some discomfort when a firm gentle stretch is maintained for 5 seconds. The arm is then lowered to the side. This is repeated 2–3 times.

Assisted Elevation with Contralateral Limb
The patient is encouraged to stretch the arm into elevation using the assistance of the contralateral limb grasping the hands together and raising the arms into elevation from supine lying (Figure 8.2). Alternatively, the

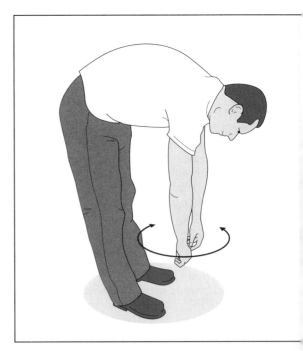

Figure 8.1 Pendular swinging exercises.

patient may hold onto a walking stick and raise the stick up in front of the body, ensuring that the stick stays parallel to the ground.

Assisted External Rotation

The patient lies supine without a pillow but with a folded towel under the humerus of the affected arm so that it is parallel to the spine with the elbow about 15 cm away from the side. The patient holds onto a walking stick with both hands, about a shoulder's width apart, and pushes the forearm away from the side, rotating the humerus and ensuring that the stick remains perpendicular to the humerus throughout the movement (Figure 8.3).

Assisted Elevation with a Pulley

This increases the elevation of the arm (Figure 8.4). It utilises more muscle activity than pure passive elevation. The pulley should be placed above the patient's head—not in front of it as this will encourage forward reaching. Using the pulley, the affected arm is passively elevated by the action of the unaffected arm. At home the pulley may be fixed in a doorway. Care must be taken with this exercise if the rotator cuff has been repaired during the arthroplasty. The physiotherapist should also check that the patient does not make unwanted secondary movements, e.g. arching the back.

Continuous Passive Motion

Some authors report the use of continuous passive motion (CPM) following shoulder arthroplasty (Craig, 1986; Neer

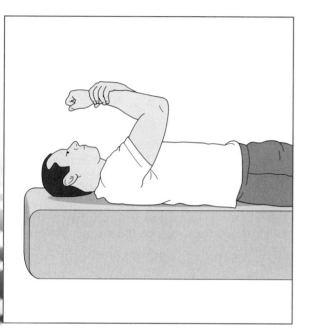

Figure 8.2 Assisted elevation with contralateral limb.

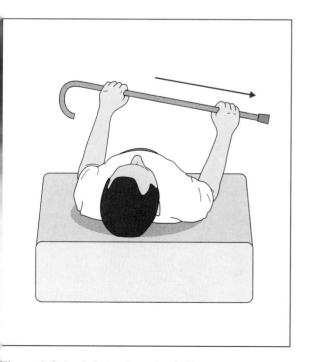

Figure 8.3 Assisted external rotation.

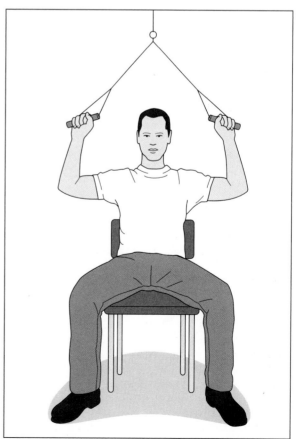

Figure 8.4 Assisted elevation with a pulley.

et al., 1987). This is usually where bilateral disease prevents auto-assisted exercises being carried out effectively. The shoulder CPM machine can provide passive movement in all three planes of the shoulder, although only forward flexion and external rotation are used initially. However, the equipment needs to be set up accurately and this is a time-consuming procedure. If CPM is initiated on the day of surgery, there will be increased wound drainage (Johnson, 1993). Most patients achieve a good postoperative recovery without the use of CPM.

Days 7–10 Postoperatively
Once the sutures have been removed, the next phase of the mobilising programme may commence, together with early strengthening exercises.

LATE MOBILISATION EXERCISES
Assisted Elevation
The patient lies supine without a pillow. Using the unaffected arm, the operated arm is lifted over the head until the fingers can reach underneath the headboard or backrest of the bed. The patient is then encouraged to relax so that the arch in the back lowers and the arms are further elevated (Figure 8.5).

Assisted Internal Rotation
Both arms are placed in the small of the back, the good arm grasping the wrist of the affected side. The arm is pulled into extension and then up the back, keeping the hand in the midline, so that the thumb tries to reach up the thoracic spine (Figure 8.6).

Assisted External Rotation
The patient stands in a doorway with the elbow held against the side and at 90°. The forearm is placed against the door frame with the unaffected arm supporting the upper arm of the affected side. The trunk is then turned, which externally rotates the shoulder (Figure 8.7).

If rotator cuff repair took place with the arthroplasty, care must be taken as the subscapularis will be sutured. External rotation should therefore be limited to 45°.

STRENGTHENING EXERCISES
The early strengthening programme aims to increase the strength of the anterior deltoid and supraspinatus muscles, assisted by gravity. Care must be taken and the programme modified in the early stages if rotator cuff repair was performed at the time of the arthroplasty. If this is the case and the anterior deltoid or supraspinatus sutured, these structures must be protected.

Strengthening in Supine
The patient lies supine without a pillow. The patient elevates the arm with the elbow flexed, moving the arm into a straight position as it is brought overhead and then slowly descending from an arc of 90° elevation. Gravity will seek to accelerate the movement of the arm between 90° elevation and 0°; control of this movement by performing the movement, slowly strengthens the muscles. The exercise is performed in repetitions of 10, progressing to using light weights sequentially up to 2 kg (Figure 8.8).

Once the patient can perform 10 controlled elevations and descents with light resistance, further strengthening exercises using gravity, and strengthening of muscles eccentrically, may commence. These exercises concentrate on the deltoid and rotator cuff muscles. The patient lifts the arm passively to a position of maximum elevation in a sitting or standing position. The arm is brought down from the elevated position in a controlled manner, preventing

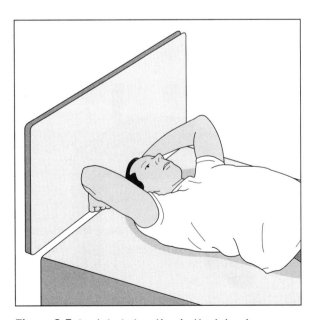

Figure 8.5 Assisted elevation in the late stage.

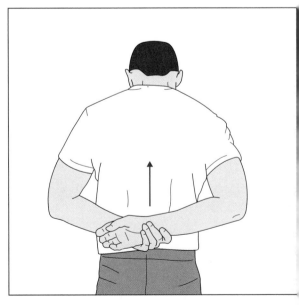

Figure 8.6 Assisted internal rotation.

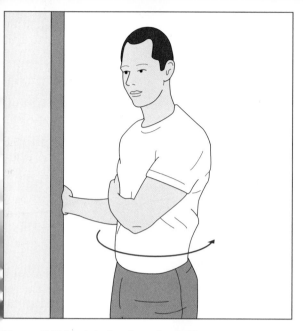

Figure 8.7 Assisted external rotation.

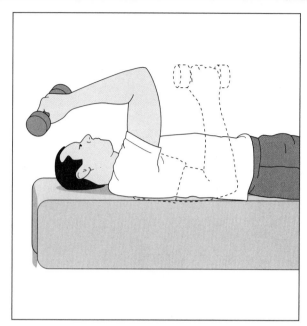

Figure 8.8 Strengthening in supine.

acceleration by gravitational forces. This is performed in repetitions of 10, adding in resistance with free weights once the exercise can be performed without fatigue. The resistance should only be increased by small increments up to 3 kg.

Elastic-Tubing Exercises

If patients have very good pre-operative strength, they may be able to commence with elastic-tubing (Cliniband/ Theraband) exercises. These strengthen the anterior, middle and posterior deltoid, subscapularis and infraspinatus muscles. Each exercise is performed against the resistance of the tubing, held for 15 seconds and repeated in sets of 10. The exercises should be carried out twice daily. Again, care must be taken if the anterior deltoid has been detached during surgery.

Anterior Deltoid

The elastic tubing is placed over the door handle. The patient stands with their back to the door. The elbow is flexed at 90° and the humerus held in the midline of the body. The tubing is pulled forwards to around 45°, held for 5 seconds and slowly released (Figure 8.9A). This is repeated 10 times.

Posterior Deltoid

The patient stands facing the door with their arm in 45° of forward elevation. The arm is pulled back to the midline, held for 5 seconds and slowly released (Figure 8.9B). Care should be taken not to extend past the midline as this puts considerable stress on the anterior capsule.

Middle Deltoid

The patient stands in front of a mirror, the elastic tubing around both arms held in front of the trunk. The patient abducts both shoulders symmetrically. This is held for 5 seconds and slowly released (Figure 8.9C). Care must be taken to prevent the shoulders externally rotating.

Internal Rotators

The elbow is held against the trunk and flexed to 90°. The arm is pulled inwards against the resistance of the tubing, no more than 45°, held for 5 seconds and slowly released (Figure 8.10A).

External Rotators

The elbow is held against the trunk and flexed to 90°. The arm is pulled outwards against the tubing by no more than 45°, keeping the elbow to the side (Figure 8.10B).

All of the muscle groups may also be strengthened by the physiotherapist using muscle strengthening techniques such as proprioceptive neuromuscular facilitation (PNF).

It is also important that the patient continues lifelong strengthening exercises of the shoulder musculature, with the emphasis on the rotator cuff and deltoid.

The rehabilitation programme will be tailored to each patient, but in all cases once the initial mobilising stage has been completed a maintenance programme must be followed. This programme allows for small gains in mobility and strength once the main rehabilitative process has finished.

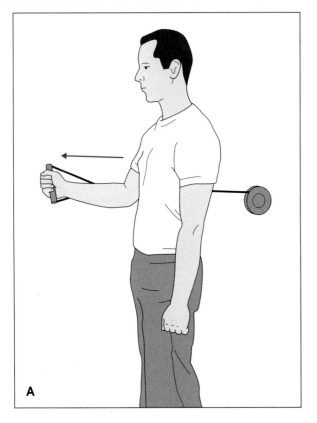

A

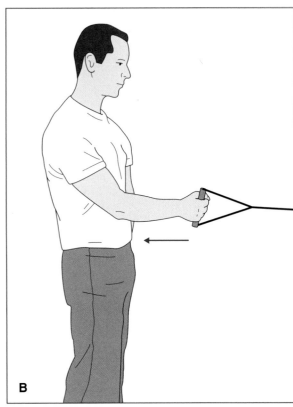

B

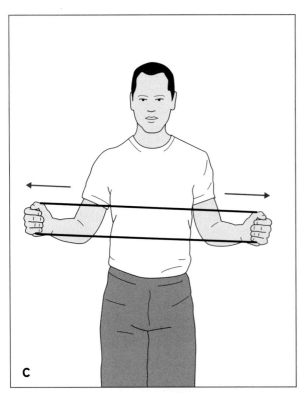

C

Figure 8.9 Strengthening exercises for the anterior deltoid (A), posterior deltoid (B) and middle deltoid (C).

Late-Stage Rehabilitation

The final stages of rehabilitation may not be possible for patients with limited range of movement, due to their underlying pathology. Few patients who have undergone arthroplasty for rheumatoid arthritis will progress this far. Exercises may be performed to achieve the last 20° of shoulder movement in all directions by:

• Assisted elevation in standing, placing the arm above the head into the corner of a room and leaning the trunk with the elbow in full extension to force the arm into full elevation (Figure 8.11A).

• Assisted external rotation in standing, with the patient standing in a doorway with their upper arms parallel to the floor and forearms on the door frame. The trunk is inclined forward to increase external rotation (Figure 8.11B).

• Assisted internal rotation, with the patient standing with their back against a shelf at waist level, the arm resting on the shelf and the thumb in the small of the back. The patient bends the knees so that the arm is forced into internal rotation.

Rehabilitation following total shoulder arthroplasty is considered successful if the main objectives of pain relief and increased function are met.

Improvements in range of movements and strength should occur, but it is unrealistic to expect the patient to achieve normal range or strength. Many patients, especially

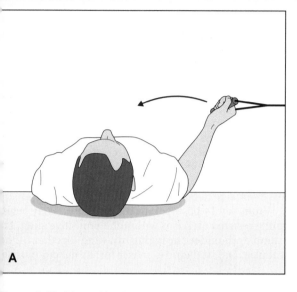
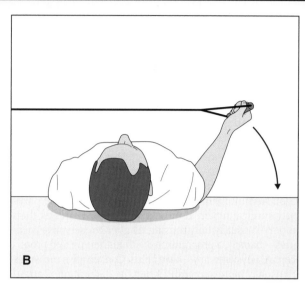

Figure 8.10 Strengthening exercises for internal rotators (A) and external rotators (B).

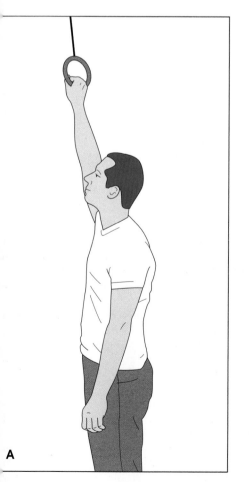
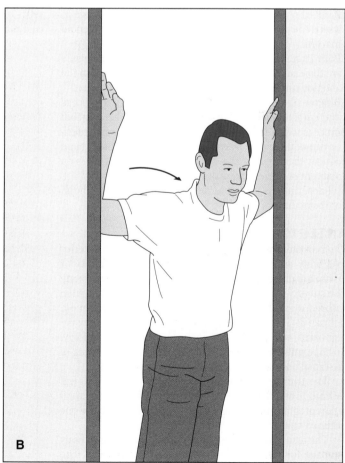

Figure 8.11 Late-stage rehabilitation exercises to increase elevation (A) and external rotation (B).

those with a lot of soft tissue involvement, will never achieve the regimens set out in late-stage rehabilitation (see page 112).

If the patients' expectations before surgery are discussed and realistic goals set, most of them are very satisfied with the outcome of their surgery.

SHOULDER STABILISATION

The most common site for dislocation is the glenohumeral joint, and the most common form of dislocation traumatic anterior dislocation, e.g. the classic antero-inferior Bankart lesion sustained during contact sports. This usually requires early surgical repair. If the instability is atraumatic then surgery is usually only considered after conservative measures—namely, a programme of strengthening and proprioceptive physiotherapy—have failed. Conservative measures are usually more successful when the dislocation is atraumatic or acquired.

Postoperatively, the rehabilitation protocol will vary according to the surgical technique and the surgeon's instructions. These techniques may be performed as either an open procedure or via arthroscopy. The wide variety of surgical techniques used shows there is no real consensus as to the best method. The most common surgical procedures are:
- Bankart repair—a repair of the glenoid fibrocartilage in which the capsule is reattached to the front of the glenoid margin.
- Putti-Platt repair—the subscapularis and anterior capsule are divided and then overlapped or reefed to shorten the anterior part of the rotator cuff and limit lateral rotation.
- Bristow repair—the origins of the short head of the biceps and coracobrachialis are transferred from the coracoid process to the scapular neck, medial to the antero-inferior rim of the glenoid cavity. These muscles act as a band across the head of the humerus when the arm is in abduction, preventing dislocation.

Full descriptions of a wide range of operations for shoulder instability are described by Copeland (1995).

ANTERIOR STABILISATION

The most common form of shoulder instability is anterior instability with stretching of the capsular ligaments or disruption of the capsulo-labral attachment (Bankart lesion). The surgery may involve the capsule being reefed and then sutured, stapled or screwed to the bony rim of the glenoid (Ellman & Gartsman, 1993). In an open procedure the subscapularis will be either detached or split horizontally. Postoperative rehabilitation must not stress the healing of the capsule to the bone or the subscapularis tendon.

The timing of each stage will vary with the surgical technique and the surgeon's preference, but the rehabilitation programme will follow a schedule similar to the one outlined below.

The arm is usually held in a close-fitting sling or body bandage for the first 24–48 hours, without moving. The patient wears a sling for 6 weeks, engaging in daily passive range of movement exercises. At 48 hours, the arm may be removed from the sling to allow supported cradling exercises (Figure 8.12). (In some centres the arm is completely immobilised for several weeks.) The patient sits cradling the operated arm with the unaffected arm, bends forward until the arms fall away from the trunk and the elbows are beyond the knees, and moves gently from side to side and then replaces the arm in the sling. While the arm is removed from the sling, full-range movements of the elbow, cervical spine and wrist joints should be performed to prevent joint stiffness. As the pain decreases, Codman's pendular swinging exercises (see page 108) may be commenced together with gentle passive flexion, abduction and minimal external rotation exercises (Jobe, 1987).

From day 14 postoperatively, the patient may begin gentle resisted exercises within the protective sling, for example, shoulder shrugging, drawing together of the scapulae, and isometric exercises for the deltoid muscle.

From Week 6 Postoperatively
At 6 weeks postoperatively, the surgical healing is more mature and isotonic strengthening and assisted range-of-movement mobilising exercises can begin. The sling is no longer worn except occasionally at night for protection if a patient is a very restless sleeper. From 6 to 8 weeks, the range-of-movement exercises should aim to achieve 90°–100° of elevation and abduction and 30°–40° of external rotation (Jobe, 1987).

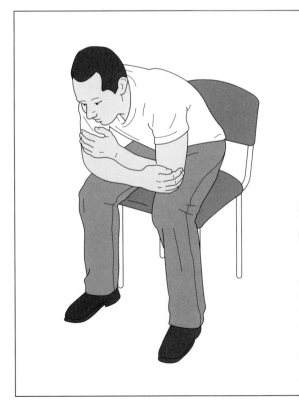

Figure 8.12 Cradling position.

Strengthening exercises of the internal and external rotators may occur with the elbow flexed at 90° and the arm held by the side. Flexion exercises at the shoulder increase the strength of the anterior deltoid, coracobrachialis, long head of biceps brachii and the clavicular part of pectoralis major. Active abduction strengthens the supraspinatus and middle deltoid.

From Week 8 Postoperatively

From 8 weeks postoperatively, resisted strengthening exercises may be commenced. These may include push-ups and bench presses, which place greater stress on the posterior structures, strengthening the pectoralis major and serratus anterior. Shoulder extension exercises will increase the strength of the latissimus dorsi and teres major, which are important in many sporting activities, e.g. tennis service and golf swing. Stretching exercises should continue until full range of movement is restored, taking care not to overstretch into external rotation. If available, strengthening via the isokinetic dynamometer may commence from 8 weeks (Figure 8.13).

From Week 12 Postoperatively

From 12 weeks postoperatively, the patient should continue to perform strengthening and mobilising exercises as part of a home exercise programme. Recreational sports may resume at 4 months and contact sports at 6 months, although elite athletes should train under supervision to regain strength, motion and endurance for up to 12 months before competition.

MULTIDIRECTIONAL INSTABILITY

Patients who have had surgery for multidirectional instability keep the arm immobilised for up to 3 months to allow the tissues to tighten and a scar to form. During this time, isometric exercises for the deltoid and the rotator cuff may be performed as described earlier. Limited activity usually occurs 6 months postoperatively and full activity by 1 year. There is little published work on the outcome of patients following such surgery, especially those who habitually dislocate.

SUBACROMIAL DECOMPRESSION (WITHOUT ROTATOR CUFF REPAIR)

This is usually performed via the arthroscope and is nowadays performed in preference to open acromioplasty (Ellman, 1987; Esch, 1993). Arthroscopic examination allows assessment of the state of the rotator cuff muscles and allows confirmation of the presence of an impingement lesion, which may then be followed by acromioplasty via the arthroscope. This technique preserves the deltoid attachment, allowing quick postoperative mobilisation, and the patient may often be treated as a day-case.

Postoperatively, the shoulder is often swollen, the swelling being worse if the surgery was lengthy. A padded dressing is applied over the arthroscope site and the shoulder rested in a sling.

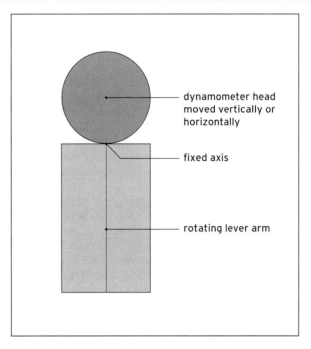

dynamometer head moved vertically or horizontally

fixed axis

rotating lever arm

Figure 8.13 Isokinetic dynamometer.

Movement will initially be limited by the swelling. The arm may be very painful immediately postoperatively and the rehabilitation of these patients is often hindered by insufficient analgesic cover. Patients must be encouraged to take their analgesics before physiotherapy. Ice may be applied immediately after surgery to control pain and swelling. Pendular swinging exercises are commenced on the first postoperative day in the same manner as those described for shoulder arthroplasty; these are frequently painful.

When pain allows, usually between 24 and 48 hours, active assisted exercises may commence using a pulley system to increase elevation, although care must be taken as this can increase impingement.

The sling will be discarded as soon as possible, usually at about 1 week. Mobilising exercises are continued from 48 hours, most patients attaining flexion and abduction to 90° by 2 weeks postoperatively.

Out-patient physiotherapy usually commences once inflammation has settled. Full range of movement may be acquired on an out-patient basis using the same techniques as detailed for total shoulder arthroplasty. This is followed by strengthening exercises, concentrating on internal and external rotation.

Final rehabilitation allowing diagonal movement patterns may be attained by using either Bad Ragaz techniques in the hydrotherapy pool or PNF techniques. The pain associated with rehabilitation will be variable but may be considerable. Most improvements in pain occur in the first 3 months postoperatively but often pain will continue for up to a year.

ROTATOR CUFF REPAIR

Acute tears of the rotator cuff are rare in young people with good musculature; it is more common for the tuberosity to be avulsed, as the tendon is stronger than the bone at this site. Where a true rotator cuff injury has occurred, early surgical repair is indicated. In the elderly, the rotator cuff may need repair due to wear and tear leading to attrition rupture. In most cases the tear will be due to a combination of an element of trauma superimposed on an already degenerated musculotendinous junction (Copeland, 1995).

A variety of surgical options may be used to repair rotator cuff tears; usually, the greater the tear, the more likely it is that an open procedure will be used. Increasingly, more complex repairs are being performed via the arthroscope. Rotator cuff repair normally always involves the supraspinatus tendon. If the tear is medium to large, it may involve the infraspinatus and teres minor and, if very large, the subscapularis.

The same principles of rehabilitation will be followed irrespective of the surgical procedure. However, the time each stage in the rehabilitation programme commences will vary with the extent of the rotator cuff tear—partial or full thickness—and with the surgeon's preference. Many surgeons only operate on full-thickness tears.

PRINCIPLES OF REHABILITATION

The main goals of rehabilitation after repair of the rotator cuff are to:
• Decrease or remove pain.
• Increase muscle strength and control.
• Increase functional activity.
• Increase range of movements.

Three stages of rehabilitation will be followed—namely, early passive motion, stretching and strengthening.

Early Passive Motion

Early mobilisation is desirable as it prevents the formation of adhesions. However, care must be taken not to disrupt the integrity of the reconstruction or delay the healing process. The tendinous insertion of the muscle should be protected against active muscle contraction for about 6 weeks. Gentle passive range-of-movement exercises, however, may be commenced as early as the first postoperative day.

Stretching

Stretching prevents the formation of adhesions, and should initially be gentle and passive. In the later stages of rehabilitation, vigorous stretching, both actively and passively, may occur.

Strengthening

Strengthening starts with simple isometric contractions progressing to active assisted movements and then movements against gravity. Progressive resistance is added until normal strength is attained. Improvements in strength may continue for up to 2 years after shoulder surgery (Ellman & Gartsman, 1993).

CONTRAINDICATIONS

Following rotator cuff repair:
• Do not place the repaired tendon in a position that lengthens it further than the position obtained at operation for at least 6 weeks.
• Do not perform isometric contractions of the repaired tendon for 4 weeks.
• Do not perform resisted exercises throughout the range of the repaired tendon for up to 12 weeks.
• Do not perform any forced lengthening of the repaired tendon for 12 weeks.
• All movements should be relatively pain free.

Positions for Lengthening Muscles

Various positions can help lengthen certain muscles, for example:
• Supraspinatus—adduction, horizontal adduction, hand behind back.
• Infraspinatus—adduction, horizontal adduction, hand behind back.
• Teres minor—elevation with internal rotation.
• Subscapularis—elevation, abduction in external rotation, abduction.

SAMPLE PROTOCOL FOR OPEN REPAIR OF FULL-THICKNESS ROTATOR CUFF TEAR

The postoperative protocol is divided into three phases—passive, active and strengthening exercises.

Day 1 Postoperatively

The patient's arm is taken out of the sling, and active elbow flexion/extension takes place with the upper arm held close to the trunk in a neutral position and the patient supine.

With the patient supine and the arm close to the side of the body, the patient's elbow may be flexed to 90° and passive external rotation commenced. Ideally, 45° of external rotation will be achieved within the first few days, but this will vary according to the surgeon's closure technique.

Passive forward flexion may also occur up to about 100°.

The patient may perform rock-a-bye exercises (see Figure 8.12).

From Day 3 Postoperatively

The patient may perform rock-a-bye (see Figure 8.12) or pendular swinging exercises (see Figure 8.1).

From Week 6 Postoperatively

Active exercises, e.g. shoulder shrugging, elevation of the arm initially supported by the contralateral arm, or using a cane, may be commenced—these are usually easier if performed from a supine position. These exercises all emphasise regaining control of the shoulder.

The emphasis should be on ensuring that there is both good mobility and control of the glenohumeral joint into elevation.

The patient may progress to pulley exercises and wall climbing, i.e. taking the fingers up a vertical surface.

From Week 8 Postoperatively

Resisted exercises may commence once the arm can move synchronously against gravity. Isometric contractions should be commenced within the subimpingement range. The exercises should not increase pain, and all are performed using Cliniband or Theraband. The exercises consist of isometric external rotation with the elbows held close to the body and pulling out against a ring of cliniband or theraband for 5 seconds (Figure 8.14A). This strengthens the infraspinatus and teres minor.

Abduction

Patients stand with their arms straight in front of them, hands at mid-thigh height. The band is stretched by pulling away from the body to about 150° (Figure 8.14B). This strengthens the deltoid and supraspinatus.

Flexion

The arms are elevated to around 60° forward flexion and the band stretched outwards (Figure 8.14C). This strengthens the lateral and posterior deltoid.

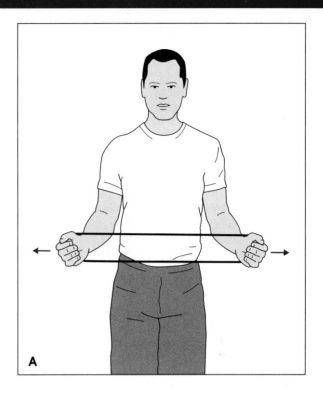

A

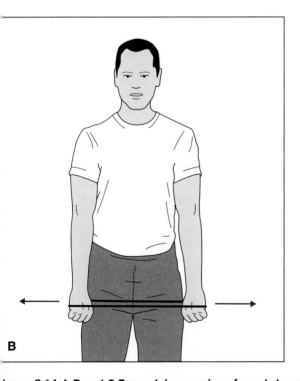

B

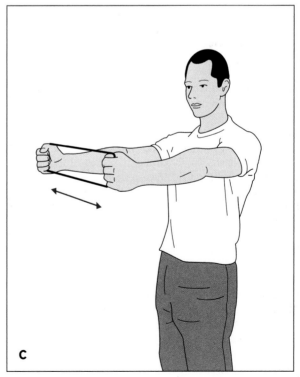

C

Figure 8.14 A,B and C Isometric exercises for rotator cuff repair.

From Week 12 Postoperatively
Free weights, wall climbing, door-jamb resistance or doorway stretches may be used. If necessary, treatment may be preceded by ice or heat packs. The speed of progression should be gauged by the patient's pain level.

Bad Ragaz techniques in the hydrotherapy pool or PNF techniques may help attain a full range of movements and increase strength.

Resisted antigravity work throughout the range of the repaired tendon may be commenced.

Isotonic and isokinetic exercises should continue for several weeks. Light non-contact sports may be resumed at 6 months, while strenuous sport or that involving activity overhead may be resumed at about 1 year. Improvements in range of movements and strength may continue for up to 2 years postoperatively.

SAMPLE PROTOCOL FOR PARTIAL-THICKNESS ROTATOR CUFF REPAIR WITH OPEN ACROMIOPLASTY
Not all surgeons repair partial-thickness tears of the rotator cuff. In this procedure the deltoid is detached coronally from its insertion and thus a small portion of the anterior deltoid will be disrupted. Six weeks should elapse before the repair is stressed by overhead elevation or contractions against gravity.

Day 1 Postoperatively
A sling is worn for the first 3 to 6 weeks. Passive mobilising exercises for forward flexion and internal and external rotation may be performed. The patient may be encouraged to cradle the arm and perform rock-a-bye movements—cradling the arm leaning forward assists in performing gentle circumduction (see Figure 8.12).

Day 3 Postoperatively
Commence pendular swinging (Codman's) exercises (see Figure 8.1), where the trunk is inclined parallel to the ground and the arm hangs perpendicular to the body. The arm is moved forwards and backwards, side to side, and in a circular pattern. The forearm may be turned into pronation and supination to achieve stretching of the internal and external rotators. These should be performed 4–6 times a day.

From Week 3 Postoperatively
This is the same as that described for full thickness repairs under the section 6–8 weeks postoperatively.

From Week 6 Postoperatively
Increasing resistance may be added to the exercises described above, progressing to exercises with free weights while prone and supine. Isotonic and isokinetic exercises may be commenced from 6 weeks. Non-contact sports may commence from 8 weeks but overhead activity should be avoided, e.g. tennis serve, overhead throwing.

From 3 months, unrestricted sports activities and strenuous overhead work may occur. Between 6 weeks and 3 months, the patient should steadily be increasing range of movements, muscle strength and exercise endurance.

TOTAL ELBOW REPLACEMENT

Elbow arthroplasty is usually performed in the patient with severe elbow pain and joint destruction caused by rheumatoid arthritis. It is not usually indicated for traumatic or degenerative arthritis since such patients place too many demands on the prosthesis because of their high level of activity. Clinical trials have demonstrated good outcomes following arthroplasty in terms of pain relief, increased range of movement and functional activity (Weiland et al., 1989).

PRE-OPERATIVE ASSESSMENT
The patient should be seen pre-operatively to discuss the rehabilitation programme and to document a detailed clinical assessment. This is particularly important when a Souter–Strathclyde prosthesis is used, as a detailed system of outcome measurement is included with the prosthesis (Souter et al., 1985).

The ulnar nerve is particularly vulnerable to injury during total elbow arthroplasty because it lies close to the posteromedial surface of the elbow as it runs through the ulnar groove of the medial humeral epicondyle. Therefore careful documentation of the sensation of the fourth and fifth digits must be made as well as the strength of the intrinsic hand muscles and the ability to adduct the fourth and fifth digits.

The majority of patients will have existing multisystem disease and so a detailed assessment of daily living activity will need to be performed to facilitate plans on discharge. Patients should be counselled that the primary objective of the operation is to relieve pain and that any improvements in range of movement or function are of secondary importance. It is important that they realise that an elbow arthroplasty is unlikely to improve a fixed flexion deformity of the elbow.

POSTOPERATIVE MANAGEMENT
After surgery the arm will be supported in a pressure bandage with a posterior plaster of Paris splint and elevated in a sling, supporting the elbow at approximately 90° of flexion. This position protects the triceps repair. The exact position used may vary according to the type of prosthesis and surgical technique. There should be regular assessment of the pulse, sensation and temperature of the digits.

Day 1 Postoperatively
The patient is encouraged to perform active finger exercises to assist in the prevention of oedema. The fourth and fifth digits should be assessed by performing active abduction and adduction to ensure that the ulnar nerve has not been damaged during surgery. It is quite common for the fingers to be slightly numb postoperatively (Dale et al., 1992).

Pain may be controlled by PCA.

Day 2 Postoperatively

Between 24 and 72 hours postoperatively, mobilisation may commence. The posterior plaster shell is removed, the wound inspected and, if satisfactory, active assisted exercises performed three times a day in short sessions lasting about 15 minutes. Between physiotherapy sessions, the plaster shell is replaced.

Once the swelling around the joint has stabilised, a thermoplastic elbow splint will be made which the patient will continue to wear for decreasing periods of time for the first 2–4 weeks.

Active assisted exercises are performed in flexion, extension, pronation and supination. Care must be taken when performing range-of-movement exercises at the elbow, to keep the arm in adduction and neutral, as abduction combined with external rotational forces apply excessive stress to the elbow and may lead to instability.

The patient can be encouraged to exercise by themselves using a frictionless board to move the hand across while performing flexion and extension. Ice, Cryocuff or moist heat may all be beneficial in relaxing the soft tissues and allowing greater movement.

The patient will usually be instructed in activities of daily living by an occupational therapist or physiotherapist, emphasis being placed on the need to avoid positions that combine shoulder abduction with internal or external rotation.

From Week 4 Postoperatively

Between 4 and 6 weeks postoperatively, the capsule will have healed and the triceps repaired, allowing the start of isometric and isotonic strengthening exercises for the biceps and triceps. The patient should be counselled to avoid placing heavy stresses on the replaced joint, for example, by carrying bags or placing a lot of pressure through the arm when using a walking aid.

The postoperative complications of total elbow arthroplasty are similar to those of other total joint replacement procedures, and the physiotherapist should be aware of them and monitor the patient during rehabilitation. Possible postoperative complications include circulatory impairment, nerve damage (particularly to the ulnar nerve), loosening of the prosthesis and infection. Patients should be advised to contact their general practitioner if they develop any systemic infection, so that prophylactic antibiotic treatment can be started.

OUTCOME MEASUREMENT AFTER UPPER LIMB SURGERY

An outcome measurement is one that uses clinical measurements, to observe and document relative changes (Pynsent et al., 1993). Outcome measures in shoulder and elbow surgery remain in their infancy compared with those of the hip and knee. They are complicated by the fact that most patients undergoing surgical procedures have polyarthritic multisystem disease, usually rheumatoid arthritis (MacDonald, 1993).

Formal outcome measurements have been applied to patients who have undergone shoulder surgery; these include those of Neer and colleagues (1982), Swanson and colleagues and the Hospital for Special Surgery (Swanson et al., 1989; Warren et al., 1982). They mostly assess a combination of pain and range of movement and function utilising activity of daily living scores. The Hospital for Special Surgery and Swanson scales give an overall outcome score, while the Neer method does not score one outcome measure but provides measurements in clinical terms.

Elbow assessments are primarily based on the type of prosthesis used. Most systems are graded as 'poor', 'satisfactory' or 'good'. The most comprehensive system is the Souter–Strathclyde assessment, designed to assess the results of the Souter–Strathclyde elbow replacement. This system has been adopted by the British Orthopaedic Association. Three complex forms are used: pre-, peri- and postoperatively. About 152 items of information are gathered on each assessment. This makes it time consuming to complete and some would argue too complex to be of use as a clinical outcome tool.

The Hospital for Special Surgery assessment (Inglis & Pellicci, 1980) scores out of a maximum 100 in categories of pain (30), function (20), sagittal movement (20), strength (10), flexion contracture (6), extension contracture (6), pronation (4) and supination (4). However, this is insufficiently detailed to be ideal as an outcome measure.

There is no one accepted measurement tool for assessing the outcome of the rehabilitation programme after upper limb surgery. However, the physiotherapists usually have extensive involvement in completing the above outcome measures where they have been adopted by an orthopaedic unit.

REFERENCES

Brems JJ. Rehabilitation following total shoulder arthroplasty. *Clin Orthop Rel Res* 1994, **307**:70-85.

Codman EA. *The shoulder*. Boston: T Todd; 1934.

Cofield RH. Uncemented total shoulder arthroplasty. *Clin Orthop Rel Res* 1994, **307**:86-93.

Copeland D. *Operative shoulder surgery*. New York: Churchill Livingstone; 1995.

Craig EV. Continuous passive motion in the rehabilitation of the surgically reconstructed shoulder: a preliminary report. *Orthop Trans* 1986, **10**:219.

Dale KG, Orr PM, Harrel PB. Total elbow replacement. *Orthop Nurs* 1992, **11**:23-29.

Ellman H. Arthroscopic subacromial decompression. *Arthroscopy* 1987, **2**:173-181.

Ellman H, Gartsman GM. *Arthroscopic shoulder surgery and related procedures*. Philadelphia: Lea and Febiger; 1993:425-452.

Esch JC. Arthroscopic subacromial decompression and postoperative management. *Orthop Clin North Am* 1993, **24**:161-171.

Harris BA, Leffert RD. The role of physical therapy in rehabilitation of the shoulder. In: Rowe CR, ed. *The shoulder*. New York: Churchill Livingstone; 1988.

Inglis AE, Pellicci PM. Total elbow replacement. *J Bone Joint Surg* (AM)1980, **62** (9):1252-1258.

Jobe FW, Moynes DR, Brewster CE. Rehabilitation of shoulder joint instabilities. *Orthop Clin North Am* 1987, **24**:161-171.

Jobe FW, Moynes DR, Brewster CE. Rehabilitation of shoulder joint instabilities. *Orthop Clin North Am* 1987, **18**:473-482.

Johnson RL. Total shoulder arthroplasty. *Orthop Nurs* 1993, **2**:14-22.

MacDonald DA. The shoulder and elbow. In: Pynsent PB, *et al.*, eds. *Outcome measures in orthopaedics*. Oxford: Butterworth Heinemann; 1993;144-173.

Neer CS. *Shoulder reconstruction*. Philadelphia: WB Saunders; 1990.

Neer CS, Watson KC, Stanton FJ. Recent experiences in total shoulder replacement. *J Bone Joint Surg* 1982, **64A**:319-337.

Neer CS, McCann PD, MacFarlane EA, Padilla N. Early passive motion following shoulder arthroplasty and rotator cuff repair: a prospective study. *Orthop Trans* 1987, **11**:231.

Pynsent PB, Fairbank JCT, Carr A. *Outcome measures in orthopaedics*. Oxford: Butterworth Heinemann; 1993.

Souter WA. Surgery of the rheumatoid elbow. *Ann Rheum Dis* 1990, **49**(Suppl.2):871-882.

Swanson AB, De Groot Swansea G, Sattel AB, Cendo RD, Hynes D, Jar Ning W. Bipolar implant shoulder arthroplasty. *Clin Orthop* 1989, **249**:227-247.

Warren RF, Ranawak CS, Inglis AE. Total shoulder replacement indications and results of Neer unconstrained prosthesis. In: Inglis AE, ed. *The American Academy of Orthopaedic Surgeons: symposium on total joint replacement of the upper extremity*. St Louis: CV Mosby; 1982;56-67.

Weiland AJ, Weiss AP, Wills RP, Moore JR. Capitellocondylar total elbow replacement: a long term follow up study. *J Bone Joint Surg* 1989, **71A**:217-222.

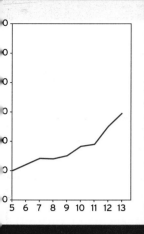

9 M Davie

OSTEOPOROSIS

CHAPTER OUTLINE

- **Bone remodelling**
- **Hormones acting on bone**
- **Osteoporosis**
- **Osteoporosis in men**

- **Mechanical consequences of bone loss**
- **Exercise**
- **Arthritis and osteoporosis**

INTRODUCTION

The skeleton contains almost all the calcium in the body. A person weighing 70 kg has about 1300 g of calcium in their bone, together with about 700 g of inorganic phosphorus, making up about 2000 g of inorganic constituents of the whole skeleton. Other constituents of bone are magnesium (~14 g) and carbonate (~200 g). The total weight of the wet skeleton in a 70 kg adult is about 7000 g. The dry skeleton is about 81% of the wet weight. Other important contributors are oxygen, carbon and nitrogen—this organic component of bone makes up about 22% of the wet weight (Nordin, 1976).

BONE REMODELLING

In land animals, the skeleton serves two structural purposes: protection of vital organs, and provision of levers for muscle function. When animals left the sea to become land dwellers, there was a need to maintain serum calcium levels. Calcium is abundant in seawater, at a concentration of about 40 mg/100 ml (10 mmol). In some fish, the concentration of free plasma calcium is 20 mg/100 ml. Plasma calcium levels are closely regulated, and the skeleton became a source of calcium to be called upon when calcium was in short supply.

Mineral is laid down in the skeleton in a well-defined sequence of events. The skeleton is continuously being remodelled and microfractures repaired. Two types of bone exist—hard cortical bone, e.g. the tibia, and soft trabecular bone, e.g. the vertebrae. The appendicular skeleton, comprising the arms and legs, has more cortical bone, while the axial skeleton, comprising the pelvis, spine and ribs, is largely made up of trabecular bone. In all bone there exist numbers of bone remodelling units (BMU). Osteoclasts start to break down bone and in so doing attract osteoblasts which start to rebuild it. During the formation phase, osteoid (unmineralised bone) is laid down and gradually calcified. Many of these processes can be detected by bone biopsy, but biochemical markers are being developed to measure products of bone metabolism in serum and urine, which will allow more frequent assessment of bone turnover. After peak bone mass has been attained, the rebuilding of bone never quite keeps up with breakdown, and bone mass declines. Bone turnover appears to increase with age, and levels of most of the biochemical markers tend to increase.

BONE CELL REGULATION

In adult bone there are three main types of cell—the osteoblast, the osteoclast and the osteocyte. The osteoblast is the main cell that makes bone and synthesises the organic collagen matrix on which the bone mineral is laid down. The osteoblast is derived from the stromal cells in the marrow cavity. Osteoblasts produce the collagen matrix and synthesise a number of other proteins, including osteocalcin and osteonectin. Osteoblasts respond to hormonal factors, the most important of which are 1,25-dihydroxycholecalciferol [$1,25(OH)_2D$](1,25-dihydroxyvitamin D), parathyroid hormone (PTH) and growth factors. An important enzyme associated with osteoblastic activity is alkaline phosphatase, which breaks down pyrophosphate, an inhibitor of mineralisation. In hypophosphatasia, a rare condition, this enzyme is absent and mineralisation is seriously impaired. Osteoblast activity can be detected by means of bone-specific alkaline phosphatase levels in blood, or serum osteocalcin levels. A number of assays which measure the formation products of collagen are also being developed.

Osteoclasts are large multinuclear cells which are derived from a haematopoietic stem cell. These stem cells, which are mononuclear, fuse to become multinucleated cells capable of secreting acid and resorbing bone. Osteoclasts have a relatively short lifespan of about 7 days. Osteoclast activity *in vivo* is usually detected either by measuring the breakdown products of collagen in urine or by bone biopsy at the iliac crest. Breakdown products include hydroxyproline, an amino acid in collagen, which, after collagen breakdown, is not reincorporated into collagen. Collagen in the diet can also be broken down in the gut to hydroxyproline, which is then absorbed and excreted in urine. This can cause spuriously high results unless the patient is on a collagen-free diet for 3 days. In recent years, the cross-links of collagen, particularly deoxypyridinoline, have been measured; this has the advantage that the patient need not be on a collagen-free diet. Osteoclasts are not particularly numerous in osteoporosis but can be present in large numbers in diseases such as Paget's disease of bone (see Chapter 1). There is increasing evidence that osteoblasts and osteoclasts can regulate the activity of each other in a process known as coupling. Osteoclasts are affected by a number of hormones and drugs, including calcitonin, which causes the cells to become markedly contracted, and the bisphosphonate group of drugs, e.g. Didronel.

Osteocytes are derived from osteoblasts entrapped in bone. They provide a rapid flux system for calcium through bone.

HORMONES ACTING ON BONE

Three main hormones act on bone—vitamin D, PTH and calcitonin.

VITAMIN D

This acts on bone through its active metabolite, $1,25(OH)_2D$ (calcitriol). Vitamin D is obtained either from the diet or through synthesis in the skin. Although vitamin D is fat soluble and occurs in foods such as butter, it is often added to foods. It is not particularly well absorbed by the intestine, and this absorption is impaired in the elderly and especially in the presence of malabsorption, e.g. coeliac disease. Vitamin D is also synthesised in the skin through the action of ultraviolet light (UVB) on 7-dehydrocholesterol. Regardless of its origin, vitamin D is carried on a specific transport protein to the liver, where it is converted to 25-hydroxyvitamin D. It is then converted specifically in the kidney to the active hormone, $1,25(OH)_2D$, and this enzymatic step is stimulated by PTH and low serum phosphate levels. In some diseases, particularly sarcoidosis, the 1-hydroxylation step in the synthetic pathway of $1,25(OH)_2D$ is undertaken by the sarcoid tissue and leads to hypercalcaemia. Vitamin D deficiency causes rickets in children and osteomalacia in adults. Patients with chronic renal failure are prone to a specific bone disease because they cannot form $1,25(OH)_2D$. In experimental systems, calcitriol seems to enhance bone resorption, but the main action of calcitriol is to increase the absorption of calcium from the intestine. There has been increasing interest in calcitriol in osteoporosis as an adjunct to increasing intestinal calcium absorption and as a means of inhibiting the output of PTH.

PARATHYROID HORMONE

Parathyroid Hormone (PTH) is an 84-amino-acid protein produced by the parathyroid glands situated alongside the thyroid gland in the neck. The output of PTH is closely regulated by serum calcium concentrations. Low levels of serum calcium increase PTH output. The resulting high hormone levels restore serum calcium by two means. Firstly, PTH acts on bone to liberate bone calcium. Secondly, PTH stimulates calcitriol production by the kidney, thereby increasing the absorption of calcium from the intestine. PTH levels tend to rise at night when the subject is starving, and for this reason dietary calcium supplements are best given in the evening. If calcium intake is low, it will not be possible to restore serum calcium levels by intestinal absorption, and calcium is liberated from bone. One of the reasons for giving oral calcium supplements is to lower serum PTH and protect the bone. In some patients, an inherited gene defect occurs in which the set level for serum calcium is higher than usual. These patients do not suffer any ill effects. It was once thought that these patients had a form of overactivity of the parathyroid glands (hyperparathyroidism), but, importantly, it is now known that this is not the case. Hyperparathyroidism occurs in three forms: primary, secondary and tertiary.

Primary Hyperparathyroidism

This involves from one, to all four of the parathyroid glands and leads to high levels of serum calcium. Usually the cause is an adenoma; carcinoma is unusual. Less commonly, a hyperplastic process affects all four glands. The high level of PTH activity also leads to loss of bone, a process which is opposed by oestrogens, and may result in osteoporosis in postmenopausal women. Surgery may be needed to remove the gland or glands.

Secondary Hyperparathyroidism

This refers to an overactive parathyroid gland responding to low levels of serum calcium. If this continues for long nough, as in chronic renal failure, the glands become utonomous (tertiary hyperparathryoidism) and very high evels of serum PTH are found. Again, surgery may be needed, although calcitriol may lower PTH levels independently of the serum calcium level.

CALCITONIN

This is not a particularly important hormone in man. It is produced by the C cells of the thyroid gland, and levels are affected by serum calcium, i.e. elevation of serum calcium leads to increased production of calcitonin. Serum calcium does not seem to be much affected by calcitonin, and removal of the thyroid gland does not lead to osteoporosis.

OSTEOPOROSIS

DEFINITION

Osteoporosis is defined by the presence of a low trauma fracture of the distal radius, vertebral body or femoral neck. Osteoporosis can also exist in the presence of a bone mineral density (BMD)—measured by dual-energy X-ray absorpiometry (DXA; see page 125)—of more than 2.5 standard deviations below the mean value for the lumbar vertebral bodies or femoral neck in healthy normal subjects.

Osteopenia is a term confined to low bone density and is usually used in a qualitative sense. Osteoporosis is sometimes divided into types 1 and 2. Type 1 refers to fractures occurring during the phase of rapid bone loss that occurs in the 15 years after the menopause, and type-2 fractures are associated with the gradual decline of bone mass with ageing (Melton & Riggs, 1983).

INCIDENCE AND PREVALENCE

The three main osteoporotic fractures start to show an increase at different times in life (Figure 9.1). The distal forearm and vertebral fractures start to show an increase in the sixth decade of life, and the hip fracture in the eighth decade of life. Unlike the forearm fracture rate, which levels off after 65 years of age, the vertebral fracture rate continues to increase. Osteoporotic fracture is considerably more common in females than in males. About one third of women can expect to have one or more of the osteoporotic fractures by the end of their life. In fracture of the femoral neck, the ratio of women to men is between 2:1 and 3:1 (Boyce & Vessey, 1985). At the distal forearm, the fracture rate is about 6:1 (Melton, 1995). The prevalence rates for vertebral osteoporotic fracture in men are less well defined. For out-patient attendances, the ratio of females

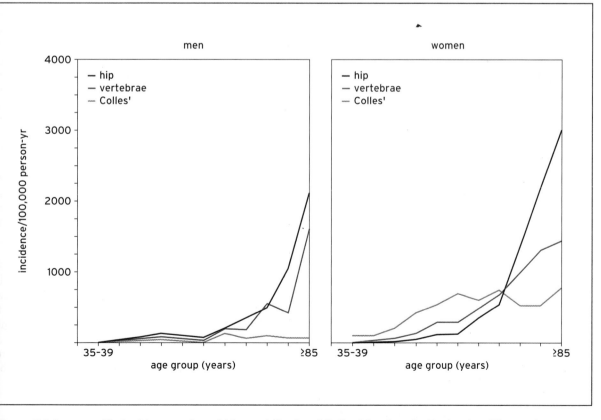

Figure 9.1 Age-specific incidence rates of hip, vertebral and Colles' fracture in Rochester, Minnesota, men and women. (Redrawn from Cooper and Melton, with permission.)

to males is about 8:1, but a lower sex ratio of 2–4:1 is found in the USA (Melton, 1995). The prevalence of vertebral body fracture was found to be about 7% among women attending their general practitioners for any cause in the UK (Cooper *et al.*, 1991). The incidence rose after the age of 50 years, and in the group aged 50–60 years was as high as 5%. Fracture of the femoral neck has achieved epidemic proportions over the past 25 years—between 1954 and 1983 in the Oxford (UK) region, the incidence per 10 000 of the population has increased in women from 10.4 to 35.4 and in men from 4.2 to 10.4 (Boyce & Vessey, 1985).

RECOGNITION

The existence of osteoporosis from an obvious fracture at the distal forearm or the femoral neck is easily recognised. A vertebral fracture, however, is less easily identified. Vertebral fractures cause back pain, loss of height and a kyphotic spine, but an X-ray film is required to identify a vertebra with a significant deformity or fracture. Since the sequelae of osteoporotic fracture result in significant morbidity, it is desirable to identify those people who have thin bones and who are at risk of fracture before they actually do fracture. For this reason there is increasing interest in identifying those people and offering treatment.

RISK FACTORS

Several studies have investigated risk factors that could identify people susceptible to fractures. The main risk factors are shown in Table 9.1. Risk factors are of value in identifying general trends through populations. There are however some well-recognised risk factors. Thyrotoxicosis at any age, previous fracture and leanness are associated with a significant increase in the risk of fracture. Patients with anorexia nervosa tend to fracture more regularly, whereas modest excess weight protects against hip fracture (Ribot *et al.*, 1993). Risk factors are easy to identify and have value in highlighting a patient's susceptibility to fracture. For example, the existence of previous fracture, such as fracture of the distal forearm, will indicate that the patient has thin bone and is at risk of further fracture. In population studies, the occurrence of a fracture after the age of 20 at most sites is associated with an increased risk of low BMD at either the lumbar spine or femoral neck (Davie, 1996). Some bones, such as the distal forearm, the rib and the foot, are better predictors of low bone density than others, and fractures of the tibia do not seem to be associated with low bone density. Since the skeleton is dependent on adequate nutrition, particularly calcium, patients who have difficulty feeding themselves, e.g. those with rheumatoid arthritis, are going to be at increased risk of fracture. This risk is enhanced by the use of drugs such as corticosteroids which also increase the risk of fracture. Disuse and spinal injury also put patients at increased risk of lower limb bone loss and fracture (Minaire *et al.*, 1974; Chow *et al.*, 1996), and patients with stroke have a higher incidence of hip fracture on the affected side.

CONSEQUENCES IN ECONOMIC AND QUALITY-OF-LIFE TERMS

Osteoporotic fracture at the femoral neck has been well investigated in terms of its economic impact. Many of these patients are elderly and require considerable support in the community after leaving hospital. About one fifth of all patients having a hip fracture will have died within a year. It is calculated that each patient with a femoral neck fracture requires resources of about £10 000. The distal forearm fracture is not a costly fracture to manage, but the function of the hand on the affected side is often considerably impaired and the fracture is associated with continuing pain. Vertebral fractures have not been investigated in great detail in terms of quality of life. Data which are available do not show a significant association between vertebral deformity and quality of life (Cook *et al.*, 1993). Loss of lung volume caused by the kyphosis results in the patient becoming short of breath, and this can be exacerbated by the presence of an hiatus hernia occupying part of the intrathoracic space. Loss of height in the lower dorsum and lumbar spine leads to a reduction in volume of the abdomen. Abdominal

Risk factors for osteoporosis
Early menopause
Amenorrhoea
Leanness
Thyrotoxicosis
Malabsorbtion e.g. Coeliac disease
Corticosteroid therapy
Rheumatoid arthritis
Maternal fracture
Increasing age
Falls
Caffeine intake*
Height loss (especially when span exceeds height by >10cm)
Alcohol
Nulliparity*
Males only
Androgen resistance
Androgen deficiency
*minor risk factors

Table 9.1 Risk factors for osteoporosis.

contents thus tend to be pushed superiorly into the thorax or inferiorly into the pelvis, leading to prolapse. Alternatively, the abdominal contents can push forward. Patients may try to counteract this by applying a corset, thereby increasing the chance of the abdominal contents being pushed into the thorax or the pelvis. The resulting indigestion from the hiatus hernia, or urinary incontinence from the prolapse, is very distressing. The relation between vertebral deformity, back pain, quality of life and other complications of vertebral fracture are in need of study.

FINDINGS ON INVESTIGATION

Osteoporosis is diagnosed by X-ray films or BMD measurements. X-ray films will show the presence of a fracture, and if the films are taken in a standardised fashion they can be quantified and small changes in vertebral dimension measured. Osteoblastic activity can be measured by exploiting serum alkaline phosphatase and osteocalcin, as well as some of the newer markers of collagen formation. When collagen is initially formed, there is a propeptide at the C terminal and N terminal ends of the collagen molecule, each of which has to be removed before the collagen can be incorporated into its helical form. These products, which are broken off at the time of collagen synthesis, are known as the collagen propeptides (P1CP and P1NP) and can be measured in serum. Low levels indicate that little collagen is being made. Bone breakdown is identified through investigation of osteoclastic activity. Hydroxyproline, an amino acid released during the breakdown of collagen, can be measured in urine and serves as a valuable indicator of total body collagen breakdown. A more specific measurement is that of the collagen cross-link, deoxypyridinoline, which is also measured in urine.

Bone biopsy through the iliac crest is a technique with limited application in osteoporosis. It is undertaken using an 8 mm trephine (not unlike a cork borer) with a serrated edge, under local anaesthetic. Osteoblastic activity can be estimated as the mineralisation rate. To measure this rate, ledermycin is taken orally for 2 days, and a fortnight later for another 2 days before the biopsy. This drug, in common with other tetracyclines, is incorporated into bone and is seen as a line when the bone is examined microscopically. If the time between the tetracycline dosing is known accurately, the distance between the two lines gives an estimation of bone mineralisation rate. Osteoclastic activity is measured either by counting these cells (usually very few) or by measuring the proportion of the bone surface which has been eroded. If the osteoporotic process has a secondary cause, e.g. myeloma, then abnormal cells are present. Bone biopsy has considerable value in osteomalacia (see page 7). In this condition, bone mineralisation is defective—large areas of bone are unmineralised and can be detected on histological examination. Ledermycin is not incorporated into bone in osteomalacia, thus no lines can be seen.

Technetium methylene diphosphonate (MDP) scanning (scintigraphy) is a technique requiring a bisphosphonate drug labelled with a radioactive isotope (Tc^{99}). The Tc–bisphosphonate complex is injected into the patient, and the bisphosphonate is taken up by bone that is undergoing rapid remodelling. The patient is then scanned with a gamma beam detector which detects the radiation, thus identifying the sites of bisphosphonate uptake. Such a state occurs in fractures, Paget's disease of bone and secondary cancer deposits in bone, as well as in many other conditions. It is a very sensitive technique, detecting areas of increased bone turnover, but is not specific, and is used to identify the presence of fractures in osteoporosis; particularly those that are too small to see on X-ray film.

BONE DENSITOMETRY

The ability to measure the amount of mineral in bone has improved our understanding of osteoporosis and its progression and management. Bone density may be measured at a number of sites using a variety of techniques. The most common methods at present are DXA, X-ray absorptiometry at the distal forearm, ultrasound attenuation at the os calcis and CT scanning at the lumbar spine. Apart from DXA, which can be used to measure bone density at any site in the body, all the other techniques are site-specific at present.

Bone mass increases with age and reaches a peak in the fourth decade of life (Haddaway et al., 1992). In women, there is a gradual decline after the age of 40 years, and this decline is accentuated after the menopause, for 10–20 years, during which time almost 20% of the spine's BMD is lost. Thus, any process associated with an early menopause, e.g. hysterectomy, may cause early loss of bone. The BMD that is equivalent to 2.5 standard deviations below the healthy adult mean—known as the fracture threshold—is described as a T score of −2.5. The World Health Organization has suggested that this level should be termed osteoporosis (Kanis et al., 1994). The majority of patients with a significant vertebral fracture will have a BMD below this threshold, and patients with a BMD below the fracture threshold who do not have fractures are still considered to be osteoporotic. Figure 9.2 shows two other factors important in the prevention of osteoporosis. Firstly, it is important to achieve as high a peak BMD as is possible, by ensuring an adequate calcium intake through the growing years. Secondly, avoiding the rapid phase of bone loss after the menopause will maintain a higher BMD for longer.

Bone densitometry is used to identify osteoporosis, to assess the risk of osteoporosis and to ensure that any treatment for osteoporosis is having a beneficial effect and that the skeleton does not continue to lose bone.

The identification of patients with osteoporosis, as measured by BMD, is important, as these patients can be targeted for treatment to prevent them losing any further bone and suffering fractures. It should become possible to scan large numbers of women to identify those at greatest risk of fracture, and to start appropriate therapy. Bone densitometers that measure density at the spine and the hip

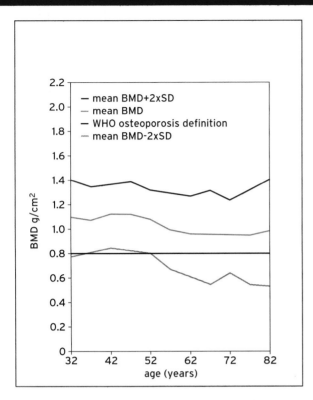

Figure 9.2 Cross sectional change of Bone Mineral Density (BMD) with age in the lumbar spine (L2-4). Note the fall of BMD in the immediate post menopausal years.

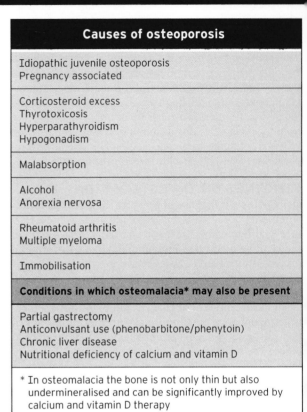

Table 9.2 Causes of osteoporosis.

are generally static, but those measuring density by ultrasonography of the heel or by X-ray absorptiometry at the forearm are smaller and more mobile and lend themselves to mass screening.

Bone densitometry has shown that certain parts of the skeleton respond to various forms of treatment more rapidly and to a greater extent than other parts. Thus, the lumbar spine tends to respond rather better than either the femoral neck or the distal forearm.

ASSOCIATED DISEASES

There are a considerable number of diseases associated with osteoporosis, and most of these can be readily excluded (Table 9.2). Of particular note is rheumatoid arthritis, in which the pathophysiology is complex. Patients with rheumatoid arthritis tend to be badly nourished because of difficulties with eating and chewing, and also relatively immobile, leading to immobilisation osteoporosis. Furthermore, corticosteroids are frequently administered and these are a potent cause of bone loss. Corticosteroids are particularly hazardous to the bone of postmenopausal women. In addition, patients with rheumatoid arthritis are more likely to suffer from thyrotoxicosis, itself an important cause of osteoporosis. Immobilisation, and particularly denervation, as seen in spinal injury patients, are common causes of bone loss; by 1 year these patients can lose

between one quarter and one third of their expected bone mass in the lower limb (Chow, 1996). Stroke is also associated with osteoporotic fracture, and the importance of mobilising patients with stroke, as much to prevent osteoporotic fractures as anything else, has been emphasised. Chronic obstructive airways disease is another condition associated with fracture, particularly as many of these patients are given corticosteroids. Smoking is associated with an increased rate of oestrogen degradation and leads to an early menopause and hence increased bone loss at an earlier age. Other important causes include chronic alcohol misuse and an increased tendency to fall—patients over the age of 70 years have an increased risk of falling, and this risk can be further increased if they are on multiple therapies or have dementia.

OTHER CAUSES OF OSTEOPOROSIS

Osteoporosis may occur in children. The most frequent associations are with osteogenesis imperfecta—a disease in which collagen molecules are not properly synthesised, and associated clinically with recurrent fractures and blue sclerae (the colour may vary in intensity)—and with leukaemia. Osteoporosis of childhood can occur during the early pubertal growth spurt and is usually self-limiting.

Other rare causes of osteoporosis include heparin administration and pregnancy. The latter may be associated

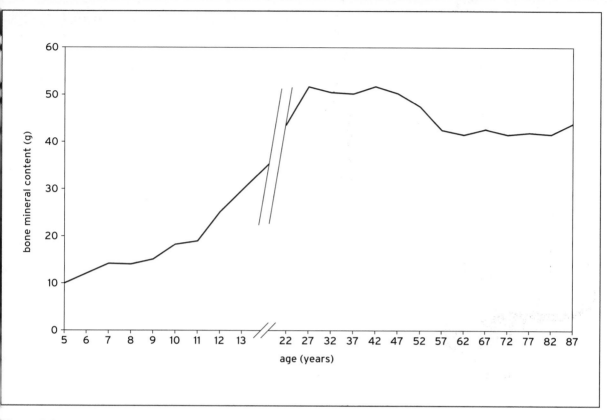

Figure 9.3 Female bone mineral change in L2-4 with age.

DIET AND OSTEOPOROSIS

Many patients are interested in learning about their diet and of devising ways to improve their chances of maintaining their skeleton. The advice, however, is not always welcome. The most important dietary constituent is calcium. It is generally agreed that the postmenopausal woman should try to achieve an intake of 1000 mg of calcium per day. There is probably no need to exceed an intake of 1500 mg per day. However, 1000 mg of calcium per day is difficult to achieve by food alone. Dairy products are the most concentrated form of calcium: half a litre of milk contains about 600 mg of calcium; 30 g of cheddar cheese about 240 mg (Paul & Southgate, 1979); and 125 g of yoghurt about 160 mg. It is important to take enough calcium, but there is no need to take an excess amount. The value of taking supplements of other minerals such as magnesium, boron and manganese is uncertain.

Calcium intake is probably most important in children and in women over 65 years of age. In children, mineral accretion is particularly rapid around the age of puberty. Over a period of about 2 years, bone mineral content in the spine increases by as much as is lost by a woman in the

with severe undiagnosed pain, most usually in the later part of pregnancy. The pain, however, frequently improves after the birth.

years following the menopause (Figure 9.3). Sufficient calcium for a positive calcium balance of as much as 500 mg per day may be required at this time for maximum growth potential.

Achieving an adequate calcium intake is important in elderly women since intestinal calcium absorption declines after 65 years of age (Birge & Avioli et al., 1990). Calcium supplements in women appear to be quite safe and do not result in the formation of renal stones. In Britain it is generally agreed that an intake of about 500 units of vitamin D per day is also beneficial. Vitamin D is either formed in the skin or ingested from food, and is necessary for the normal intestinal absorption of calcium. In the winter, many elderly people in Europe have low vitamin D levels (Lawson et al, 1979), and the resulting tendency to hypocalcaemia induces secondary hyperparathyroidism which further increases the rate of bone loss.

In recent years there has been increasing interest in the adverse effects of high-protein diets on calcium balance (Barzel et al., 1995). There are some compelling data to suggest that high-protein intakes lead to a negative calcium balance, i.e. calcium is lost from the skeleton, and that this can be reversed by lowering the protein intake. In general, about 1 g of protein per kilogram of body weight is a reasonable goal. There are also some data to suggest that vegetable protein is more bone sparing than animal protein.

Fibre and roughage often feature in the diet of the elderly. Both may bind calcium in the gut and prevent it being absorbed. Calcium is best taken separate from fibre and at night, when it will overcome the nocturnal surge of PTH. A good daily diet for bone preservation in women would include 1000 mg of calcium, 500 units of vitamin D, not more than 40 g of protein and sufficient calories (energy) to prevent weight loss. Concentrated foods may be best, particularly in patients who have poor appetites or who cannot chew properly.

PREVENTION AND TREATMENT

Management of osteoporosis is directed towards the prevention of fractures. The prevention of bone loss is frequently used as a substitute for fracture incidence, as measured by bone densitometry. The two main drug treatments for the management of osteoporosis are hormone replacement therapy (HRT) and the bisphosphonate group of drugs.

Hormone replacement therapy refers to the replacement of oestrogen and progestogen in women after the menopause. With the onset of ovarian failure at the menopause, oestrogen levels decline and bone is lost (see Figure 9.2). HRT aims to produce oestrogen levels adequate for the woman to maintain bone mass. If the patient has an intact uterus, it is necessary to give a progestogen in addition to the oestrogen so that a regular monthly bleed occurs, ensuring that the lining of the uterus (endometrium) is shed. If the endometrium is allowed to proliferate under the influence of oestrogen in the absence of a progestogen, it becomes hyperplastic and the risk of malignancy increases. Newer forms of HRT give the progestogen continuously and are intended to do away with the monthly bleed. These are, however, often not successful. Nevertheless, the endometrium rarely becomes hyperplastic (this can be checked by ultrasonography) in patients on this continuous combined regimen. If the patient has had a hysterectomy, oestrogen alone can be given. The amount of oestrogen that is necessary to prevent bone loss is uncertain. If a woman has had an ovariectomy in the fourth decade of life, she will probably need the equivalent of 0.625 mg Premarin daily. However, women after the age of 55 years show an improvement in BMD at the lumbar spine on low levels of oestrogen replacement. The lowest dose of oestrogen is administered by a transdermal patch containing 25mcg oestrogen (Estraderm 25 or Evorel 25). A conventional patch to prevent menopausal symptoms releases 50 mg oestradiol daily. In elderly women, the use of conventional dosages of oestrogen can lead to several side effects, including painful breasts, abdominal bloating, nausea, ankle swelling and headaches. The breast tenderness usually improves after about 3 months. Studies are now showing a significant antagonistic affect of Estraderm-25 patches on bone loss in women from their late 50s into the ninth decade of life (Evans & Davie, 1996).

In elderly women, there is probably no need to use more oestradiol than is contained in a 25 mcg patch. The anxiety about HRT in the long term concerns a possible increase in the risk of breast cancer. Many early studies of breast cancer in women taking HRT showed no risk up to 5 years on HRT and an increased risk after 10 years. The recent American Nurses' Study (Colditz et al., 1995) has shown that an increased risk exists in women who have been on HRT for 5 years or more. However, case-control studies published at the same time have failed to show any increased risk of breast cancer with HRT (Stanford et al., 1995). It seems reasonable to give every woman a chance of going onto HRT for 5 years, and it is logical to begin to count those years from the average age of menopause (51.7 years). Thus, any woman having an early menopause or a hysterectomy early in life can go onto HRT and continue until the age of 52 years before she starts to count the number of years she has to stay on the treatment. Other benefits do, however, accrue from the use of HRT and these include protection against heart attack and stroke. Overall, women on HRT live about 2 years longer than those who have not had HRT. Oestrogens also have beneficial effects on the skin and on mental function. HRT should not be regarded as interchangeable with bisphosphonates as the latter only have an effect on bone.

The bisphosphonates have a basic core structure (Figure 9.4), and the central carbon atom can have a large number of side chains. Didronel was the first commercially available bisphosphonate. Bisphosphonates, like oestrogens, act to inhibit the action of osteoclasts although the actions are not the same. For example, the bisphosphonates clearly have an action in Paget's disease of bone, whereas the oestrogens do not, and it is yet to be established whether oestrogens and bisphosphonates have additive effects. Bisphosphonates act slightly differently according to the type of side chain on the central carbon atom, but

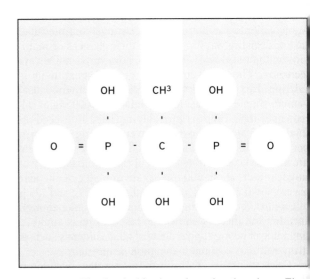

Figure 9.4 The basic bisphosphonate structure. The HCM_3 attached to the central carbon atom is the side chain which determines the activity of the bisphosphonate.

ley all share the basic property of inhibiting osteoclasts. Bone mineral density increases with the administration of bisphosphonates, and fracture incidence in the spine falls. When given in excess, some bisphosphonates, notably Didronel, can inhibit the proper mineralisation of bone; for this reason, Didronel PMO (post-menopausal osteoporosis) is given in a cyclical dosage. Other bisphosphonates, e.g. alendronate, do not have this effect. Bisphosphonates are taken up by bone and have a long half-life—often 12 or more months. They seem to be very effective in preventing bone loss and have been shown to increase the mechanical strength of bone in primates. They are relatively free of side effects, the main ones being nausea and indigestion. There are no contraindications to their administration, although Didronel is generally not used within 6 months of a long bone fracture because of the risk of the inhibition of mineralisation. All bisphosphonates are badly absorbed from the gut (only 0.7% of Alendronate is absorbed) and need to be taken on an empty stomach.

Other treatments for osteoporosis include sodium fluoride, calcitonin, anabolic steroids and 1,25-dihydroxyvitamin D. Sodium fluoride is very effective at increasing BMD but may build up bone density at the spine at the expense of bone density at the femoral neck; bone density may fall at this site. It is nevertheless a valuable means of increasing BMD in some patients, particularly when combined with a bisphosphonate to avoid any removal of bone at the femoral neck.

Calcitonin is valuable in the management of acute osteoporotic fracture of the spine. It has an analgesic effect and directly prevents bone breakdown. Its effects are, however, comparatively brief, and it has a short half-life so needs to be given either daily or on alternate days at a dosage of 20–40 units per day for 6 weeks. Intranasal preparations of calcitonin have been used on the continent but are not available in the UK. Calcitonin has also been used with effect in osteoporosis of pregnancy. Its use seems to be safe, in contrast to bisphosphonates, which increase the fetus' bone density and reduce growth. Calcitriol (1,25-dihydroxyvitamin D) has been used to increase the intestinal absorption of calcium, particularly in the elderly, in whom the intestinal absorption of calcium is impaired. There is a significant risk of hypercalcaemia, which may occur quite suddenly, since 1,25-dihydroxyvitamin D is also a comparatively potent absorber of bone. Except when there is a well-documented deficiency of 1,25-dihydroxyvitamin D, e.g. the bone disease of chronic renal failure, 1,25-dihydroxyvitamin D is generally not used.

Specific causes of osteoporosis can be treated. Thus, multiple myeloma is treated with chemotherapy (often together with pamidronate), thyrotoxicosis is treated by antithyroid drugs and radio-iodine therapy, and steroid excess by lowering the oral steroid intake. Immobilisation osteoporosis is currently of much interest. Patients in spinal injuries units are liable to fracture bone in the lower limb. This loss is not affected by sex steroids but preliminary work suggests that bisphosphonates may prevent bone loss. With the recent emphasis on walking in spinal injury patients, preservation of skeletal integrity is increasingly important.

OSTEOPOROSIS IN MEN

This is a relatively neglected branch of osteoporosis (Scane et al.,1993). It does seem to be getting more frequent, with hip fractures showing a marked increase over the past 25 years. The prevalence of osteoporotic vertebral fracture is more difficult to ascertain. At present about one male osteoporotic patient is seen for every eight females in our clinics at Oswestry.

Osteoporosis in men tends to present at an earlier age than in women. In Europe, the average age of presentation is 50–60 years. Bone mineral density is usually very low, but not all investigators have confirmed this. Results of bone biopsy in idiopathic osteoporosis are variable, but many reports show a low bone formation rate or reduced osteoblastic activity. Other studies have suggested that markers of collagen synthesis may be low.

Most cases of osteoporosis in men are idiopathic, accounting for up to 40% of patients. Family studies may show other family members with low bone mass in the absence of fracture. Hypogonadism in the male will also lead to osteoporosis, and about 15% of all male cases of osteoporosis are associated with significantly low testosterone levels. Multiple myeloma must always be considered in men with osteoporosis, and prostate cancer may also be present with back pain and fracture. The most important other secondary cause is corticosteroid excess, usually as a result of treatment with corticosteroids for other diseases. High dosages of corticosteroids are prescribed after cardiac transplantation, and osteoporotic fracture is a serious complication. In the USA, alcohol misuse is as frequent a cause of osteoporosis in men as corticosteroid therapy.

Other conditions which are associated with osteoporosis in men have a multifactorial aetiology. Rheumatoid arthritis is frequently associated with osteoporosis—immobility, poor nutrition and corticosteroid therapy, as well as the rheumatoid process, can all be implicated. Recent observations have suggested that the female sex hormone, oestrogen, has an important role in the development of bone in men. Oestrogen is required to fuse epiphyses in both sexes, and a deficiency of the oestrogen receptor in men is associated with osteoporosis and tall stature (since the epiphyses are late in fusing). The enzyme that forms oestrogen may be deficient in certain inherited disorders, and the resulting low levels of oestradiol are an insufficient stimulus for bone growth.

There is no well-established therapy for osteoporosis in men. Since many men with osteoporosis exhibit hypercalciuria, calcium supplements have to be given with care. Didronel is licensed for vertebral osteoporosis in men, and testosterone can be given to men with hypogonadism. Effective treatment is becoming available with newer bisphosphonates, but these are still at the trial stage.

9

MECHANICAL CONSEQUENCES OF BONE LOSS

The loss of bone in the vertebrae that accompanies the menopause totals almost 20% before the rate of bone loss subsides. A number of studies have examined the relation between bone mass and the mechanical properties of bone, with particular reference to changes in bone density in the spine of post-mortem specimens.

Mechanical properties of bone, particularly yield energy, show a greater measure (about 2–2.5 fold) than does bone density with ageing (Britton & Davie, 1990). Measures to preserve density are thus particularly valuable in terms of maintaining the mechanical integrity of bone.

EXERCISE

Exercise is considered to be beneficial to the skeleton under most circumstances. Patients confined to bed or immobilised as a result of a spinal injury, lose bone. In the latter case, it is not at present clear whether the spinal injury causes bone loss over and above the immobilisation. Nevertheless, the bone loss in these patients can be considerable, with almost one third of the bone in the calcaneus being lost in the first year. Considerable loss of bone also occurs in the femur. In the past this loss was not important, but the development of technology that allows the paraplegic patient to walk means that the mechanical integrity of the skeleton in the lower limbs should be maintained. Immobilisation of bone in a plaster cast will also lead to loss of mineral and predispose to further fracture.

Exercise can be shown to have a positive effect on bone mass in teenagers. However, excessive exercise, especially long-distance running, may lead to weight loss and amenorrhoea. This combination in its fully expressed form leads to anorexia nervosa, in which bone is lost and fractures occur. Exercise cannot substitute for oestrogen at this age. In tennis players, exercise on one side of the body can cause an increase in bone mass by as much as 11% in the playing arm compared with the non-playing arm (Huddleston et al., 1980). Other studies have confirmed that lifetime exercise and current exercise are associated with better femoral neck density (Greendale et al., 1995).

In elderly patients, especially women, exercise has a number of beneficial effects; and it does not have to be hard. Walking 1 mile per day can have a useful effect on preserving bone mass. Increased BMD has been found to accompany both exercise alone and the use of HRT concurrently. Indeed it has been suggested that the two have independent additive effects. Exercise in the elderly can also preserve muscle mass, thereby helping to preserve muscle function and rendering a fall less likely. It has further been suggested that exercise prevents the basal metabolic rate (BMR) from falling. If BMR is maintained, food intake remains at a reasonable level, thereby securing the daily requirement of essential nutrients that exist in low concentration in foods.

ARTHRITIS AND OSTEOPOROSIS

There is often much interest in the relation between these two conditions. Osteoarthritis is often associated with increased skeletal bone density (Dequecker, 1985), and rarely co-exists with osteoporosis. However, deformity in the spine following a change of vertebral shape due to osteoporosis, can progress to arthritis of the posterior facet joints. This condition is a good example of the hidden seriousness of osteoporosis, which, although itself causes comparatively little pain (except in the acute stage), can result in serious pain or morbidity arising from complications (Table 9.3). Many patients can gain pain relief from heat, transcutaneous electrical nerve stimulation (TENS) machines or non steroidal anti-inflammatory drugs, e.g. Brufen. Other diseases affecting joints or bone around joints which interact with osteoporosis include systemic lupus erythematosus, rheumatoid arthritis and reflex sympathetic osteodystrophy. Systemic lupus erythematosus can deteriorate or even appear for the first time in women taking HRT for osteoporosis. Rheumatoid arthritis (see above) may be associated with dietary deficiency, calcium malabsorption from the intestine and corticosteroid therapy. Reflex sympathetic osteodystrophy is a poorly understood condition, characterised by pain and bone resorption, often close to a joint following trauma that is often quite minor. Treatment is unsatisfactory and includes early movement, guanethidine blocks, systemic calcitonin or a bisphosphonate. None are ideal. A similar painful condition can affect diabetic patients particularly their feet, and may respond to intravenous pamidronate.

Complications of osteoporosis
Kyphosis can lead to:
Vertebral insufficiency due to entrapment of the vertebral arteries on hyperextension of the neck Reduced lung volume and shortness of breath Lung infections being more difficult to treat
Loss of height in lower dorsal/lumber spine can lead to:
Abdominal distension Hiatus hernia (and further loss of chest volume) Prolapse
NB Girdles to 'hold in the stomach' may worsen hiatus hernia and prolapse
Thin bone can lead to:
Easy fracture (care with chest physiotherapy) Pain and deformity (e.g. Colles' fracture) Death (1:5 patients with fracture of femoral neck will be dead within 1 year) Restriction of living and quality of life

Table 9.3 Complications of osteoporosis.

REFERENCES

Barzel US. The skeleton as an ion-exchange system: Implications for the role of acid base imbalance in the genesis of osteoporosis. *J Bone and Mineral Res* 1995, **10**:1431–1436.

Birge SL, Avioli LV. Pathophysiology of calcium and phosphate absorptive disorders. In: Avioli LV, ed. *Metabolic bone diseases and clinically related disorders.* Philadelphia: WB Saunders; 1990:206.

Boyce WJ, Vessey MP. Rising incidence of fracture of the proximal femur. *Lancet* 1985, 1: 150–151.

Britton JM, Davie MWJ. Mechanical properties of bone from iliac crest and relationship to L5 vertebral bone. *Bone* 1990, **11**:21–28.

Chow YW, Inman C, Pollintine P, Sharp CA, Haddaway MJ, El Masry W, Davie MWJ. Ultrasound bone densitometry and dual energy X-ray absorptiometry in patients with spinal cord injury: a cross sectional study. *Spinal Cord* 1996, **34**:736–741.

Colditz GA, Hanjinson SE, Hunter DJ, Willet DJ, Manson JE, Stampfer MJ, Hennekens C, Rosner B, Speizer FE. The use of estrogens and progestins and the risk of breast cancer in postmenopausal women. *New Eng J Med* 1995, **332**:1589–1593.

Cook DJ, Guyatt GH, Adachi JD, Clifton J, Griffith LE, Epstein RS, Juniper EF. Quality of life issues in women with vertebral fractures due to osteoporosis. *Arthritis and Rheumatism* 1993, **36**:750–756.

Cooper C, Melton LJ III. Epidemiology of osteoporosis. *Trends in Endocrinology and Metabolism* 1992, **314**:224–229.

Cooper C, Shah S, Hand DJ, Adams J, Compston J, Davie M, Woolf A. Screening for vertebral osteoporosis using individual risk factors. *Osteoporosis International* 1991, **2**:48–53.

Davie MWJ. Fractures at specific sites indicate low bone mineral density at lumbar spine and femoral neck in women. *J Orthop Rheum* 1996, **9**:41–45.

DeQuecker J. The relationship between Osteoporosis and osteoarthritis. *Clinics in Rheumatic diseases* 1985, **11**:271–296.

Evans SF, Davie MWJ. Low and conventional doee transdermal estradiol are equally effective at preventing bone loss in spine and femur at all post-menopausal ages. *Clin Endocrinol* 1996, 44:79–84.

Greendale GA, Barret-Connor E, Edelstein S, Ingles S, Haile R. The Rancho-Bermardo study. *Am J Epidemiol* 1995, **141**:951–959.

Haddaway MJ, Davie MWJ, McCall IW. Bone mineral density in healthy normal women and reproducibility of measurements in spine and hip using dual-energy X-ray absorptiometry. *Br J Radiol* 1992, **65**:213–217.

Huddleston AL, Rockwell D, Kulund DN, Harrison RB. Bone mass in lifetime tennis athletes. *JAMA* 1980, **244**:1107–1109.

Kanis JA, Melton LJ III, Christiansen C, Johnston CC, Khaltaev N. Perspective: The diagnosis of osteoporosis. *J Bone and Mineral Res* 1994, **9**:1137–1141.

Lawson DEM, Paul AA, Black AE, Cole TJ, Mandal AR, Davie M. Relative contributions of diet and sunlight to Vitamin D state in the elderly. *BMJ* 1979, **2**:303–305.

Melton LJ III. Epidemiology of fractures. In: Riggs BL, Melton LJ III, eds. *Osteoporosis: Etiology, Diagnosis and management,* 2nd Ed. Philadelphia: Lippincroft-Raven; 1995;10.

Minaire P, Meunier P, Edouard C, Bernard J, Courpron P, Bourret J. Quantitative histological data on disuse osteoporosis: comparison with biological data. *Calcified Tissue Research* 1974, **17**:57–73.

Nordin BEC. *Calcium, Phosphate and magnesium metabolism.* Edinburgh: Churchill Livingstone; 1976.

Paul AA, Southgate DAT. The composition of Foods. In: Paul AA, Southgate DAT, eds. *McCance and Widdowson's,* 4th Ed. London: HMSO; 1979.

Ribot C, Tremollieres F, Pouilles JM, Albarede JL, Mansat M, Uthesa G, Bonneau M, Bonnissent P, Ricoeur C. Risk factors for hip fracture. MEDOS study: Results of the Tolouse centre. *Bone* 1993, **Suppl 1**:77–80.

Riggs BL, Melton LJ III. Evidence for two distinct syndromes of involutional osteoporosis. *Am J Med* 1983, **75**:899–901.

Scane AC, Sutcliffe AM, Francis RM. Osteoporosis in men. *Bailliere's Clinical Rheumatology* 1993, **7**:589–601.

Stanford JL, Weiss NS, Voight LF, Daling JR, Habel LA, Rossing MA. Combined estrogen and Progestin hormone replacement therapy in relation to risk of breast cancer in middle aged women. *JAMA* 1995, **274**:137–142.

GENERAL READING

Woolf AD, Dixon AStJ. Osteoporosis: A Clinical Guide. London: Martin Dunitz; 1988.

Riggs BL, Melton LJ III, eds. Osteoporosis: Etiology, Diagnosis and Management. Philadelphia: Lippincott-Raven; 1995.

SECTION 3

PAEDIATRIC CONDITIONS

rthopaedics (orthopædix). That part of
rgery which deals with the
normnalities, diseases and injuries of
e locomotor system

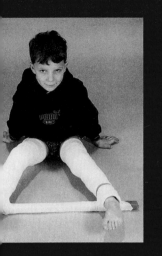

10

G A Evans & R Jones

CHILDHOOD DISORDERS OF THE HIP AND LEG

CHAPTER OUTLINE

- **Developmental dysplasia of the hip**
- **Perthes' disease**
- **Slipped upper femoral epiphysis**

- **Coxa vara**
- **Inequality of leg length**

DEVELOPMENTAL DYSPLASIA OF THE HIP

EPIDEMIOLOGY

This condition occurs more frequently in females than in males, with a ratio of 3:1 at neonatal diagnosis. The reported incidence at birth is between 3 and 5 cases per 1000 live births. The left hip is affected more frequently than the right, and it is bilateral in 20% of cases (Figure 10.1). Familial and environmental factors predispose to this condition. It is probable that the most important familial factor is excessive generalised joint laxity, and, if one parent has suffered from congenital dislocation, the risk of presentation in a child is 12% (sons, 6% ; daughters, 17%) (Wynne-Davies, 1973). Antenatal environmental factors associated with an increased incidence of a dislocation are a first-born child, breech presentation and lack of amniotic fluid.

It is possible that intrauterine compression or fetal position, or a combination of the two, results in a dislocation in those babies with a genetic predisposition. The joint laxity may be further increased in the perinatal period by maternal hormones responsible for relaxing the ligaments of the birth canal. These hormones cross the placenta, affecting the baby. The majority of unstable hips undergo spontaneous resolution in the postnatal period (Barlow, 1962). However, if the hips are maintained in an unfavourable extended and adducted position, spontaneous resolution does not occur, with the result that the incidence of dislocation appears much higher in societies in which it is customary to 'swaddle' infants.

PATHOLOGY

Neonatal hip instability varies in severity and has three different presentations. These are:
- Frank dislocation, when the femoral head is completely displaced from the acetabulum but can be gently relocated by the Ortolani manoeuvre (see page 136).
- The dislocatable hip, when the femoral head is in the acetabulum but, with a provocative manoeuvre of backward pressure on the adducted thigh, can be completely displaced from it (Barlow, 1962). Once the leg is released, the femoral head usually reduces spontaneously.
- A subluxable hip, the most difficult to diagnose and associated with the least capsular laxity. Subluxation occurs when the femoral head can be moved significantly, but not completely, out of the acetabulum.

The shape of the femoral head and acetabulum is virtually normal in the neonatal period, but persistence of the instability results in a secondary abnormality. The acetabular labrum becomes deformed and may become inverted between the head and acetabulum (limbus). When a dislocation has been present for a prolonged period, the inferior capsule and psoas tendon develop contractures, which prevent relocation of the femoral head. The femoral head begins to lose its spherical shape and the anteversion of the femoral neck tends to increase rather than decrease as in the normally located joint. The acetabulum becomes shallow through lack of growth of its lateral and anterior margins (see Figure 10.1). These features are progressive with the persistence of the dislocation. It is therefore important to diagnose and treat the condition at birth to prevent the development of the soft tissue and bony changes described, and to reduce the magnitude and morbidity of the treatment. Rarely, there may be irreducible dislocation in utero, which is usually associated with other joint problems such as arthrogryposis. In these circumstances, the secondary changes will be present at birth.

CLINICAL PRESENTATION

All newborn infants should be examined to try to identify dislocation or abnormal laxity of the hip. Frank dislocation is associated with shortening of the leg, a high- riding prominent trochanter, a relative emptiness of the femoral triangle and telescoping on proximal pressure. The head can be felt to relocate on performing the Ortolani manoeuvre, which involves abducting and raising the flexed thigh gently forwards. Occasionally on performing this manoeuvre, the sensation of a click can be elicited from the joint. In the absence of displacement of the femoral head, this is of no serious significance. With such neonatal screening, Barlow (1962) claimed that he was able to diagnose all cases in the newborn period, and eradicate the late presentation of hip dislocation. However, in most centres worldwide, we have not been able to reproduce this success, and a small number of cases continue to present later in life. Ultrasound examination demonstrates the unstable hip and is now used for the diagnosis and monitoring of treatment. Apart from failure to recognise a neonatal dislocation, a further possible explanation for late presentation is that the occasional neonatal subluxation, which is difficult to detect

clinically, may result in progressive acetabular dysplasia and displacement of the femoral head (Kepley & Weiner 1981).

In the older infant, the classic clinical signs of dislocation include limited abduction, a high-riding greater trochanter and relative femoral shortening. The dislocation is no longer reducible by the Ortolani manoeuvre. At the age of walking, there is a noticeable limp with a positive Trendelenburg test. Bilateral cases present with a symmetrical waddling gait, which may not be recognised as being abnormal until the child has grown out of the toddler stage.

TREATMENT

The objective is to reduce the femoral head into the acetabulum without producing damage to it or its blood supply by forceful manoeuvres. The specific treatment depends on the age of the child at diagnosis. It is advantageous to start treatment in the neonatal period, before the onset of secondary soft tissue and bony changes. For this reason, all children are screened for congenital dislocation as part of the neonatal examination, and at the developmental screening usually undertaken by the community physician at approximately 6 weeks and 6 months of age.

When the diagnosis is made in the newborn infant, the principle of treatment is to retain the hip in flexion and abduction so that the femoral head is reduced in the acetabulum. The initial capsular laxity regresses and after approximately 3 months' treatment the joint is stable, requires no further treatment and the prognosis for a normal joint is excellent. Treatment usually starts immediately once the diagnosis has been made, although in some centres it is deferred for 2–3 weeks because, as mentioned earlier, a large number resolve spontaneously, leaving only a minority of hips with residual instability to be treated. There are many different devices available to maintain the flexed and abducted posture of the hips, and these include the Von

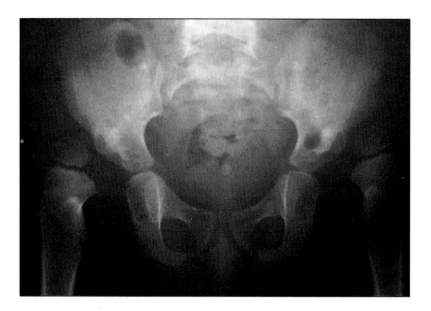

Figure 10.1 Bilateral hip dislocation in a 3-year-old, resulting in secondary acetabular dysplasia and a straight femoral neck-shaft angle due to excessive anteversion.

Rosen splint and the Pavlik harness. The former holds the hips in one position, whereas the latter allows motion within a constrained range (Figure 10.2).

When treatment is started later, up to 6 months of age, the Pavlik harness achieves reduction in the majority of cases. When the harness is first applied, the hip is still dislocated, but the relaxation of the child within the constraints of the harness achieves a spontaneous reduction. The complications of this treatment in terms of damage to the femoral head are negligible. When successful, the reduction is achieved within 3 weeks, but the harness is usually retained for up to 6 months depending on the appearance of the bony growth and remodelling on ultrasound and X-ray examination. The treatment described so far can be undertaken as an out-patient.

If diagnosed after 6 months of age, or if any of the previously mentioned treatments have failed to achieve reduction, the child requires in-patient treatment. At this stage there is relative shortening of the soft tissues adjacent to the hip joint, and skin traction is usually applied before manipulative or operative reduction. This prevents excessive pressure on the head and damage to it following reduction. There are several different techniques of

applying traction to the legs, some of which attempt to obtain reduction during the period of traction. Other forms, e.g. overhead divarication 'gallows' traction (Figure 10.3), are primarily used to stretch the soft tissues for 2 weeks, followed by a gentle manipulative reduction under general anaesthesia. This is called a 'closed reduction'. An arthrogram of the hip joint may be performed at the same time to demonstrate absence of soft tissue interposition between the femoral head and acetabulum, because in a small infant the majority of the femoral head and acetabulum is made of cartilage and does not show up on a plain X-ray film.

If a closed reduction cannot be achieved, an operation is necessary to remove the obstructive factors. This is called an 'open reduction'. The most common obstructive factors are persistent contracture of the inferior capsule, a tight psoas tendon and an inverted limbus.

Once the reduction has been achieved, by either manipulation or operation, it is maintained by application of a plaster of Paris spica. The regimen thereafter depends on the preference of the treating surgeon. In general terms, hip abduction is maintained either by a plaster cast or splint until there is evidence of satisfactory bony

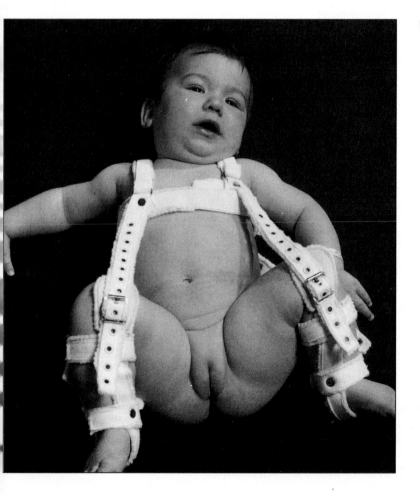

Figure 10.2 The Pavlik harness.

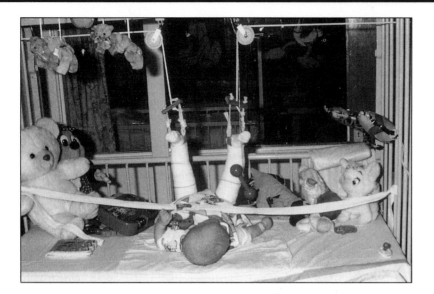

Figure 10.3 Gallows traction.

remodelling of the joint on the X-ray film. Plaster casts are changed at intervals depending on the rate of growth of the infant, with short periods of physiotherapy at the time of admission for plaster change. Stiffness is more likely to be a problem after open rather than closed reduction.

Additional operative procedures may be required in an older infant when there is less potential for bony remodelling following reduction of a dislocation. It may be elected to correct either the excessive femoral anteversion or the dysplasia of the acetabulum to improve the stability of the reduction while the leg is in the weight-bearing functional position. This reduces the need for prolonged splintage in abduction and flexion. The anteversion is corrected by de-rotation osteotomy of the proximal femur (Figure 10.4A and B), and the acetabular dysplasia by a pelvic osteotomy (Figure 10.5A and B) (Salter, 1961). After such surgery, the child is immobilised in a plaster spica for 6 weeks until the osteotomy has united, and then requires physiotherapy to assist progressive mobilisation. In the very occasional case presenting after 3 years of age, both the femoral anteversion and acetabular dysplasia may require surgical correction. The whole correction can be performed at one operation but there is an increased risk of postoperative joint stiffness.

Very occasionally, a patient may present for the first time during adolescence with a limp or discomfort in the hip due to subluxation and acetabular dysplasia (Figure 10.6). If the subluxation is irreducible, as is frequently the case at this age, the position is accepted and the cover of the femoral head improved with a pelvic osteotomy. At this age a Chiari osteotomy is appropriate, dividing the ilium immediately above the level of the head and displacing the lower fragment with the head medially under the cover of the upper fragment. The superior joint capsule remains between the articular surface of the femoral head and the exposed bone of the osteotomy surface (Chiari, 1974). Unlike the Salter osteotomy performed at a younger age, this does not place normal articular cartilage over the head, and is therefore regarded as a salvage rather than a recon-

structive operation. Sometimes a bony shelf is constructed over the femoral head rather than performing the Chiari osteotomy. After a period of immobilisation in plaster to allow the osteotomy to unite, the patient requires physiotherapy to mobilise the joint and to strengthen the abductor and extensor muscles.

PHYSIOTHERAPY

Physiotherapy has only a small part to play in the early stages of the treatment, dealing with the application of splints mentioned previously. As with all treatments, careful assessment should be made, looking for clinical signs such as limited range of abduction and apparent inequality of limb length.

Should splintage not achieve its objectives, or if the infant has been diagnosed after 6 months of age, it will be necessary for the infant to be treated as an in-patient. They will be on traction for 2 weeks, and during this time the physiotherapist will gain the co-operation of the patient. The infant is encouraged to perform active movements of the feet and isometric contractions of the feet and gluteal muscles. Treatment will take the form of play, and parents and nurses should be encouraged to attempt to achieve this aim during their stay with the patient. When reduction of the hip has been achieved, the infant is immobilised in a plaster of Paris double hip spica.

Further physiotherapy is undertaken after a variable period depending on the hip anatomy and the surgeon's preference. Once the plaster spica is bivalved following a 'closed reduction' of the hip, the infant is fitted with a removable flexion–abduction hip splint usually incorporating plastic thigh cuffs (Figure 10.7). This allows movement of the hip within a constrained arc of flexion and abduction, enhancing remodelling of the hip with growth. It is important to remember that before applying the splint it must be moulded around the hip to avoid extreme abduction, ensuring that the blood supply to the head of the femur is not impaired. The infant takes a few days to adjust to the splint, during which

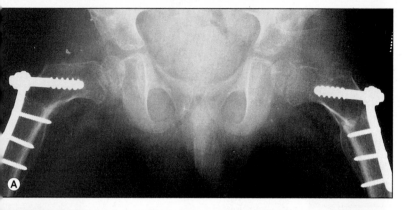

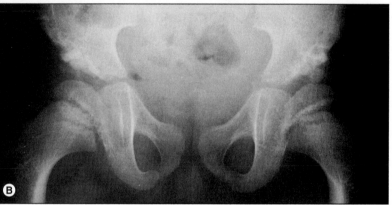

Figure 10.4 (A) Open reduction with additional femoral derotation osteotomy bilaterally to correct the anteversion (same patient as Figure 10.1). (B) The surgical plates and screws have been removed and the acetabula are slowly remodelling as the child grows.

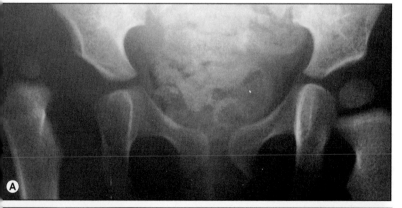

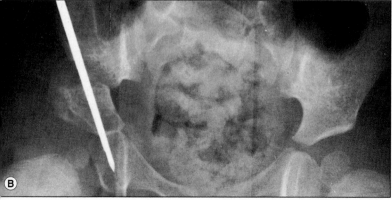

Figure 10.5 (A) Unilateral hip dislocation in a 22-month-old child. (B) The same child, following combined open reduction of the limb dislocation and a Salter pelvic osteotomy which turns the acetabulum over the reduced femoral head.

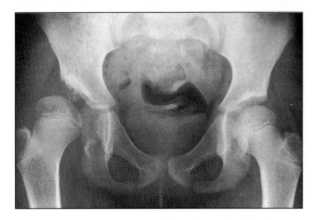

Figure 10.6 An adolescent presenting with unilateral subluxation and acetabular dysplasia.

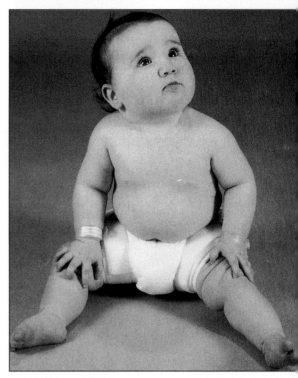

Figure 10.7 Baby with flexion-abduction splint applied to encourage acetabular remodelling during growth following a closed reduction.

time gentle active movements of the knees and ankles are encouraged. Careful positioning on pillows, with the infant alternating between supination and pronation, gives greater comfort and a more contented patient. Gradually, over a few days, the infant learns to sit unaided. The parents are advised on handling, and care of the skin within the splint. The period of splintage depends on the surgeon and the radiological appearance of the acetabular remodelling.

On removing the plaster spica after an 'open reduction', exercises are commenced to regain mobility of the hips and knees, combined with muscle strengthening, especially of the gluteals. Wherever possible, mobilisation should include hydrotherapy. A gradual weaning out of the plaster halves will take about 10 days. Weight bearing is commenced once the hips and knees are mobile and have active control. It is important to discourage any asymmetry of gait which, if left uncorrected, may become habitual.

PERTHES' DISEASE

EPIDEMIOLOGY

Perthes' disease is a transient ischaemic necrosis of the capital femoral epiphysis which occurs in children between the ages of 2 and 12 years, but mainly between 4 and 8 years of age. Males are affected four times more frequently than females, and the condition is bilateral in about 12% of affected children. It was described almost simultaneously at the beginning of the 20th century by Legg from the USA, Calvé from France and Perthes from Germany. There is no obvious pattern of inheritance. Many children appear to be undersized and skeletally immature at the time of developing Perthes' disease. There is also a slightly higher incidence of minor congenital anomalies in these children compared with a control population. Many have abnormal blood coagulation. It is speculated that there may be a congenital abnormality affecting skeletal development which in some way makes the hip susceptible to Perthes' disease. The precise aetiology, however, is unknown.

PATHOLOGY

The pathological process involves bone necrosis of part or the whole of the capital femoral epiphysis followed by gradual revascularisation. The articular cartilage is normal or, at most, shows faint signs of degeneration in its basilar layers. At an early stage, an X-ray film will show flattening and increased density of the femoral head (Figure 10.8A). On microscopic examination there is pronounced necrosis of the bone with grossly distorted marrow trabeculae, and the bone fragments are of a soft consistency. Later, the X-ray film seems to show the femoral head broken up into areas that are comparatively dense, interspersed with areas of radiolucency. This represents the resorption of the dead bone with added areas of osteoid and new bone. The femoral head may become distorted, flattened and extruded laterally from its normal location under the acetabulum. There is a gradual increase in the amount of living bone and on the X-ray film the femoral head usually regains its homogeneous density over 2–4 years. In the meantime, it may lose its normal spherical shape and become flattened superiorly. This is important as the final shape of the head influences the long-term prognosis of the joint. If the head remains spherical, even if it is slightly larger, the prognosis is good. Increasing loss of sphericity and congruity predispose to a proportionate increase in the severity of secondary osteoarthritis during adult life (Lloyd-Roberts & Ratliff, 1978).

CLINICAL PRESENTATION

The most frequently observed symptom is a limp, which may or may not be associated with pain in the groin and inner thigh. Occasionally the pain may be referred to the distal thigh and knee. Muscle spasm is usually present and limits abduction and internal rotation of the hip. The absence of pyrexia, with normal haematological investigations, excludes the differential diagnosis of pyogenic arthritis or osteomyelitis of the femoral neck.

TREATMENT

Perthes' disease is a self-limiting condition, and all affected femoral heads heal. The objective of treatment is therefore to try to minimise the deformity during the active stages of the disease to reduce the incidence of osteoarthritis during adult life. The age of onset of the condition, and the amount of femoral head involved, seem to be the two major prognostic factors. Children under 5 years of age usually do very well, especially if the femoral head is only partly necrotic. However, onset after 5 years of age has a less favourable prognosis. When the child first presents, it is generally agreed that the appropriate treatment consists of bed rest and skin traction to relieve the muscle spasm and regain the range of hip motion. The majority of children will have regained full abduction and internal rotation after 2–3 weeks' treatment. The management thereafter varies widely throughout the world. There has been a general trend to try to select the appropriate cases which will benefit from further treatment. For example, the prognosis for presentation under 4 years of age with partial head involvement, and without lateral displacement of the head, is excellent and does not justify the imposition of restricted activities or surgical intervention.

Although there are many different specific methods of managing Perthes' disease, there are two basic treatment principles. These may be applied individually or in combination. The first principle is weight relief and the second is containment. The latter principle refers to the fact that if the femoral head can be maintained deeply within the acetabulum during the soft vulnerable phase of the disease process, the acetabulum will function rather like a mould, and a more normal femoral head will result. Since it is the lateral portion of the capital epiphysis which becomes uncovered, the containment can be achieved by abduction of the hip (Figure 10.8B).

Non-weight-bearing treatment includes bed rest with or without traction, and was traditionally applied on a Robert Jones frame. Bed rest for longer than is necessary to regain motion in the hips is now no longer considered practical. Weight relief is also achieved with a Snyder sling or with ischial weight-bearing braces. The hip usually remains adducted and the results of treatment are inferior to those of containment methods. There are several methods of treatment which rely on containment of the femoral head but allow weight bearing. These include plaster casts to maintain the abduction and internal rotation, so-called broomstick or Petrie plasters (Figure 10.9), abduction splints and surgical intervention.

Surgical containment of the femoral head can be produced either by a proximal femoral varus osteotomy (Figure 10.10), or by altering the acetabulum to provide further lateral coverage. The acetabulum may be redirected by a Salter osteotomy, or its cover enlarged by a bone graft (Shelf operation). Surgery is more often needed when the prognosis indicates that the healing phase may be prolonged, as in older children. It can also be used for patients who will not tolerate a bracing programme. The range of movement must be almost normal before surgical treatment.

PHYSIOTHERAPY

If bed rest is advised as a method of symptomatic treatment, an assessment of the range of hip movements is necessary, as frequently there is limitation of abduction and internal rotation due to muscle spasm. Bed rest will relieve this over 2 weeks and therefore the range of movement will be regained. Static exercises are taught, especially for the quadriceps and gluteals. Hydrotherapy may be of value after the first week of bed rest to regain movement, maintain strength, gradually introduce weight bearing and retrain gait.

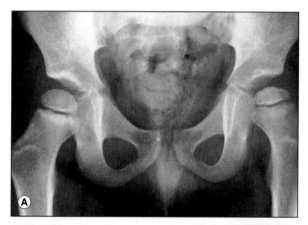

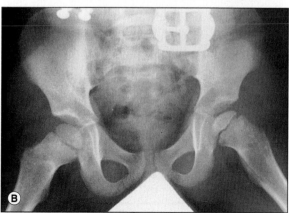

Figure 10.8 (A) Early flattening and displacement of the femoral head (right side of illustration) due to Perthes' disease. (B) Femoral head 'contained' in the acetabulum by abduction.

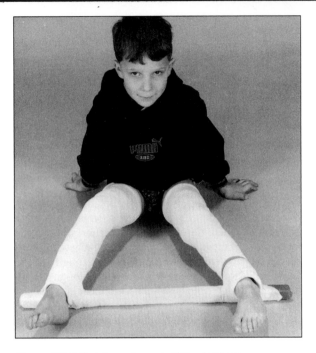

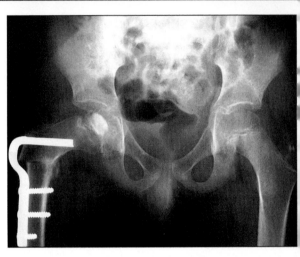

Figure 10.10 Perthes' disease presenting with a dense infarcted capital epiphysis which has been treated by femoral varus osteotomy.

Figure 10.9 Petrie or broomstick plasters.

One method of treatment is the application of Petrie plasters (see Figure 10.9). These are long leg plaster cylinders, keeping the knees flexed approximately 15°. By attaching a broomstick at the lower ends of the plaster cylinders, with the hips abducted 30° and internally rotated 20°, containment is achieved. This method does not allow reciprocal hip flexion and the child has to be taught to stand in the plasters, eventually becoming reasonably independent. Such children are admitted at regular intervals, when the plaster is removed for a period of hip and knee mobilisation. Hydrotherapy has proved invaluable at this time. Once a full range of movement at the hip and knee has been regained, the plasters are re-applied and the child discharged. This process is repeated until, based on radiological findings, adequate healing has occurred.

Following surgical intervention, either after a femoral osteotomy or a Shelf procedure, the child usually spends 6 weeks in a double hip spica. The child is discharged home for this period. On readmission, the plaster is bivalved and the child weaned out of it over a few days, gaining hip and knee joint ranges and increasing muscle power. Weight bearing is commenced when there is adequate strength and control of the leg.

SLIPPED UPPER FEMORAL EPIPHYSIS

This term refers to displacement of the femoral neck in relation to the head, usually during adolescence. The femoral neck rotates externally and slides upwards, causing the radiological appearance of a femoral head which is displaced posteriorly and inferiorly (Figure 10.11A).

EPIDEMIOLOGY

Males are more frequently affected than females, and because of the delayed growth spurt in boys the condition occurs on average about 2 years later than in girls. The age range for boys is 10–17 years, with an average of 11–12 years. The black population is apparently more frequently affected than the white population. The skeletal age is usually below chronological age, and approximately half the patients have body weight at or above the 95th percentile. The condition occurs bilaterally in approximately one fifth of cases. There is occasionally a positive family history of the condition.

AETIOLOGY

The precise aetiology is still unknown. The plane of separation is at the bone–cartilage junction of the growth plate and it is thought that there may be increased structural weakness at this site during the adolescent growth spurt. There are some interesting mechanical factors which have been observed. The growth plate normally changes from a horizontal to an oblique position during the early adolescent period, and the periosteum of the femoral neck, which is the main stabiliser of the epiphysis, atrophies at the same time. In addition, there may be hormonal factors which relate to the balance of pituitary growth hormone and sex hormones. The sex hormones induce growth-plate closure at skeletal maturity, and growth hormone stimulates the proliferation of the cells of the growth plate. A frequent condition associated with a slipped epiphysis is the adiposo-genital syndrome, a condition characterised by obesity and deficient gonadal development, which suggests that the slip may be due to excessive loading of the comparatively weak growth

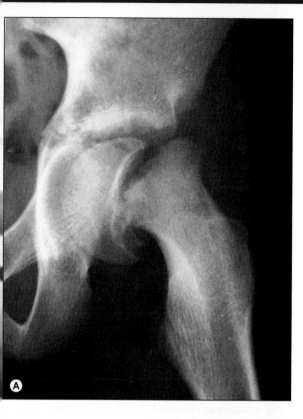

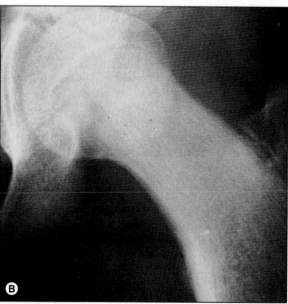

Figure 10.11 (A) Slipped upper femoral epiphysis which occurred suddenly after a history of an ache and occasional limp. (B) Improved position of the epiphysis as the result of skin traction applied with progressive abduction and internal rotation of the hip.

plate. Less frequently, it occurs in a very tall, thin boy, which may indicate a relative excess of growth hormone and weakness of the rapidly proliferating growth plate. When the slip is bilateral and symmetrical, other conditions such as hypothyroidism should be excluded.

CLINICAL PRESENTATION

There are three classic presentations. These are:
- The acute slip. This is the result of significant injury with no previous history of pain. It is usually severe enough to prevent weight bearing.
- The acute on chronic slip. This presents with some aching in the hip or distal thigh for weeks or even months before an acute episode (see Figure 10.11A).
- The chronic slip. This is the commonest presentation, the child complaining of a limp, pain and loss of motion which may have been present for several weeks (Figure 10.12A). Occasionally, the only symptom is pain referred to the knee.

Examination reveals restriction of internal rotation and abduction, and as the thigh is flexed it tends to roll into external rotation and abduction. There is frequent shortening of the leg, which tends to lie in external rotation. X-ray examination will confirm the diagnosis and indicate the severity of the displacement. In chronic cases there is remodelling of the inferior and posterior aspects of the femoral neck adjacent to the growth plate, which begins to develop a slight hook. The opposite hip should be examined carefully for early involvement, which may simply be a widening of the epiphyseal line.

TREATMENT

Once the diagnosis has been made, the child should not be allowed to weight bear, and arrangements should be made to admit the child to hospital for treatment directly. This is to prevent any further displacement. The child is placed in bed with skin traction on both legs to reduce spasm and relieve discomfort.

If the slip is acute, the displacement can be corrected with skin traction by slowly and progressively abducting and internally rotating the leg (Figure 10.11B). Alternatively, the reduction can be achieved by gentle manipulation under general anaesthesia. If the acute slip has been present for more than a day, there is considerable risk of avascular necrosis from manipulation, and because of this problem, opinions are divided as to whether manipulative treatment should be used at all. If an acute slip has occurred on a pre-existing chronic slip, it is important that the repositioning only reduces the acute aspect of the slip. The greater threat to the hip is avascular necrosis, and not incomplete reduction. Further displacement is prevented by surgical insertion of pins or a screw along the femoral neck into the epiphysis.

The objective of treatment in the child with a chronic slip is to stabilise the femoral head *in situ* and maintain the range of motion. Further displacement is prevented by

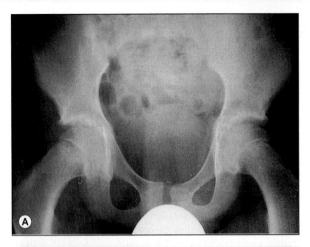

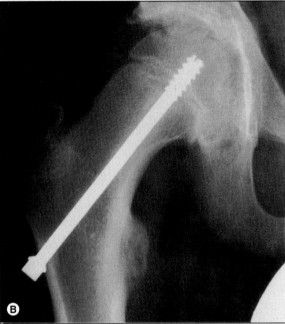

Figure 10.12 (A) A chronic slip of the capital epiphysis (left side of the radiograph). The growth plate is widened and the epiphysis displaced slightly. **(B)** Surgical fixation of the epiphysis.

operative insertion of pins or a screw along the femoral neck into the epiphysis (Figure 10.12B). In cases with severe displacement, this may be technically very difficult. Operations have been devised either to correct the displacement at the level of the open growth plate (Dunn's osteotomy) (Dunn & Angel, 1978) or to compensate for the deformity with a subtrochanteric osteotomy (Southwick, 1976). There seems to be an increased risk of avascular necrosis with the former procedure and chondrolysis with the latter.

If the opposite hip shows widening of the growth plate, or early slip, it should also be fixed. There is debate as to whether prophylactic fixation of the contralateral hip

should be undertaken routinely. As surgery can be associated with complications, it is probably better reserved for selected cases such as those with predisposing hormonal abnormalities or with femoral neck retroversion.

The main complications of this condition and its treatment are avascular necrosis and chondrolysis. Avascular necrosis occurs as a result of tension and occlusion of the retinacular vessels passing along the femoral neck to the capital epiphysis. This causes necrosis and collapse of the femoral head with loss of sphericity. The potential for retaining a spherical head is very much poorer at this age than in young children with Perthes' disease, and usually results in secondary osteoarthritis during early adult life. Chondrolysis presents with acute pain and restricted motion of the hip joint. The precise cause is not known. There is loss of articular cartilage, which is later replaced by fibrocartilage—this does not have the same properties of wear, and predisposes to secondary osteoarthritis. The initial treatment is to try to reduce the joint reaction with traction and anti-inflammatory medication and to retain a range of motion with physiotherapy. This is followed by a prolonged period of non-weight bearing and motion exercises. Despite this treatment, the range of motion may be very limited. The natural history of even the most severe slips is that they do well into middle life before the development of osteoarthritis, if there has been no avascular necrosis or chondrolysis. This therefore suggests that simple methods of treatment that decrease or eliminate the risk of avascular necrosis or chondrolysis should be used most commonly.

After fixation of the femoral epiphysis, the patient is encouraged to regain active control of the hip and, in particular, the ranges of abduction and internal rotation. When this has been achieved, the patient is allowed to partially weight bear with the aid of crutches; the decision when to allow full weight bearing will vary according to the degree of displacement and security of fixation. The growth plate usually fuses prematurely, which prevents any further possibility of displacement, and it is usual to remove the metal at this stage.

PHYSIOTHERAPY

After surgery it is important to commence early active assisted movements to the hip to regain, in particular, the ranges of abduction and internal rotation. Gradually over a few days the child will achieve active control and then is allowed to partially weight bear with crutches.

In cases with severe displacement, following surgery, e.g. Dunn's osteotomy, the child may require a longer period of bed rest, such as on slings and springs. During this period it is important that the child continues with exercises to increase and maintain a full range of movement of the affected hip. Isometric exercises to the muscles around the hip and to the quadriceps are taught. During treatment it is necessary to exercise the sound hip. Very occasionally this epiphysis may slip and, as the result of handling the patient on several occasions, it is often the physiotherapist who first detects this.

COXA VARA

Coxa vara is an abnormality of the proximal end of the femur which is characterised by a decrease in the neck shaft angle. This angle normally measures approximately 150° at 1 year of age and gradually decreases to 120° in the adult. A neck shaft angle of less than 120° in a child is arbitrarily labelled as coxa vara.

ETIOLOGY

There are many different causes of coxa vara. Infantile coxa vara is regarded as a distinct entity and is characterised by a triangular bone defect in the inferior part of the metaphysis of the femoral neck (Figure 10.13). It is sometimes bilateral but is not associated with any other developmental defect. Several reports of a family history suggest that the condition has a genetic transmission.

Other focal forms of coxa vara include children with a congenital short femur, which may sometimes be associated with lateral bowing of the proximal femoral shaft and sclerosis on the concave side (Figure 10.14). In the more severe forms, a pseudarthrosis may be present between the femoral neck and shaft, and this is known as proximal focal femoral deficiency. Other causes of coxa vara include any skeletal disorder or dysplasia which results in softening or weakening of the bones. Examples include osteogenesis imperfecta and metaphyseal chondrodysplasia.

CLINICAL PRESENTATION

In infantile coxa vara, the deformity is diagnosed when the child first walks—usually with a painless limp or waddling gait. The Trendelenburg test is positive and hip abduction limited. The greater trochanter is elevated sometimes, so that the tip of the trochanter impinges upon the ilium, resulting in profound gluteal deficiency. In unilateral cases there is usually a leg length discrepancy.

TREATMENT

Treatment depends on the degree of deformity, the functional impairment and evidence as to whether the deformity is progressive. Conservative treatment may be employed in mild cases where the varus deformity is not progressing and the neck shaft angle approaches normal. However, in the majority of patients with the infantile variety of coxa vara, early surgery provides the best opportunity to achieve a painless and fully mobile hip without further shortening of the limb. The indications for surgery are the presence of a vertical defect in the femoral neck, a neck shaft angle of less than 100° and progression of the coxa vara, which may or may not be associated with discomfort. An intertrochanteric or subtrochanteric valgus osteotomy accompanied by internal fixation is the preferred form of treatment (see Figure 10.13). The goal of surgery is to place the proximal femoral growth plate in a normal alignment, perpendicular to the resultant weight-bearing force acting across the hip joint. This in turn improves the hip abductor function and reduces the leg length discrepancy. Postoperatively, a plaster spica is applied for approximately

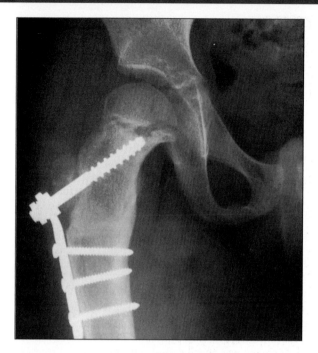

Figure 10.13 Bilateral coxa vara which has been corrected on one side by a valgus osteotomy. On the other side, the triangular bone defect persists at the inferior margin of the metaphysis.

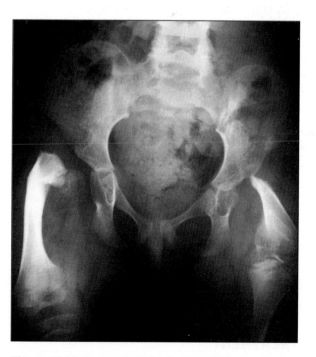

Figure 10.14 Congenital shortening of the femur with coxa vara. On the opposite side there is congenital absence of the femoral head and proximal shaft.

6 weeks until the osteotomy has united. Mobilising and strengthening exercises are prescribed.

PHYSIOTHERAPY

After surgery the patient is immobilised in a plaster spica for 6 weeks. After this time the plaster is bivalved, and gentle active exercises are undertaken to mobilise the hip and knee joints. Hydrotherapy and strengthening exercises are introduced, with particular attention to strengthening the hip abductors and achieving hip abduction range. Often, the posterior part of the plaster is retained as a night splint until the patient is able to control active leg movements adequately. Weight bearing is started as soon as union of the osteotomy is confirmed by X-ray films and the patient is able to control the limb fully. Gait re-education may be necessary.

INEQUALITY OF LEG LENGTH

AETIOLOGY

The problem of leg length discrepancy is common despite the fact that the aetiological factors have changed considerably during the past 30 years. Before the advent of poliomyelitis vaccine, the most common cause of shortening was muscle paralysis from the polio. Other causes of leg length discrepancy have now assumed greater importance. These may result in either shortening or lengthening of a limb. A short leg may be caused by a congenital abnormality (Figure 10.15A and B), infection of the bone and joint, and fractures of the long bones, especially those which result in damage and tethering of the growth plate. Neurological conditions such as spinal dysraphism and spastic hemiparesis may also cause shortening. Overgrowth of a limb may be associated with haemangioma or arteriovenous malformation, neurofibromatosis and fibrous dysplasia. Rarely, significant overgrowth may occur due to stimulation of bone growth after fracture of the femur or tibia, or the stimulus of osteotomy and subsequent plate removal.

CLINICAL PRESENTATION

The child may present with a limp and other symptoms or signs which relate to the aetiology. The inequality of leg length does not cause pain. When standing with both feet flat on the floor, there is a pelvic obliquity and compensatory scoliosis, without symptoms, which the child tolerates (see Figure 10.15A). Alternatively, the child may stand with a level pelvis either by flexing the knee on the longer leg or by weight bearing on the forefoot of the shorter leg. If the condition is not associated with weakness, the gait may seem remarkably normal. The child frequently vaults on the forefoot of the short leg to compensate for the discrepancy.

TREATMENT

The degree of discrepancy is the most significant factor in deciding the management. Differences of less than 2 cm are usually accepted by the patient and can be treated by non-surgical methods, e.g. shoe raise. At the other end

of the scale, any projected inequality exceeding 20 cm usually in excess of the amount that any combination operations can be employed to equalise effectively or pr dictably. These cases usually require the application of prosthesis. For the most part therefore, only discrepan cies between 2 and 20 cm warrant serious consideratio of surgical equalisation. These are not rigid values b

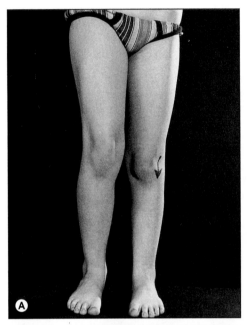

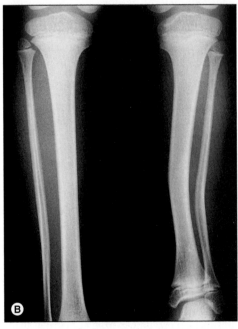

Figure 10.15 (A) Inequality of leg length. The child stands with pelvic obliquity and compensatory scoliosis. **(B)** Radiograph showing the short and slightly bowed tibia and fibula.

they represent practical guidelines which may be modified by the many other factors involved in the aetiology. It is assumed for the purpose of the following discussion that the problem is a true discrepancy of length rather than an apparent shortening or lengthening of the limb produced by a fixed adduction or abduction contracture, respectively, at the hip.

In addition to the severity of the discrepancy, the other factors which influence the nature and timing of treatment include the skeletal age, anticipated adult height and sex. The progression of discrepancy can be measured accurately by taking serial X-ray films or CT scans. These also allow assessment of the relative discrepancy within the femur and tibia. Serial X-ray films of the hand will allow an assessment of bone age and development, which may precede or lag behind chronological age by up to 2 years. Serial measurement of height on a percentile chart will allow prediction of the anticipated adult height. These measurements are important to help decide the most appropriate treatment, and to monitor its effect if started before skeletal maturity.

Surgical equalisation of limb length can be achieved by either shortening the long side, lengthening the short side or a combination of shortening and lengthening.

A limb can be shortened in one of three ways:

- The growth plate of the distal femur and/or the proximal tibia and fibula can be arrested prematurely by epiphyseodesis (Phemister, 1933).
- The same centres can be arrested temporarily or permanently by epiphyseal stapling (Blount, 1958).
- The femur or tibia can be shortened by resection of bone.

Epiphyseodesis is performed on the longer leg at an appropriate time before skeletal maturity, and if successful, the shorter limb continues to grow and will exactly correct the discrepancy by the completion of growth. It is critical to time the operation correctly, and this depends on the information gained from serial pre-operative grid films and bone age assessment. Epiphyseodesis is usually reserved for discrepancies not exceeding 5 cm. It is now a relatively simple operation involving drilling the growth plate under X-ray guidance. The operation is without significant complications,

and the rate of acceptable correction is high. Stapling of the epiphysis has a similar effect, and convalescence is more rapid. Theoretically, the principal advantage that this operation offers over epiphyseodesis is that it can be reversed by removal of the staples if overcorrection is occurring. However, experience has shown that the response of the growth plate to staple removal is not predictable and the reliability of this procedure is not really proved. The operation is also technically demanding, and if the staples are not inserted in precisely the correct manner there is a risk of producing asymmetrical growth arrest and deformity. Unlike the former two procedures, bone-shortening operations can be performed after completion of growth. Up to 6 cm of bone can be resected from the femur without causing permanent weakening of the limb. Shortening below the knee requires resection of a portion of the tibia and fibula. These operations are usually associated with internal fixation of the bone fragments.

Correction of inequality can also be achieved by lengthening of bone. The current techniques of lengthening apply the principles of division of the bone while retaining soft tissue continuity, especially of the periosteum (corticotomy), and delaying distraction for 7 to 10 days to allow formation of early callus (callotasis). Distraction is undertaken by adjusting the external fixator at the rate of 1 mm per day until the desired length is achieved. For most discrepancies, electromyographic study of the lengthened muscles indicates that a 10% lengthening of the bone's initial length is a safe limit, with 15% being the absolute maximum. Slow lengthening protects the soft tissues, in particular the peripheral nerves, and during distraction, daily clinical assessment should be performed to detect early neuropraxia. If present, further distraction is temporarily discontinued until nerve function has recovered, and then further gradual lengthening is usually possible until the desired length is achieved (Figure 10.16). Clinical guidelines helpful in governing the rate of distraction are the degree of pain, the development of sensory or motor neurological deficit, alterations in local circulation, and any significant elevation of the diastolic blood pressure. Once the desired length is achieved, the fixator is locked until the newly formed bone

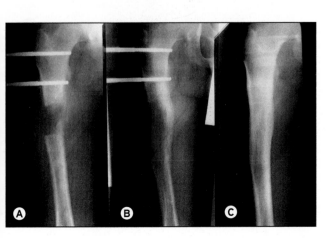

Figure 10.16 X-rays of a femur showing it (A) being lengthened by an external fixator; (B) the desired length has been achieved; and (C) the bone has consolidated and the fixator removed.

strengthens sufficiently to allow removal of the fixator. This usually takes at least 3 months. With a monolateral fixator, the new bone can be allowed to take axial loading while still protected for angular loads for the last 2 months (dynamisation). Circumferential fixators, e.g. the Ilizarov, are less rigid and do not require this feature. They are also more versatile for correcting deformity at the same time as lengthening.

The lengthening operations are more extensive surgical interventions than the shortening operations, and are accompanied by greater morbidity. Lengthening is therefore reserved for patients who either have a short stature and would be unsuitable for shortening, or have a discrepancy which cannot reasonably be corrected by shortening procedures alone.

There is one situation where the cause of discrepancy may be remedied. Following a fracture across the germinal layer of the growth plate, a bony tether sometimes forms between the epiphysis and metaphysis. This retards growth, and if the tether is not central it causes angular deformity. An operation may be performed to resect the bony bridge or tether. This operation was first described by Langenskiold (1981). The surgical defect created is then filled with inert material, e.g. a fat plug or bone cement, to prevent the bone from growing into the defect and retethering the growth plate (Figure 10.17A). Minor angular deformities will correct spontaneously with further growth (Figure 10.17B), and the operation may be of benefit for tethers which affect up to 40% of the growth plate. After this procedure, the leg is initially protected in a plaster. Subsequently, physiotherapy is required to mobilise and strengthen the limb. A brace is sometimes applied to protect the leg until the weakened area of bone has remodelled.

PHYSIOTHERAPY
Leg Shortening
Following epiphyseodesis, the patient is immobilised in a removable knee-extension splint. This allows the physiotherapist to begin active knee flexion on the second postoperative day, together with static quadriceps exercises. This splint is worn at all times other than during physiotherapy sessions. As soon as the patient has achieved 90° of knee flexion and is able to straight leg raise, they may partially weight bear with crutches with the knee splint applied. The patient is taught to continue the exercises at home twice a day, maintaining 90° of knee flexion. The patient returns to the clinic 4 weeks postoperatively, when the knee immobiliser is removed permanently. If the knee flexion has not been maintained at 90°, then a period of out-patient physiotherapy will be necessary.

It is important to point out to the child and parents that at the end of the 4 weeks the limb length will be the same as pre-operatively and a shoe raise, if worn previously, will still be necessary. Gradually the size of the raise will be reduced as the discrepancy becomes less. This occurs until growth has been completed.

Leg shortening can also be achieved by simple bone resection of the femur or tibia, with internal fixation.

Immediately following femoral shortening, a system of slings and springs may be applied to both legs to relieve any muscle spasm and encourage free movements. These are used for approximately 5 days and then discarded as more intensive physiotherapy is given. Gradually the patient is taught non-weight bearing on crutches. Most patients require non-weight bearing for a month, followed by a further month of partial weight bearing, by which stage the osteotomy will have united sufficiently to allow full weight bearing. An active exercise programme is then prescribed— for example, to strengthen the thigh muscles after femoral shortening to correct the quadriceps lag.

Leg Lengthening
This is carried out by means of a distraction device. Close observation of the limb is of vital importance postoperatively, and the physiotherapist should be aware of the complications, e.g. interference with the nerve supply to the limb. Immediately postoperatively, a graduated programme of active exercises is begun and continued, especially during the period of lengthening. Intensive physiotherapy is necessary to stretch the soft tissues around the site and to maintain the length of the surrounding muscles parallel with the bone length.

During lengthening of the tibia, the posterior tibial group of muscles must be stretched frequently, to prevent a secondary equinus deformity of the foot. A full-length night splint with the foot included should be worn throughout the lengthening period to help maintain full knee extension and a plantigrade foot.

With the callotasis techniques of lengthening, the patient is encouraged to weight bear with the aid of crutches. A programme of regular home exercises is given to each patient, and the importance of compliance emphasised. The patients are monitored regularly in clinics.

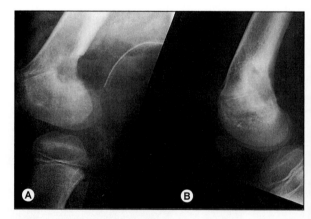

Figure 10.17 (A) Postoperative appearance following resection of a bony tether. (B) The appearance 9 months later showing continued growth of the femur and realignment of the growth plate to a more transverse position.

REFERENCES

Barlow TG. Early diagnosis and treatment of congenital dislocation of the hip. *J Bone Joint Surg* 1962, **44B**:292-301.

Blount WP. Unequal leg length in children. *Surg Clin North Am* 1958, **38**:1107-1123.

Chiari K. Medial displacement osteotomy of the pelvis. *Clin Orthop Rel Res* 1974, B:55-71.

Dunn DM, Angel JC. Replacement of the femoral head by open operation in severe adolescent slipping of the upper femoral epiphysis. *J Bone Joint Surg* 1978, OB:394-403.

Eeply RF, Weiner DS. Treatment of congenital dysplasia-subluxation of the hip in children under one year of age. *J Paed Orthop* 1981, 1:413-418.

Langenskiold A. Surgical treatment of partial closure of the growth plate. *J Paed Orthop* 1981, 1:3-11.

Lloyd-Roberts GC, Ratliff AHC. *Hip disorders in children*. London: Butterworths; 1978.

Phemister DB. Operative arrestment of longitudinal growth of bones in the treatment of deformities. *J Bone Joint Surg* 1933, **15**:1-15.

Salter RB. Innominate osteotomy in the treatment of congenital dislocation and subluxation of the hip. *J Bone Joint Surg* 1961, **43B**:518-539.

Southwick WO. Osteotomy through the lesser trochanter for slipped capital femoral epiphysis. *J Bone Joint Surg* 1967, **49A**:807-835.

Wynne-Davies R. *Heritable disorders in orthopaedic practice*. Oxford: Blackwell Scientific; 1973.

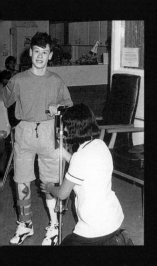

11 R Jones & A Roberts

GAIT PROBLEMS IN CEREBRAL PALSY

CHAPTER OUTLINE

- **The child with cerebral palsy**
- **Gait analysis**
- **Formulating a treatment programme**

- **Monitoring the result**
- **Physiotherapy**

INTRODUCTION

Cerebral palsy is a constellation of conditions resulting from a fixed injury of the central nervous system (CNS) associated with a significant amount of remaining growth. A hemiplegia in an adolescent will not differ greatly from an ischaemic stroke in an elderly person. However, the clinical picture produced by an identical injury sustained at birth is very different, with torsional skeletal deformities and contractures, which are impossible to correct even with intensive physiotherapy. In the child, the physiotherapist is often struggling to maintain ranges of movement against growth. There is certainly development occurring in the child's injured brain, and education of posture, balance and movement are all worthwhile. There comes a point, however, when physiotherapy is struggling against increasing contracture during the adolescent growth spurt, with little prospect of success. Then, the application of a carefully planned surgery–physiotherapy package can remove contractures and enable further maintenance physiotherapy.

THE CHILD WITH CEREBRAL PALSY

WHO BENEFITS FROM SURGERY?

Before commencing any treatment in a child with cerebral palsy, it is important to establish a reasonable objective and then formulate a plan to achieve that objective. In deciding whether to offer such patients a complicated series of procedures for total correction of the lower limbs, followed by a programme of rehabilitation, a mental checklist needs to be consulted to identify potential problems that may limit or prevent success (Table 11.1).

Spastic cerebral palsy produces deformity by preventing the normal growth of muscle by movement and stretching. The epiphyseal plates in the long bones are not affected by this, and skeletal growth leads to increasing contracture in the limbs. The velocity of skeletal growth equates with the rapidity of onset of tightness and deformity. Clearly, if corrective surgery to the soft tissues and skeleton is undertaken too early, further growth will lead to the development of more deformity, and repeat soft tissue surgery needs to be avoided wherever possible as it leads to weakness and scarring. There are occasions where surgery has to be performed in the young infant. In such cases, temporising measures, e.g. injections of phenol and botulinum toxin, may be used to enable a physiotherapy programme of stretching. In addition to contracture and deformity, growth disturbs the child's power-to-weight ratio. This is high in the infant, tailing off as weight increases with the cubed power of height while strength increases as the square of height. This deterioration in the power-to-weight ratio, and the progression of contracture and deformity, stop at skeletal maturity.

	Checklist for correction of lower limb abnormalities	
	Criteria	**Optimal situation**
A	Age	Only during the adolescent growth spurt
B	Balance	Must be able to high kneel
C	Cognition	Must be able to understand instructions for physiotherapy and be able to follow the reasoning behind the physiotherapy programme
D	Disability	Must have sufficient strength and control that when joints are realigned and the soft tissues released the child would be able to benefit from surgery
E	Emotion	Must be sufficiently mature to be able to undergo the stress involved in extensive surgery and rehabilitation, which may last up to a year

Table 11.1 Checklist when considering a child with cerebral palsy for correction of lower limb abnormalities.

REQUIREMENT FOR BALANCE

No matter how satisfactory the child's muscle control, if the child lacks balance control he or she will be limited to using a Kaye walker or another restricted appliance, and will not be able to progress to sticks or fully independent mobility. At the very least, the child should be able to balance in a high-kneeling position and be stable. Methods are being developed to enhance and train balance skills in children with cerebral palsy, but these are currently mostly used for the potential sitter rather than the child on the borderline of independent walking.

INTELLECTUAL FUNCTION

Cognition is essential if a child is to gain the maximum benefit from a physiotherapy programme. A mild degree of mental handicap, however, does not necessarily preclude a successful rehabilitation programme, provided there are no adverse emotional features. Where there are doubts regarding a child's ability to co-operate with a rehabilitation programme, an in-patient physiotherapy assessment period can be helpful. This will allow an understanding of the potential for difficulties and establish a working relationship between the physiotherapist, the child and the family.

DISABILITY CONSIDERATIONS

The level of the child's disability must be taken into account when making decisions about surgery. An 8-year-old child with marked knee flexion contractures and hip flexion contractures, coupled with muscle weakness and poor control, is quite possibly not going to be able to walk at skeletal maturity. It is more reasonable to accept this and adopt a strategy which leads to surgery for the ability to use a standing frame and transfer, rather than the child enduring a prolonged programme of surgery aimed at walking, which has little hope of success. Energy consumption

estimations are helpful in identifying those children at very high risk of failure of walking at skeletal maturity (Rose et al., 1989). A physiological cost index of greater than 3. extra heart beats per metre progressed has been suggested as a useful cut-off point above which the child is likely to be unable to walk at skeletal maturity even after surgery (Evans, 1996). Where the levels of disability suggest that walking ability will not be maintained, then the objective of walking should be reconsidered. If a different, achievable objective other than walking is agreed, then surgical treatment can still be undertaken on that basis if necessary.

EMOTIONAL AND BEHAVIOURAL CONSIDERATIONS

Many children with cerebral palsy have a labile personality and do not have the maturity of their normal peers. Epidemiological studies suggest, that compared with age-matched populations of healthy children, a child with cerebral palsy without intellectual handicap will have an approximately fivefold increased incidence of behavioural problems, while a child with intellectual handicap will have an eightfold increased incidence (McDermott, 1996). Not only does this lead to difficulty with compliance while these children are in-patients receiving their rehabilitation, but a difficult family situation may be exacerbated once they are discharged. The psychological effects of complex surgical and rehabilitation programmes have yet to be fully researched in children with cerebral palsy. Again, where problems are anticipated, it is worth arranging for an in-patient assessment period before deciding on surgical treatment.

GAIT ANALYSIS

A clinical assessment and observation of gait are essential. Before admission, all patients will have had a gait analysis giving a complete assessment of the patient's abnormalities.

of gait. After a clinical assessment, the surgeon will be able to treat the orthopaedic problems using the gait analysis information.

The advantage of gait analysis is that it allows a systematic appraisal not possible with the time constraints and equipment of clinics or physiotherapy treatment rooms. It has to be emphasised that the gait analysis is only a component of the assessment. Numbers, tracings and graphs are only of use integrated into a rational treatment package (Figure 11.1).

PARAMETER MEASUREMENT

The perception that gait analysis is a complex and highly technical subject is not strictly correct, as there is a considerable amount of useful information which can be collected with a video camera, tape-measure, stop-watch and some coloured paint applied to the sole. Gait parameters such as velocity, cadence, stride length and step length are derived by timing the patient's progress along a level surface between two markers. Paint applied to the sole of the feet allows the step and stride lengths to be calculated.

Video Recording

A good-quality video camera is invaluable. The ability to replay the videotape frame by frame in either direction is an absolute must. The gait can be examined by viewing and reviewing the taped motion in all three planes, and can be watched many times—long after the patient would have become exhausted. Each joint can be examined in turn and in each of the planes. The main limitation of video recording is that it only gives a two-dimensional representation of a three-dimensional movement; for example, what may seem like a very valgus knee is simply a combination of flexion (sagittal plane) and rotation (transverse plane) in a knee which is in normal alignment in the coronal plane.

Three-Dimensional Analysis

The next stage in sophistication is to record the progress of the limbs in all three dimensions. Several systems are available which allow the position of segments in space to be followed as the limbs move across the laboratory floor. The study of these segment positions and joint angles is known as kinematics. Simply, kinematics documents the position of the levers during gait. A variety of sensing systems use either passive markers to reflect infrared or coloured light back to an array of sensors, or active markers which emit light or radiation. The great weakness of these systems is that they model skeletal movement by extrapolating the position of the joints from the position of markers attached to the patient's skin. Particularly in the thigh and in obese patients, skin movement does not mirror the underlying skeletal movement because of the inertia of the soft tissues and the action of the intervening muscles. Even when a skin marker is ideally placed, there is considerable variation in marker placement, which means that the normal database of joint angles and range is slightly different for each operator, regardless of their experience.

Kinetic Analysis

A final step towards understanding the mechanics of the skeleton is to record the forces it generates. This branch of gait analysis is kinetics. A force platform is necessary for kinetic analysis. A force platform is a sensitive balance which, as a patient walks over it, measures the magnitude, point of application and direction of forces applied. By combining the kinematic and kinetic data, the relation between the levers and the forces is known enabling a calculation of

Figure 11.1 The gait analysis process.

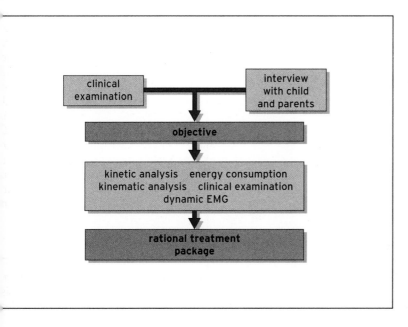

the moments around the joints (Figure 11.2). Further, these data can be combined with the angular acceleration at the joint concerned, to calculate the net power generated or absorbed at that joint. It is tempting to ascribe the power curves to the action of specific muscles, or to believe that the power generated or absorbed is a true reflection of the work being done at a joint. To do this is to misunderstand the limitations of this type of data. Certainly, power and moment graphs give useful data about the function of triceps surae at the ankle and the activity of the hip abductors. Generation of power at the hip, knee and ankle is vital if the patient is to have a means of forward progression. Thus, if a patient lacks power at the hip, caution is needed before surgery is performed at the knee and the ankle which might compound that deficit and immobilise the patient.

The video vector generator is a simplified analysis of the forces acting around joints, and is ideally suited for use by the physiotherapist. The video vector generator superimposes the position of the ground reaction vector on a video image of the patient walking across a force platform, allowing instantaneous visualisation of the relation between the limb and the forces which the body transmits to the ground. The immediacy of the image showing the forces allows the physiotherapist or orthotist to alter an orthotic or splint and then re-record the gait pattern to see if their objective has been met. With time it is possible for the physiotherapist to learn to predict what the forces are likely to be around a

joint and to develop a way of thinking which takes this dimension into account when treating patients.

Dynamic Electromyography

A final common component of a gait analysis in cerebral palsy is a dynamic electromyogram (EMG). This should enable useful analysis of the timing and relative intensity of muscle activity through the gait cycle. Unfortunately, the EMG signal is not quantitative—it is like listening to the roar of a football crowd from outside the stadium; it is possible to tell whether the game is exciting or dull but not what the score is or even who is winning. A dynamic EMG is very helpful in the understanding of the activity of the rectus femoris and gastrocnemius. These muscles pass across two joints where the lack of muscle control in cerebral palsy leads to inappropriate timing of muscle contraction.

ANALYSIS OF THE DATA

Once the child's gait has been assessed, the clinician has to process the information to produce a coherent and practical treatment package. Each clinician practising gait analysis has their own method of arriving at a plan. The method outlined below may suit some individuals but not others.

If walking is the goal, then the child's energy consumption should be checked. If this is within normal limits, then the objective is a cosmetic improvement in gait

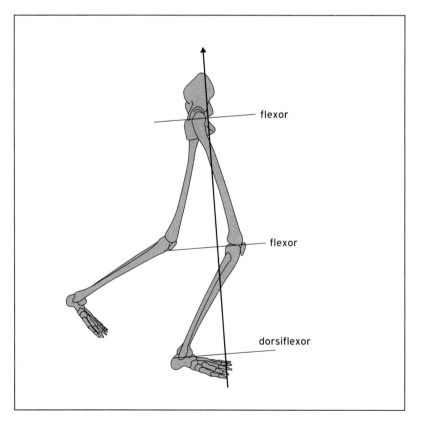

Figure 11.2 Moments around joints.

Those children with high energy consumption, however, have some functional benefit to be gained. Where the energy consumption approaches four times normal, then a very serious reappraisal of the objective should be undertaken as there are limits to what is feasible, and extensive surgery and rehabilitation without eventual benefit is inappropriate.

The next step is to assess the gait abnormalities in each of three planes, working methodically from the lumbar spine down to the toes. Perry (1992) has stated the prerequisites of normal gait and these represent features of the deformity of gait which may be recognised (Table 11.2). Each of these areas of function may be affected by several abnormalities in each of the three planes. In addition to the prerequisites for normal gait, the skeleton may be seen as a series of levers with muscle motors, and the abnormalities classified as those of power, control or alignment. Whether the clinician is thinking of prerequisites for normal gait or the biomechanical features, the next step is to assemble the data gathered for each plane.

Coronal Plane

This is the view from the anterior or posterior aspect of the patient. Scoliosis and leg length discrepancy affect the assessment in this plane. Hip abduction and adduction ranges are noted. A common area for difficulty is the weakness which often affects the gluteus medius muscle, leading to a Trendelenburg gait. While a physiotherapy programme may give a grade of power improvement, weakness of grade 3 (as defined by the Medical Research Council) or worse cannot be addressed and results in a continued Trendelenburg gait or dependence on walking aids long term. Where there is less than 15° of hip abduction and a leg length discrepancy, the child is bordering on a limp because of inadequate abduction. In such cases, correction should be considered. The contribution of the gracilis muscle is assessed by flexing the knee and assessing the increase in hip abduction. At the knee, the relation between the mechanical axis running between the centre of the hip and the talus and the knee joint is examined, but it is uncommon to encounter a significant abnormality resulting from cerebral palsy. At the level of the subtalar joint, there may be either a varus or valgus malalignment. Generally, varus is seen in the hemiplegic limb whereas

valgus is a feature of diplegia. The hindfoot valgus in the diplegic child allows the heel to contact the ground during stance. The disadvantages are that there is instability in stance following the poor pre-position at initial contact and, from a biomechanical perspective, the foot is not in the normal alignment in the transverse plane and thus the power generated by the triceps surae is wasted. In the adolescent, varus or valgus instability may be controlled by an extra-articular arthrodesis with a screw across the tarsal sinus. Where deformity is excessive or the patient is skeletally mature, a triple arthrodesis may be the best option.

The kinematic data are checked and will then give information about the behaviour of the pelvis and hips during the gait cycle. Some valgus does seem to occur in the human knee during the first half of swing, when the knee is in a loose pack configuration, but during the stance phase of the cycle there should be very little change in alignment.

Sagittal Plane

The next step is to examine the sagittal plane, where contracture has a major influence on step length and thus the efficiency of gait. From the clinical examination, the state of the lumbar lordosis is noted and the presence of hip flexion contractures identified both by the Thomas test (Thomas, 1895) and the Staheli test. The knee is examined for contracture and the presence of hamstring tightness. With the patient supine, the knee to be examined is stabilised by one hand holding the femur vertical, while the other hand extends the knee by lifting the ankle. Once the knee has extended to its limit, and providing the lumbar spine is flat, the extension deficit in the knee is the popliteal angle. A value of greater than 50° is abnormal. An abnormally tight hamstring will be reflected in a deficit of knee extension at initial contact as well as by an oscillation of the pelvis. This is due to the interplay of the tight stance psoas and the tight swing hamstrings. The Duncan Ely test, performed by flexing the knee sharply with the patient prone, will reveal spasm in the rectus femoris leading to the pelvis rising off the examination couch. This, coupled with significant amounts of rectus EMG activity in the first half of the swing phase and a poor rise in the knee flexion angle in pre-swing and early swing, leads to a diagnosis of rectus spasticity, which usually requires correction if a stiff leg gait pattern is to be avoided. The term 'co-spasticity' is often used for this condition; however, inspection of the hamstring EMG traces in the same limb usually fails to show any close relation between the firing of the rectus femoris and the hamstrings. At the ankle, the video film will reveal where the patient has initial contact. Normally this should be with the heel, with the tibialis anterior muscle acting eccentrically to 'pay out the rope' and lower the forefoot to the floor, rather than a slapping gait. The segment of normal stance during which the forefoot is being lowered to the floor is called first rocker, and during this period the loading response occurs in the limb to decelerate the body smoothly on impact, storing energy in ligament, tendon and muscle ready for the next step. Second rocker starts when the metatarsal heads contact the floor and ends when the gastrocnemius joins the

Prerequisites of normal gait
Stability in stance
Clearance of the foot in swing
Pre-positioning of foot in swing
Adequate step length
Energy conservation

Table 11.2 Prerequisites of normal gait.

soleus to provide a propulsive spurt of energy to lift the heel and move the body forward. The soleus is the muscle of second rocker, acting eccentrically to control the advancement of the tibia over the now stationary talus. By controlling the forward movement of the tibia, the soleus ensures that the knee joint centre does not deviate too far from the line of the ground reaction force so that the quadriceps does not have to work excessively. Again, clinical examination allows the differentiation of gastrocnemius contracture and triceps contracture, indicating that a release of the gastrocnemius alone rather than of the heel cord might be appropriate. Dynamic EMG and the power graphs may show inappropriate activity and power generation at the ankle in the early stance, resulting from a spastic reflex contraction of the gastrocnemius at initial contact.

Transverse Plane

The final step in the analysis is to examine the transverse plane, i.e. the 'bird's-eye' view of the patient. Clinical examination of the ranges of movement and the torsional deformity of the femora and tibiae allow the findings of the kinematic analysis to be cross-checked. This cross-checking is important as most of the kinematic systems are least reliable at recording transverse plane motion. Video recording is of little use for examining deformities in the transverse plane. While the sagittal plane is disturbed by muscle contracture and poor control, the transverse plane is principally affected by the skeletal deformities seen in cerebral palsy. Where there is significant asymmetry in the torsional deformity, the patient often adopts a strategy of walking with the pelvis retracted (further back) on the side of the greatest internal torsional deformity, so that the foot progression angles are more symmetrical. The pelvic rotation kinematics identify this, and further graphs allow the examination of segments further down. One useful way of sorting out what needs to be done is to assess the degree of deformity in the foot progression angles relative to one another, allowing for a normal external foot progression angle of 10°. This gives the total amount of rotation to be performed throughout the lower limbs. Once this has been established, the tibial torsion is addressed and tibial osteotomies performed to correct any deformity of greater than about 15°. After this, the femoral anteversion is corrected; the remaining amount of rotation is distributed between the femora according to the kinematic analysis, supplemented and cross-checked by the femoral anteversion and ranges of movement. At the end of the process, the balance sheet should add up. The objective of this component of a correction is to restore the relation between the knee joint axis and the direction of progression, and to normalise the femoral neck to the outer table of the ilium, allowing the hip abductors to work as efficiently as possible. A more cosmetic appearance to the gait will also result from correction of the rotational abnormalities.

The graphs in Figure 11.3A–C represent the kinematic and kinetic analysis of an 11.5-year-old child with cerebral palsy diplegia. The child first walked independently at the age of 3 years but is now increasingly tending to fall, and

tires after a long day. The physiological cost index is abnormal at 0.82 extra beats per metre (upper limit of normal =0.6) and the child has a relatively short step length of 40 cm on the right and 46 cm on the left. The coronal plane data (see Figure 11.3A) show that the right hip has a tendency to be adducted during stance with respect to the normal. In addition, the abduction moment graph shows that the child is adopting a Trendelenburg gait by shifting the trunk over the hip during stance, thus reducing the moments around the hip. Video recording of the feet during gait in the coronal plane shows no particular problem that could not be dealt with by orthotic management.

The child has 15° of hidden flexion in each hip in the sagittal plane (see Figure 11.3B), shown by both the Staheli and the Thomas test—this is reflected in a tendency to sacrum up during gait and end-stance hip flexion contracture. At the knee level, a degree of hamstring tightness is combined with co-spasticity of the rectus femoris, giving a very flat trace on either side. The graph is typical of a crouch gait. At the ankle and foot level there is marked dynamic equinus in swing. This leads to difficulty with foot clearance on the left, and the ankle moment on power graphs indicates that there is an abnormality in the triceps surae during the loading response and, later on during stance, there is very little useful propulsive power in pre-swing; usually provided in a spurt by the gastrocnemius. Normally, the gastrocnemius, a fast twitch muscle, fires in the latter half of stance. It joins with the soleus to turn what is initially eccentric power absorption in the second rocker into the concentric generation of power in the third rocker.

Finally, the transverse plane data (see Figure 11.3C) show that the foot progression angle on either side is relatively internal, and this is in part explained by mild internal rotation deformities in each hip and internal torsional deformity in the subtalar joint on the left side.

This child is too young for staged surgery, although it will clearly be beneficial later on once the adolescent growth spurt has established itself. It can be predicted that the child's energy consumption will deteriorate during that time. Then, a programme of staged bony derotational surgery with soft tissue releases of the right adductors, the psoas muscles and the hamstrings, along with transfers of the rectus femoris, will provide a useful reduction in energy consumption and improve endurance, provided there is an appropriate package of orthotic and physiotherapy rehabilitation postoperatively.

FORMULATING A TREATMENT PROGRAMME

Once the three planes have been studied, recommendations can be made for treatment. It is important not to regard surgery as the automatic outcome of gait analysis. Orthotic management can be enhanced dramatically by the use of video vector analysis of the relation between the ground reaction force and the patient's joints. Physiotherapy treatment can be monitored and guided by gait analysis, particularly where kinetics are available.

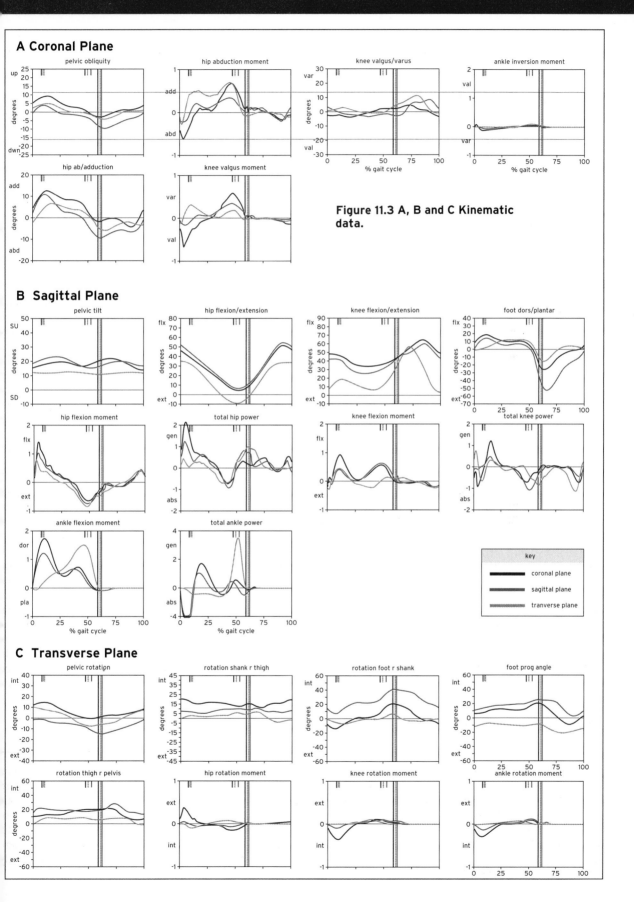

A Coronal Plane

pelvic obliquity · hip abduction moment · knee valgus/varus · ankle inversion moment

hip ab/adduction · knee valgus moment

Figure 11.3 A, B and C Kinematic data.

B Sagittal Plane

pelvic tilt · hip flexion/extension · knee flexion/extension · foot dors/plantar

hip flexion moment · total hip power · knee flexion moment · total knee power

ankle flexion moment · total ankle power

key	
	coronal plane
	sagittal plane
	tranverse plane

C Transverse Plane

pelvic rotation · rotation shank r thigh · rotation foot r shank · foot prog angle

rotation thigh r pelvis · hip rotation moment · knee rotation moment · ankle rotation moment

For the purposes of this chapter, however, the role of gait analysis in guiding a surgery–physiotherapy treatment programme is outlined. While some centres perform single-stage surgery for total correction of gait abnormalities, it has been our practice to stage the surgery with bony surgery and lengthening of the Achilles tendon 6 weeks before the soft tissue correction. The rationale of this two-stage surgery is that as soon as pain allows after the second stage, the rehabilitation programme can begin. This prevents recontracture and scarring, which might diminish the result. Without the initial surgery, the physiotherapy cannot succeed, but without the physiotherapy, soft tissue surgery is generally futile.

BONY SURGERY

As mentioned previously, bony surgery is usually for deformities in the transverse plane. In the femur, derotation procedures should if possible be performed in the intertrochanteric region, as the external rotation of the lesser trochanter leads to a small but useful lengthening of the psoas tendon which supplements later soft tissue surgery. Modern forms of internal fixation are sufficiently stable that they do not require plaster spicas to protect the child during the healing process. A spica is useful, however, in providing some protection from the painful muscle spasms which most children with cerebral palsy seem to have after surgery. Where a child has a significant amount of spasm pre-operatively, an indwelling epidural catheter inserted by the anaesthetist at the time of operation can be used to dramatically lessen the pain and subsequent spasm. Derotation surgery in the tibia is performed either in the metaphyseal region distally or with a plate in the diaphysis. The former is less stable, particularly where there is a tight heel cord, but has the advantage that the fixation wires are removed at the time of the second operation without the need for reopening the wound. The plate in the tibial diaphysis should be removed a couple of years after the corrective surgery and this can be done at the time of femoral plate removal. A subtalar arthrodesis is a common requirement for providing stability in stance, and is performed by removing the fatty tissue from the tarsal sinus and introducing bone graft between the inferior surface of the neck of the talus and the extra-articular aspect of the calcaneum (Dennyson & Fulford, 1976). A screw is passed through the neck of the talus into the calcaneum. This stabilises the joint in a neutral alignment while the bone graft is incorporated. In the child near skeletal maturity, a triple arthrodesis may be the most appropriate form of stabilisation in the foot, as this deals with all aspects of deformity and only leads to a small deficit in growth.

SOFT TISSUE SURGERY

Soft tissue surgery is generally for contractures in the coronal and sagittal planes. The key to contracture correction is to perform a procedure which maintains as much of the function of the muscle as possible but which allows the skeleton to be aligned in a functionally efficient fashion. At the hip, the iliopsoas is lengthened by performing an intramuscular release at the pelvic brim. This is done through an incision just medial to the anterior superior iliac spine, and requires the tendon to be divided at a point where there is muscle attached both proximal and distal to the tendon cut. The cut ends of the tendon retract but are linked by the muscle fibres passing across the gap. With time, scar fills the gap between the tendon ends, and the continuity of the tendinous portion is restored. One of the disadvantages of this procedure in children with cerebral palsy is that before surgery the psoas is efficient at working in an inner range, which makes the climbing of stairs relatively easy, whereas after surgery, stair climbing becomes more difficult, as the muscle is working in a range more suited to normal gait and is not accelerating the thigh into flexion from a relatively flexed position.

A similar lengthening procedure is performed at the distal end of the hamstrings to lengthen the superficial tendon of the biceps femoris and semimembranosus. Three diagonal incisions are made through the thin tendon, leaving the underlying muscle intact. By using three parallel incisions, the strain on the intervening muscle is much reduced and the fibres remain in continuity rather than rupturing.

Lengthening-surgery at the triceps surae has justifiably gained a poor reputation with physiotherapists who regularly treat children with cerebral palsy, because the tightness of the heel cord often protects the child from developing a crouch gait. Where the heel cord is overlengthened, the tibia has a tendency to fall forward in stance, allowing the centre of the knee joint to advance in front of the ground reaction vector. The moments acting about the knee are then strongly flexing, and from that point onwards the child is destined to a high-energy gait resulting from cerebral palsy. Although this situation can be rectified in the early stages with a rigid foot orthosis, later on the foot becomes so deformed that a triple arthrodesis is the only option for a stable foot. When the child has a tight heel cord, attempts should be made to apply serial holding casts after stretching sessions. If attempts at achieving a splintable foot fail, then the orthopaedic surgeon may help, but only if he is prepared to have the child in a rigid ankle–foot orthosis after surgery, to prevent the development of a crouch gait.

Occasionally there is evidence suggesting that tightness of the calf is confined to the gastrocnemius rather than all three muscles. Firstly, the relation between the tightness of the heel cord and knee joint flexion will be evident if there is an isolated gastrocnemius problem. Dynamically, EMG studies of the gastrocnemius will show a burst of electrical activity early on in the stance phase in response to the initial contact—generally with the forefoot on the ground. Kinetic analysis using a force platform will show a burst of power early on in the stance phase, which is the mechanical expression of the electrical activity seen on the EMG. Where the gastrocnemius is an isolated problem, this can be addressed by selectively lengthening the gastrocnemius at the musculotendinous junction.

Because cerebral palsy is very much a condition of failed control, the muscles requiring the most control are those which cross two joints—sometimes called the strap muscles. The hamstrings, the rectus femoris and the gastrocnemius are examples of strap muscles in the lower limb. The rectus femoris has the action of hip flexion as well as knee extension, and transmits force in an efficient way along the limb. The control strategy for this action is complex and requires precise timing if it is to be to advantageous to the patient. Where control is deficient, the rectus femoris serves its proximal joint and acts as a hip flexor, attempting to accelerate the thigh into flexion in the swing phase. This leads to a knee extension force at a time when the knee must flex rapidly to about 60° to allow the swinging foot to clear the ground. The surgeon can influence this by altering the function of the rectus femoris distally, by transference of the tendon from the patella to the flexor compartment, so that the inappropriate burst of knee extension is converted into a more appropriate flexion.

MONITORING THE RESULT

After surgery, the techniques of gait analysis can be used to monitor progress and adjust orthotics. Where the hamstrings have been lengthened, and perhaps the rectus femoris removed from the quadriceps mechanism at the knee, there is a need to augment the midstance extension of the knee. This is performed by analysing the moments around the knee joint either with a three-dimensional kinematic analysis or by means of video vector analysis. If the ground reaction vector falls behind the knee, then there is a flexing moment acting across the knee, and an equinus pitch is required on the ground reaction orthosis. Conversely, where the ground reaction vector lies in front of the knee joint, there is an extending moment acting and there is a need to elevate the shoe beneath the heel or recast the ground reaction orthosis in more calcaneus.

Clearly, the multilevel surgery undertaken as a result of gait analysis needs careful appraisal to ensure that patients really benefit. Furthermore, it is the techniques of gait analysis which promote the development of increasingly sophisticated treatments for motor handicap. Gait analysis has become a valuable component in the multidisciplinary treatment of movement disorder resulting from cerebral palsy.

PHYSIOTHERAPY

In the USA, some centres perform the bony and soft tissue surgery in one operation. Patients may have up to 12 incisions, and they are discharged from hospital approximately 3 weeks postoperatively. Their rehabilitation is undertaken as out-patients, and they are seen 2–3 times a week for about a year. The parents are instructed on a rehabilitation programme, including positioning of the child. The patient also returns to school very quickly.

The centre this author works in uses a two-stage surgical procedure, and physiotherapy plays a large part in its success. A pre-operative physiotherapy assessment before the first stage of surgery is very important. It is essential that both the child and parents have confidence in the proposed routine. They gain this in part by understanding the physiotherapy involvement and the rehabilitation programme. This also helps in the psychological preparation of the child for the procedure.

A pre-operative clinical assessment, including level of function and observation of gait, is essential. This provides a baseline for comparison after surgery. Before admission, all patients will have undergone gait analysis. With this information, and after a clinical assessment, the surgeon will be able to treat the underlying orthopaedic problems.

PRE-OPERATIVE PHYSIOTHERAPY

Physiotherapy plays a large part in the success of multilevel surgery. A pre-operative physiotherapy assessment before the first stage surgery is very important. Confidence must be given to the child and parents. They must have an understanding of the physiotherapy which represents the rehabilitation programme. This understanding also helps to psychologically prepare the child and family.

Assessment
Observation of Gait
Observe the abnormalities of gait and the major prerequisites for normal gait that are lacking. Note:
• The stability in stance.
• The clearance of the foot in swing.
• Appropriate pre-positioning of the foot in swing.
• Adequate step length.
• Energy conservation.
• If the child uses a walking aid, e.g. crutches, stick.
• The distance the child walks.

Measurements
The passive and active ranges of movement of the hips, knees and ankles are documented. These are a useful guideline for assessments pre- and postoperatively.

Muscle Contractures
These limit the ability of the muscles to reach their full length due to the presence of spasticity and abnormal gait patterns. Stretch is the stimulus which causes muscle growth. In a child whose muscles are growing, muscle stretching during normal daily activities maintains muscle growth in proportion to bone growth (Ziv et al., 1984). For example:
• Hip flexion muscle contracture limits the range of active and passive extension of the joint. The presence and extent of the effect of this contracture can be evaluated using the Thomas test. Matsuo and colleagues (1986) demonstrated that in shortening of the iliopsoas muscles in children who have spastic diplegia, lengthening of the psoas major tendon corrected the flexion contracture of the hip.
• Adductor muscle tightness limits the range of abduction in the hip joint. The patient may demonstrate the presence of this contracture by using a scissor-type gait.
• Hamstring muscle tightness results from the imbalance of muscle spasticity between the hamstrings and quadriceps (co-spasticity), leading to the knee-flexed posture. This leads to a very stiff legged gait and consequently difficulty in foot clearance in swing. It must be noted also that if a child sits

with a posterior pelvic tilt and a resultant compensatory flexion of the trunk, the tilt is increased when the child is in the long sitting position.

- Tendocalcaneal tightness results from the tightness and shortening of the calf muscles, thus limiting the ability of the patient to produce a plantigrade foot. It is particularly obvious in weight bearing, as the child stands on tiptoe with the heels clear of the ground. The gastrocnemius and the soleus muscles can be evaluated by noting the difference between the measurements of dorsiflexion with the knee in flexion and extension. Any loss in dorsiflexion is an indication of shortening of the gastrocnemius (Silverskoid test). Spasticity in the rectus femoris muscle is determined by the Duncan Ely test or the prone rectus test (Gage, 1991).

Bony Deformities

These are frequently observed in children with cerebral palsy. Some common deformities are:

- Femoral anteversion.
- Tibial torsion.
- Foot deformity.

It is necessary to document upper body strength, as this varies from patient to patient. The patient's social and medical history must also be recorded.

The first stage of surgery may include:

- Unilateral or bilateral derotational femoral osteotomy.
- Unilateral or bilateral derotational tibial osteotomy.
- Fusion of the subtalar joint.
- Lengthening of the tendocalcaneus, the combined tendon of the gastrocnemius, the soleus and the plantaris (if present).

POSTOPERATIVE PHYSIOTHERAPY

During the early postoperative period, the patient will experience pain. Analgesia and a muscle relaxant, e.g. diazepam, may be given to relieve the pain.

On the first postoperative day, the physiotherapist encourages breathing exercises and checks on the patient's comfort and position. On the second day, the patient's legs are suspended using an arrangement of slings and springs (Figure 11.4). This gives greater comfort to the patient, allowing them to move more easily. While suspended by the slings and springs, the patient is encouraged to perform active assisted exercises of the legs, progressing to active movements of the hips and knees. The slings are removed in a few days, when comfort allows and there is sufficient controlled active range of movement to enable the patient to sit out of bed.

The child is taught to transfer from bed to wheelchair. Non-weight-bearing walking with crutches is maintained for 6 weeks, while the bone is healing. The child is also encouraged to lie prone for a period during each day as soon as this is possible.

Most patients are discharged between the first and second stages of surgery. Before discharge, they are taught a few simple exercises to perform daily at home.

Six weeks after the first stage of surgery, the patient is readmitted to hospital for the second stage. Before the second operation, a cast for a ground reaction orthosis is taken.

The second stage of surgery may include:

- Psoas muscle release.
- Adductor muscle release.
- Rectus femoris muscle transfer.
- Lengthening of the hamstring muscles.

Generally, the patient will be in hospital for up to 6 weeks postoperatively and sometimes even longer. The physiotherapist explains the procedures to both the child and the parents to prepare them for the rehabilitation programme. The time spent at the beginning of the rehabilitation programme is invaluable. It reinforces a new gait pattern and teaches the importance of maintaining and improving on the achievements to date. Patients also learn to take responsibility for continuation of the exercise programme after discharge. Improvement may continue for up to 2 years postoperatively.

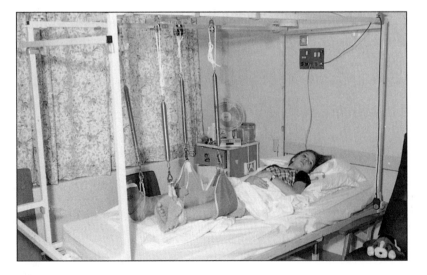

Figure 11.4 Demonstration of the application of slings and springs postoperatively.

HYSIOTHERAPY AFTER THE SECOND
TAGE OF SURGERY

fter surgery, the patient is nursed supine with long leg
obilisers *in situ* and without pillows supporting the
ees. An abduction wedge may be placed between the
gs to maintain hip abduction following the adductor mus-
e release. The patient lies flat with one or two pillows
der the head for 5 days and then starts to sit up for short
eriods. Small-range gentle passive movements of the
ees and hips are commenced. Initially, the range is
nall, but is gradually increased. Active movements are
mmenced as postoperative muscle spasm reduces. When
e patient has active control of hip and knee movements,
e long leg immobilisers may be removed during the day.
atients continue to wear the immobilisers at night for
any months, to ensure maintenance of knee extension.

Quadriceps exercises are encouraged from the second
stoperative day, ensuring active knee extension is main-
ined. Prone lying is encouraged as soon as comfort
lows. Patients are expected to maintain this position for
hour each day and night, when they will also be wearing
e long leg immobilisers.

Five to seven days postoperatively, the patient is encouraged to sit in long sitting, to stretch the hamstring muscles.
When comfortable, the patient can start sitting out of bed
for short periods without wearing the long leg immobilisers. This stage is reached approximately 7 days after
surgery. The patient should be wearing the orthosis, and
good supportive footwear is essential. Maintenance of a
good sitting posture is important.

After approximately 5 days, the patient will be ready to
start standing. Additional support may be given by using
the tilt table or parallel bars. The knee immobilisers and
ground reaction orthosis must be worn. Once the patient is
used to maintaining an erect posture at the parallel bars, re-
education of gait commences (Figure 11.5). It is important
to spend time encouraging an improved gait—for example,
knee bracing in standing, progressing to hip flexion and
clearance in swing, and heel strike on initial contact. This
prevents the development of bad habits.

The patient progresses to walking with a rollator or posterior walker (Figure 11.6). The latter is preferable as it
encourages a more upright posture. The physiotherapist
must continue gait re-education at every opportunity.

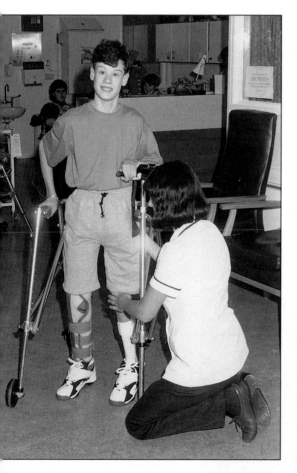

gure 11.5 Gait re-education.

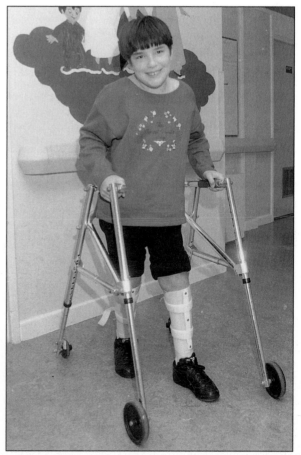

Figure 11.6 Walking with a posterior walker.

Once the surgical wounds have healed, hydrotherapy is started. Water is a useful medium for general mobilising and strengthening exercises (Figure 11.7).

Mat work is started, if possible in a class. The children tend to work harder in groups and the introduction of games can also add a fun element to the exercise regimen (Figure 11.8).

The patient is encouraged to walk everywhere, using a walker, to build up muscle strength, and may progress to sticks when able, provided a good gait pattern is maintained.

It is essential to encourage good gait. The prerequisite for this include:
- Restoration of stability in the stance phase.
- Gaining foot clearance in the swing phase.
- Appropriate positioning of the foot before striking the ground.
- Adequate step length.

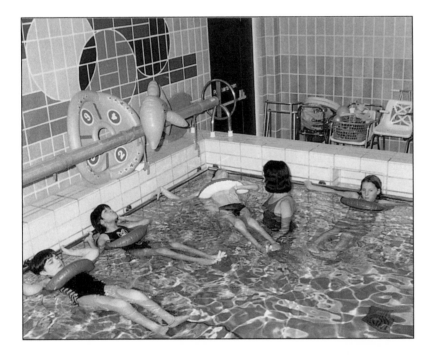

Figure 11.7 Patients in the hydrotherapy pool.

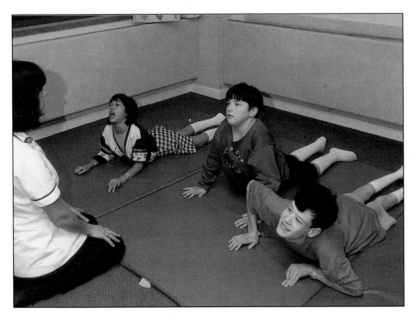

Figure 11.8 Patients participating in an exercise class.

• Reduction of energy expenditure, which will result from successful implementation of the prerequisites above.

The static bicycle is introduced for strengthening the muscles, and also helps with reciprocal leg movements. The patient is discharged when satisfactory progress has been made. The exercise programme is continued at home under the supervision of the domiciliary physiotherapist.

Good communication between the hospital-based physiotherapist and the community-based physiotherapist is essential. Co-operation with the parents is essential too, as they will be required to encourage the child to continue exercising at home. Both the child and the parents must fully understand the demanding nature of the rehabilitation programme.

One-year postoperatively the child will have a further gait analysis to determine progress. If the surgeon considers the child would benefit from further physiotherapy, arrangements are made for readmission for a 1-week or 2-week intensive programme of physiotherapy.

REFERENCES

Evans GA. Personal communication, 1996.

Dennyson WG, Fulford GE. Subtalar arthrodesis by cancellous grafts and metallic fixation. *J Bone Joint Surg.* 1976, **58B**:507-510.

Gage JR. *Gait analysis in cerebral palsy.* MacKeith Press with Blackwell Scientific Publication Ltd; 1991:14-15.

Matsuo T, Hara H, Hiromichi S, Tada S. Selective lengthening of the psoas and rectus femoris and preservation of the iliacus for flexion deformity of the hip in the cerebral palsy patients. *J Paediatr Orthop* 1986, **6**:690-698.

McDermott S, Coker AL, Mani S, *et al.* A population based analysis of behaviour problems in children with cerebral palsy. *J Paediatr Psychol* 1996, **21**:447-463.

Perry J. Phases of gait. In: *Gait analysis: Normal and pathological function.* New Jersey: Thorofare Slack; 1992.

Rose J, Gamble JG, Medieros J, Burgos A, Haskell WL. Energy cost of walking in normal children and in those with cerebral palsy—comparison of heart rate and oxygen uptake. *J Paediatr Orthop* 1989, **9**:276-279.

Thomas HO. *Hip knee and ankle,* 2nd ed. Liverpool: Dobbs; 1895.

Ziv I, Blackburn N, Rang M, Koreska J. Muscle growth in normal and spastic mice. *Develop Med Child Neurol* 1984, **26**:94-99.

GENERAL READING

Bleck EE. Management of the lower extremities in children who have cerebral palsy. *J Bone Joint Surg* 1990, **72A**:140-144.

12 D C Jaffray

DEGENERATION OF THE LUMBAR SPINE

CHAPTER OUTLINE

- Degeneration of the lumbar spine
- Pain patterns
- Investigations

- Treatments
- Facet arthritis
- The 'back school'

INTRODUCTION

In 1934 WJ Mixter and JS Barr described disc prolapses. Fifty years later they concluded:

The diagnosis of a herniated lumbar disc started all the damn trouble. WJ Mixter.

I am sorry that the discovery of herniation of the disc has led to so high an incidence of back cripples. ... They [the patients] are more common and more severely disabled after surgery than they would have been had no surgical treatment been pursued. JS Barr.

The structure of the lumbar intervertebral disc has been well described. For over a decade it has been known that the outer annulus is innervated by nerve fibres. More recently, proprioceptor organs have been identified in the annulus. There can be no doubt that because the disc has an innervation it must have a proprioceptive function. There is much controversy over the precise function of the lumbar disc, but, whatever the nature of its mechanical function, given its innervation, there is no excuse for thinking that the disc is of little functional importance. For years it was thought that the lumbar intervertebral disc was of little importance—just like the menisci of the knee, if needed the disc was to be excised. Slowly, knee surgeons realised the importance of the menisci and that random excision could lead to a crippling arthritis of the knee. Not every unnecessary menisectomy led to arthritis and not every unnecessary

discectomy led to a patient with a crippled back, but enough did to encourage surgeons to be selective.

The discovery of the nerve supply to the annulus helped to explain why the lumbar disc can be a source of pain after injury or surgery. It is no surprise that unnecessary or careless surgery to the lumbar disc can result in patients with a crippled back. That the disc can be a source of pain is graphically demonstrated in patients with an infected disc. Such patients are in extreme pain, and the pain will only resolve with successful treatment of the infection, either by antibiotics or by surgery. That fusion can resolve discogenic pain is clearly seen in disc infection when a spontaneous fusion or ankylosis occurs. If it is necessary to confirm that a disc is a source of pain—for example, if a fusion is contemplated—the best way to do this is using lumbar discography. This has been much criticised, but in the hands of an expert radiologist or surgeon it is invaluable in the assessment of severe back pain (Figures 12.1 and 12.2). Magnetic resonance imaging (MRI) scanning cannot yet confirm or refute a source of pain in the lumbar disc.

The function of the lumbar spine depends on the integrity and health of the intervertebral discs. The disc has a blood supply to its outer rim only. Once the vertebral endplates ossify in adolescence, the blood flow between the vertebral body and the disc stops. Thereafter, the nutrition and health of the disc are precarious. The loss of the integrity of the disc, whether acute or chronic, is responsible for most of the common disorders in the lumbar spine.

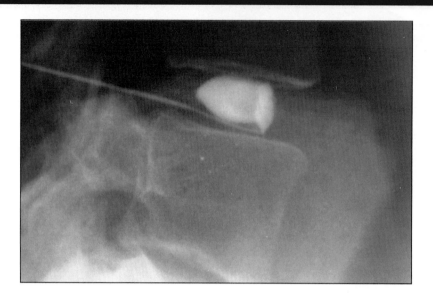

Figure 12.1 Normal disc on discography at L4/5. This was painless.

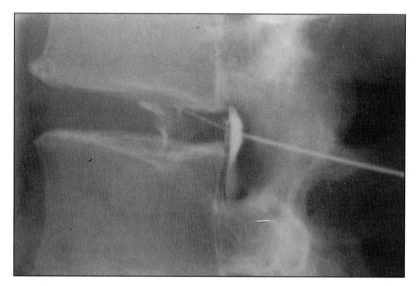

Figure 12.2 Traumatic tear of the L4/5 disc with leakage of the dye into the spinal canal. This reproduced the patient's symptoms.

DEGENERATION OF THE LUMBAR SPINE

Even in adolescence, early degeneration of the lumbar discs can be seen (Figures 12.3 and 12.4). Why this should occur in some individuals remains unknown. Perhaps there is a genetic predisposition. Some authors—this one included—describe another condition, known as isolated disc resorption, in the young adult. This usually occurs in the lumbosacral disc, with the rapid disintegration producing a distinct pattern on X-ray film.

This author likens disc resorption to a rapid advance of the normal degenerative process. Whereas normal slow degeneration is painless or merely a nuisance in most cases, rapid degeneration in the young can be very painful.

Trauma can lead to rupture of the disc with subsequent complications, e.g. pain, prolapsed disc. Common sense

dictates that if the disc is degenerate it will tear easily. However, if the spine is unprotected, the force required to rupture even a normal disc is surprisingly small. Obviously not every torn disc is painful. The disc has a limited ability to heal, but this is more than enough for most of us. It is now thought that much of the pain is not mechanical but a significant inflammatory component due to chemicals leaking out of the disc causing irritation of the posterior annulus and a chemical radiculitis. Traditional treatment has focused upon only the mechanical element of the problem, but now perhaps we need to address both elements.

Slow degeneration of the lumbar discs is usually painless (Figure 12.5). There is no correlation between symptoms and X-ray film appearances of the lumbar spine. About 8% of the UK population suffer an episode of back pain each year; few become chronic back pain sufferers. The slow degeneration of the lumbar discs in itself may not be that painful, but it

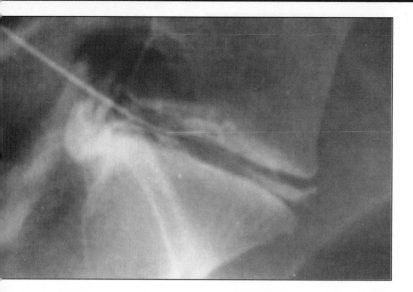

Figure 12.3 Early resorption of the L5/S1 disc with reproduction of pain at lumbar discography.

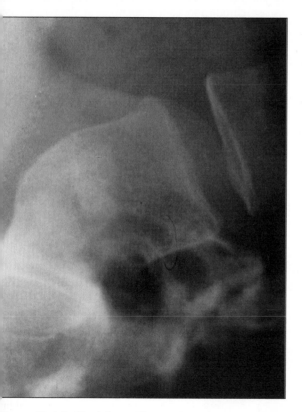

Figure 12.4 Patient from Figure 12.3 after interbody fusion to restore the disc height. Note the enlargement of the L5/S1 root foramen.

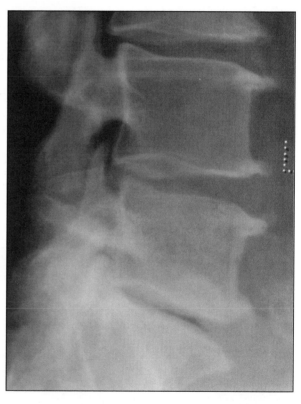

Figure 12.5 Widespread disc degeneration, most marked at L5/S1.

rings an unwelcome process. As the disc collapses, it bulges into the spinal canal. At the same time, the facet joints become arthritic because the disc no longer keeps the joint surfaces apart. As the facet joints become arthritic, they grow large osteophytes which protrude into the spinal canal and into the root canals. The laminae approximate posteriorly, forcing the ligamentum flavum to bulge into the spinal canal. Thus, as a consequence of the discs collapsing through degeneration, spinal stenosis, both central and foraminal, follows (Figure 12.6).

Thus, the disc is a culprit in both early and late adult life. In early adult life it is a source of pain, causing back pain with referred pain usually to the thigh, or root pain where there is a sequestrated disc prolapse. In later life, disc collapse leads to spinal stenosis. The major source of severe back pain is the disc. Primary symptomatic arthritis of a facet joint adjacent to a normal disc with good height is uncommon. Osteoarthritis of a facet joint is virtually always secondary to collapse of the adjacent disc. Many authorities dispute that the facet joints are ever painful. Although the pain from facet arthritis is not as significant as discogenic pain, it brings a new pattern of pain, which will be described later.

PAIN PATTERNS

There are three pain patterns as a result of disc degeneration—root pain, discogenic pain and facet pain. Often, there are combinations of these pain patterns.

ROOT PAIN

This can be acute, as in disc prolapse, or chronic, as in lateral recess stenosis.

Acute Root Pain

Despite the huge numbers of discectomies performed daily around the world, a true disc prolapse with only leg pain is uncommon. The huge discrepancies between the rates of discectomies in various countries confirms that the diagnosis is wrong in many cases. Probably the main failure is the confusion between referred leg pain with a painful back and true root pain with no back pain.

The history is acute by definition. This author does no believe that there has to be pre-existing obvious degenera tion before a disc prolapse occurs. The pain is sharp, sever and unrelenting. Women who have gone through chil birth and who have also suffered root pain will tell you th the latter is the worse. No relief comes with rest, positio or time of day. The pain may initially be a consequence of pressure, but a chemical inflammation of the root from disc materials is increasingly thought to have an importan role in chronic discs. The L4/5 and L5/S1 disc spaces ar by far most commonly involved, and therefore the pain i acute disc prolapses goes to the foot.

Chronic Root Pain

Usually this occurs in lateral recess stenosis and is not a severe as acute root pain. It is related to walking, whic makes it worse, and relieved by lying. Because the L4, L and S1 roots are most often involved, the pain is felt belo the knee. Unlike claudication through peripheral vascula disease, chronic root pain is not worse at night. As flexio of the lumbar spine increases the diameter of the spina canal, patients can cycle further than they can walk.

DISCOGENIC PAIN

This causes back pain which is mechanical in nature Some would call it instability. This means that the pai is made worse by movement and eased by rest; th forms the basis of some tests used by surgeons to see fusion could work. Immobilisation of the spine in a plas ter hip spica or using external fixators into the pedicle of the affected segment should relieve discogenic pain Few pain patterns, however, are that pure. Nearly a

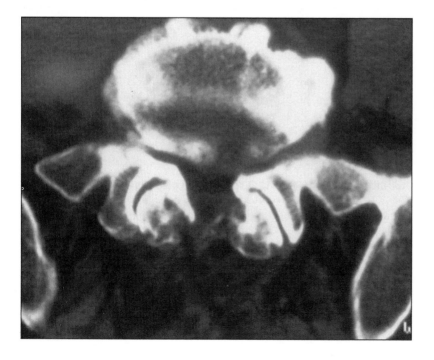

Figure 12.6 Computerised tomogram showing massive hypertrophy of the L5/S1 facets in the patient from Figure 12.3. Both lateral recesses and the central canal are narrowed, causing spinal stenosis.

patients with discogenic pain will have referred pain to the legs, but seldom below the knee. There will be no root signs. Straight leg raising will be painful but will cause back and not leg pain.

FACET PAIN

Before facet pain is evident, by definition the disc has usually collapsed already to a degree; so discogenic or instability pain exists. Facet pain is usually superimposed on an instability pattern. The pain is made worse by rest and relieved by movement—the opposite to discogenic pain—and night pain is common. A spica will worsen the pain. Referred pain to the leg can occur in facet arthritis. Usually root pressure is eventually associated with facet osteoarthritis and introduces yet another pain pattern.

Life is never simple. Often patients have a combination of all the pain patterns.

INVESTIGATIONS

The clinical history and examination should provide the diagnosis. Listen and look—it is all too easy to forget to use our eyes and ears, and instead process patients through high-technology scans, hoping for a diagnosis. These techniques, in particular MRI scanning, will show some abnormality, but you must relate these findings to the patient. If your clinical examination has been brief, mistakes will follow. For example, myelography will always show disc bulges. These bulges, often mistaken for disc prolapses, disappear on flexion films. This author wonders how many discectomies have been carried out on this basis. You should make your diagnosis on a clinical history and examination, with the various imaging techniques and blood tests simply reinforcing your diagnosis. If they do not, then re-examine the patient.

If it is necessary to confirm that a disc is a source of pain—for example, when a fusion is contemplated—the best way to do this is with lumbar discography. MRI scanning cannot yet confirm or refute a source of pain in the lumbar disc. Lumbar discography has been much criticised, yet in the hands of an expert radiologist or surgeon, it is invaluable. The findings of discography must be considered in conjunction with other clinical findings.

TREATMENTS

All pain patterns from lumbar degeneration are benign and not life threatening; most are self-limiting. The outcome of disc prolapses, whether treated surgically or conservatively, is the same. Surgery carries risks, particularly discectomy, e.g. the wrong level, the wrong side, root damage. So, conservative treatment and 'mother nature' will do for the majority of patients.

TRUE DISC PROLAPSE (SEQUESTRATION)

Apart from a cauda equina syndrome, there is no need for urgent surgery, as most conditions will settle. If the pain cannot be controlled, then discectomy must be considered. This author has scheduled patients for surgery, only to find that their acute severe pain has disappeared by the time they are admitted. Far too much surgery is performed for this condition.

DISCOGENIC PAIN

The principles of conservative treatment are analgesia and strengthening the muscles. Given that movement makes discogenic pain worse, strengthening the muscles presents problems. Prescribing supports, such as corsets, is an admission of defeat—lumbar supports do little to help strengthen the abdominal or lumbar muscles. Restoring flexibility to a source of instability pain flies in the face of logic. In this author's experience, patients never complain of stiffness—he has yet to see a patient with solid ankylosing spondylitis complain of stiffness provided that the spine is ankylosed in a straight position and there is good hip function.

SURGERY

The aim of surgery is to stabilise a painful mobile segment, and this is left to a very small population. Most patients with back pain have illness behaviour and unrealistic expectations. Fusion does not restore normality but will hopefully decrease the pain. Therefore patients must receive a clear explanation of the aims, risks and expectations of surgery, and must understand and consent to that treatment (perhaps by video recording to avoid future litigation).

Fusion must be reserved for a very small percentage of people with a severe pain pattern. How the fusions are carried out varies, although interbody fusion makes most sense in discogenic pain. This type of surgery is major, however, and many surgeons prefer to perform a posterior or onlay fusion, which may be less efficient on mechanical grounds but less challenging surgically.

There have been two recent changes to treating discogenic pain. The first is disc replacement, in which an artificial disc replaces the affected disc. Disc replacement has been performed for over a decade. Whether the prosthesis simply acts as a jack separating the vertebrae or is a true 'disc' is debatable. This author has experienced remarkable results with this procedure. However, the disadvantage is that a foreign material is implanted into the spine, with all the risks (Figures 12.7 and 12.8).

The other more recent development is to stabilise but not fuse the spine. In this procedure, screws are inserted into the pedicles and connected by bands. The principle behind this technique has slowly emerged. The aim is to slow the degeneration down to that of the normal ageing process. Although earlier attempts, using nylon to join the spinous processes together, were a failure, this technique may be different. By definition the spine is extended. Treating discogenic pain by extension of the spine will not help facet pain or the nerve roots passing closely by. Both disc replacement and flexible stabilisation have been developed because of the failings of fusion. Careful patient

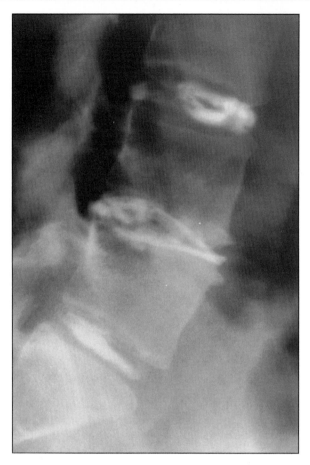

Figure 12.7 Painful disc degeneration at all three levels in a 30-year-old woman. An example of failed conservative treatment.

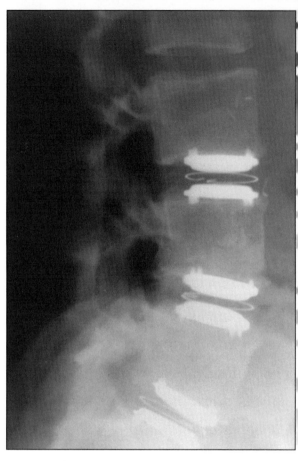

Figure 12.8 Return to work following disc replacement. The outcome of spinal surgery in back pain, however, remains unpredictable.

selection and meticulous technique in fusion surgery are still the best options.

FACET ARTHRITIS

Facet arthritis in the presence of a normal disc (i.e. primary) is uncommon, and is nearly always secondary to disc disease. The natural history of osteoarthritis of a synovial joint is ankylosis, usually in a degree of flexion. This is universal to synovial joints. Thus, osteoarthritis of a hip in the Third World ends up as an ankylosed hip with a fixed flexion deformity. Nature's way is to stiffen the joint in the position of rest, so attempts to restore mobility go against nature. Attempts to treat advanced osteoarthritis of facet arthritis by manipulation are likely therefore to be of very short-term benefit. The only facet pathology that this author manipulates as a spinal surgeon is facet dislocation in the cervical spine. Conservative treatments should help, not hinder, nature.

Injections of Marcaine and steroid into the facet joint—performed using an image intensifier and confirmed by arthrography—give meaningful relief of facet pain for months. Some authorities believe that the Marcaine simply diffuses into the adjacent painful abnormal disc. Nevertheless, meaningful relief can be obtained. Other treatments aimed at the inflammatory component of facet arthritis are logical.

Given that facet arthritis is nearly always secondary to disc pathology, spinal fusion for facet arthritis should address the levels concerned. Often, facet problems are multilevel in the middle aged or elderly, and surgery is not a viable proposition.

THE 'BACK SCHOOL'

This chapter has discussed the conservative and surgical managements of disc degeneration of the lumbar spine. Conservative treatments cover the vast majority of procedures, while surgery is aimed at a selective few. There are a group of patients whose pain will not resolve but who are not suitable for surgery, maybe because their pain pattern does not justify surgery, or they are too old, unfit or choose not to undergo surgery. This author refers these patients o the 'back school', where they are instructed in how best o cope with their disability. For each 100 patients seen in his author's clinic, 5 undergo surgery, 80 are discharged and 15 are referred to the back school. An audit of those eferred to the back school demonstrated an improvement n over 80%. The surgeon must know the type of patient hat the back school can help.

Every year about 8% of the adult population experience an episode of significant back pain. Few go on to develop chronic pain. Treatment should be aimed at helping nature resolve the problem promptly. If resolution is not achieved quickly, then the cost to the patient and society is high. In the Oswestry back pain clinic, 60% of patients with acute back pain that failed to resolve within 3 months never worked again.

Chronic low back pain is real and not imagined. The illness behaviour and non-organic signs often associated with the condition are evidence that conventional treatments, whether conservative or surgical, are likely to have limited success. These patients deserve our sympathy: more often than not they get the reverse. Hopefully, in the future, treatments will be of more help.

GENERAL READING

O'Brien JP. Mechanisms of Spinal Pain. In: Wall, Melzack, eds. *Textbook of Pain*. Churchill Livingstone; 1984: 240-251.

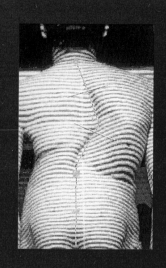

13 S Eisenstein & R Jones

SPINAL DEFORMITIES

CHAPTER OUTLINE

- Deformities
- Causes
- Diagnosis and assessment

- Treatment
- Role of the physiotherapist

INTRODUCTION

The management of spinal deformity represents a return to the origin of orthopaedic philosophy and the earliest traditions of orthopaedic practice: the achievement of 'straight children'. In those early days, almost all of orthopaedics was conducted by external splintage rather than by surgery, as exemplified by the many representations of Andry's crooked sapling lashed to a stake (Figure 13.1) (Andry, 1743). Modern surgical treatment for spinal deformity often requires the insertion of a 'stake' alongside the crooked spine, in a remarkable re-creation of Andry's illustration. The badges of orthopaedic professional associations around the world proudly display this emblem.

For the newcomer to the practice of spinal deformity, there is a new language to learn. This should not be regarded by novices as a deterrent, but as a challenge on joining a fascinating and rewarding clinical endeavour.

DEFORMITIES

SCOLIOSIS

Scoliosis is a side-to-side 'S' bend in the spine, or part of an 'S' bend, produced by more than just temporary asymmetrical posture (Figure 13.2). The term implies an element of permanence because of some structural abnormality inherent in the spine of a particular individual. In addition, there is almost always some degree of

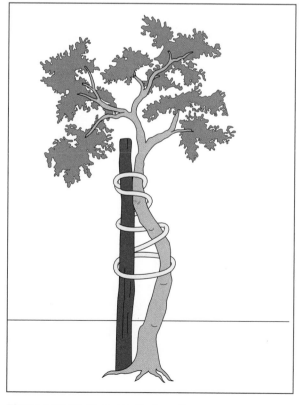

Figure 13.1 Andry's crooked sapling.

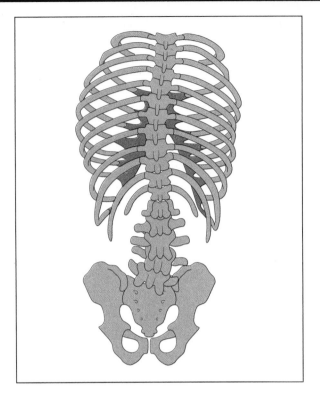

Figure 13.2 Scoliosis.

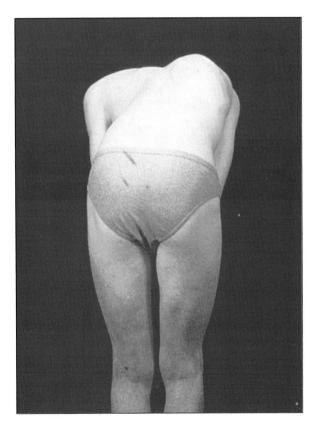

Figure 13.3 Rib hump of scoliosis.

twist in the spine (rotation), where several vertebrae are permanently turned about their vertical axis so that the spinous processes point into the concavity of the bend. This rotation can be the most important feature in a scoliotic spine because it is the rotation of thoracic vertebrae which causes the unattractive rib hump. It is the rib hump (Figure 13.3) that is usually the obvious deformity in the patient, and not the curved spine. The ribs are attached to the sides of the vertebrae: as the vertebrae rotate with the development of scoliosis, the ribs rise up on one side to form the hump (Figure 13.4).

KYPHOSIS

Kyphosis is a smooth forward bend of the spine. The thoracic spine has a normal forward bend of up to 40°, so that in this instance the kyphosis is normal or physiological. In clinical practice, the term implies an excessive forward bend (Figure 13.5). Kyphosis may be found together with scoliosis, called kyphoscoliosis.

KYPHOS (OR GIBBUS)

Kyphos (or gibbus) is a sharp forward bend but more like a kink or a knuckle in the spine. Traditionally, the term applied to the deformity resulting from the destruction caused by tuberculosis (Figure 13.6), but kyphos can be found wherever vertebrae have collapsed into wedges such as in osteoporosis, cancer, injury, infection, and disease which weakens bone. It is also rarely found at birth or soon after, in infants born with imperfectly formed vertebrae (congenital kyphos).

LORDOSIS

Lordosis is the opposite of kyphosis. It is a smooth backward bend of the spine, found as normal posture in the cervical and lumbar spine, to balance the thoracic kyphosis, but again usually indicating an excessive or pathological

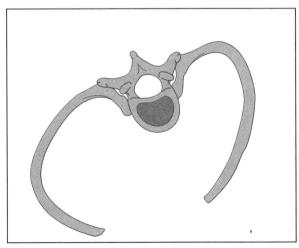

Figure 13.4 Ribs rise up on one side to form the hump.

condition. It may be found in the lumbar spine as compensation for a pathological kyphosis in the thoracic spine. A relative lordosis of the thoracic spine (loss of normal kyphosis) is frequently associated with idiopathic scoliosis.

SPONDYLOLISTHESIS

Spondylolisthesis is a horizontal shift of a vertebra in relation to another, as if the vertebra slides along the one below it, in any direction, to take up a new but abnormal position (Figure 13.7). The direction of shift is usually forward. (Spondylolisthesis must not be confused with similar-sounding words such as spondylosis—degenerative changes in the spine—and spondylolysis—an un-united fracture of the lamina of a vertebra.)

NATURE OF THE DEFORMITY

It is sometimes held that spine deformities are 'only cosmetic', as if they did not matter much, because they are usually painless and no longer associated with a diminished life expectancy. The fact is that there is a degree of deformity which is so pervasive as to go well beyond a question of vanity. If severe, scoliosis and kyphosis are just such deformities. The whole body shape may be altered to a degree which is simply unacceptable to the patient and materially affects the patient's perception of their place in society. Moreover, the deformity is very likely to be progressive and may indeed cause disabling pain in adult life.

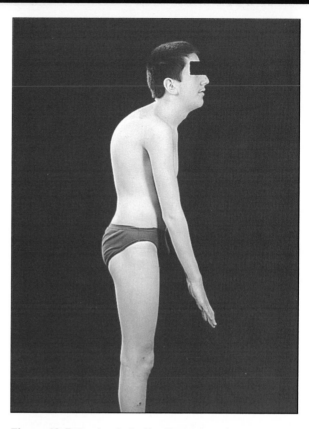

Figure 13.5 Kyphosis in the thoracic spine: example of 'juvenile osteochondrosis'.

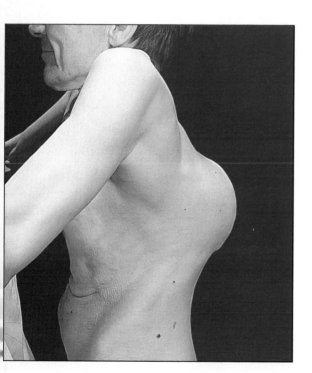

Figure 13.6 Kyphosis or gibbus in spinal tuberculosis.

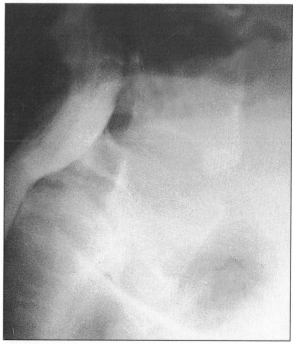

Figure 13.7 Spondylolisthesis: L5 has shifted forwards on S1, resulting in a kink in the contrast column within the dural sac.

CAUSES

SCOLIOSIS

By far the most common spinal deformity to require treatment is scoliosis. There are several types of scoliosis, classified according to cause, and each type needs a different treatment programme.

Idiopathic ('Cause Not Known')

This is the most common diagnosis (ironically, in a condition classified by 'cause'), affecting mostly adolescent girls and producing a thoracic curve to the right, with a right-sided rib hump. The spine appears perfectly normal at birth but deforms in the adolescent years of rapid growth, for reasons not yet understood. Because the curve is associated with a loss of the normal thoracic kyphosis, the deformity is more correctly termed 'lordoscoliosis' (Professor Robert Dickson, Leeds). Despite the term 'idiopathic', we know that this type of scoliosis runs in families: there must be a genetic influence of varying importance.

Less commonly, idiopathic scoliosis can appear in infants and juveniles. Then it presents major management problems because of the early start of the deformity.

Extensive research worldwide over many years, has failed to produce a convincing and conclusive answer to the cause of the disease. Theories are many, based on suspicions of genetic tendencies, hormone imbalances, neuromuscular imbalance and the various stresses of childhood, both physical and emotional (Goldberg et al., 1997). The answer is likely to be found in a gradual realisation that all these factors are relevant, in varying proportions, in all cases of 'idiopathic' scoliosis.

Congenital

The spine is deformed from the start of its development in the fetus, either through failure of the vertebrae to form symmetrically, or through failure of the vertebrae to separate completely from each other (Figure 13.8). The worst of these deformities are found when the two types of failure occur together. This type of scoliosis presents the greatest treatment challenge of all because of its tendency to increase from birth despite major and repeated attempts to achieve correction.

Neuromuscular ('Paralytic')

The spinal column may be normal at birth but one of the many paralysing conditions will affect the stabilising muscles of the spine, and scoliosis develops. These paralysing conditions are spinal injury, cerebral palsy, poliomyelitis, transverse myelitis and the muscular dystrophies (Figure 13.9) (Mehdian et al., 1989). The paralysis of myelodysplasia

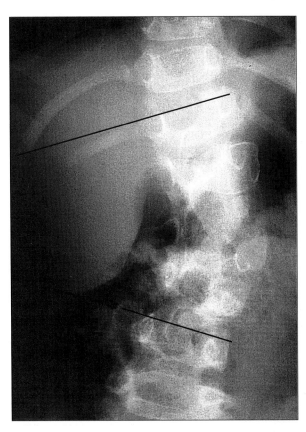

Figure 13.8 Congenital scoliosis. Note the jumble of asymmetric upper lumbar vertebrae between the black lines.

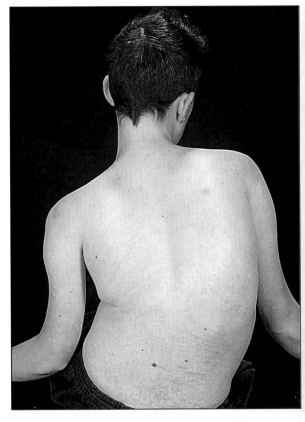

Figure 13.9 Collapsing 'C'-shaped curve of neuromuscular scoliosis, specifically Duchenne muscular dystrophy in this case.

spina bifida) will be present at birth and any scoliosis may be compounded by the presence of congenital abnormalities, as described on page 176.

Other Causes

This is a disparate group of rarer causes, such as the scoliosis secondary to spinal tumours, acute back strains, disc prolapse, advanced lumbar spondylosis and, very rarely, hysteria.

KYPHOSIS

Kyphosis is far less common than scoliosis, but successful treatment may be more difficult to achieve.

Juvenile Osteochondrosis (Scheuermann's Disease)

This is a mysterious condition and probably the most common cause of mild-to-moderate kyphosis in developed countries (Scheuermann, 1920). The endplates of the thoracic vertebrae of teenage boys are damaged in some way that produces anterior wedging of the vertebral bodies and results in the 'round shoulders' which parents sometimes blame on bad posture in a lazy child. Patients often complain of low back pain in a compensatory lumbar lordosis.

Infection

Infection in the form of tubercular destruction of one or more adjacent thoracic vertebrae is probably the most common cause of a pathological kyphosis in developing countries. The deformity is likely to be sharply angled (a gibbus) and cause spinal cord compression with paralysis (Figure 13.10).

Spinal Injury

This is a frequent cause of kyphosis because the injury is so often a crush of one or more vertebral bodies, and is associated with paralysis through direct damage to the spinal cord at the level of the crush (Figure 13.11).

Osteoporosis

Osteoporosis associated with the menopause, alcoholism and dietary inadequacy, is the most important cause of kyphosis in adults. The loss of mineral content of the bone so weakens the vertebral bodies that they collapse into wedges under the normal loads of daily living. The pain produced in this condition is severe and almost incurable.

Congenital Abnormalities

These occur less frequently in the sagittal plane, but they can cause a severe and progressive kyphosis with the likelihood of paralysis if left untreated.

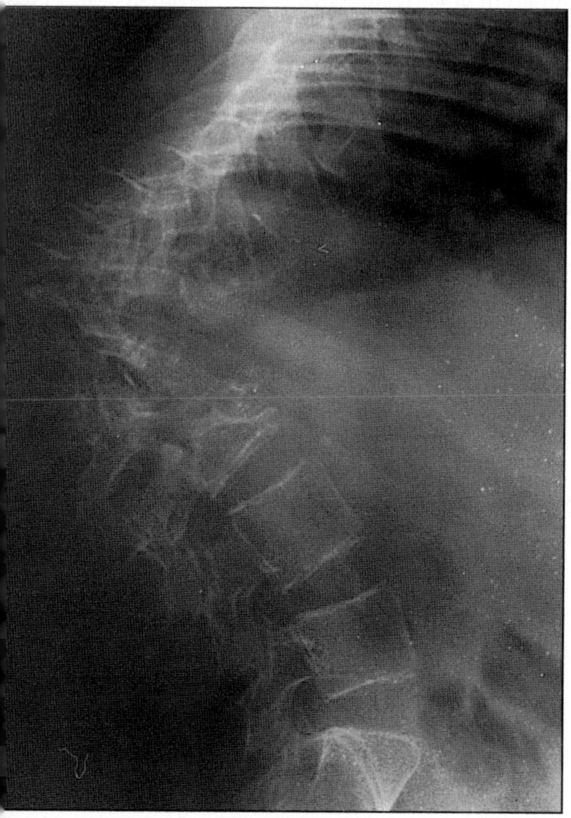

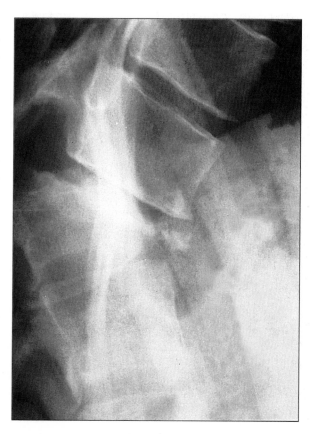

Figure 13.10 Lateral X-ray showing tuberculosis kyphosis (gibbus) at the thoracolumbar junction.

Figure 13.11 Spinal injury causing kyphosis (and paralysis). Note one vertebra crushed into a wedge shape.

Rheumatoid Disease

Rheumatoid disease of the spine, as exemplified by anky-losing spondylitis, can produce a kyphosis and loss of for-ward gaze in young adults (Figure 13.12).

Idiopathic Kyphosis

This is rare and is probably the forward-deforming coun-terpart of idiopathic lordoscoliosis. The thoracic vertebrae are all very slightly wedged, as are the disc spaces between them.

Degenerative Changes

Degenerative changes of ageing in the discs of the cervical and lumbar spine are frequently associated with a relative kyphosis (loss of lordosis) in these areas, producing the typ-ical stoop of the elderly.

LORDOSIS

Lordosis is almost always a deformity to compensate for a primary kyphosis deformity elsewhere in the spine. It is also the logical response to fixed flexion deformities at the hip. In the thoracic spine it is seen as a relative loss of the normal kyphosis in idiopathic scoliosis.

SPONDYLOLISTHESIS

Spondylolisthesis may result from: disc degeneration (spondylosis), especially at L4/5 in obese women in mid-dle life; an un-united fracture in childhood of the lamina

between the facet joints (pars interarticularis); a weakness (dysplasia) in the growing bone of the lamina which allows the lamina to stretch and the vertebral body of L5 to slide forward; or a violent spinal injury which may disrupt the neural arch so severely that the vertebral body is free to slide forward.

Degenerative disc disease may cause a vertebra to slide backward (retrolisthesis) or to twist and slide off to one side (rotatory subluxation).

Spondylolisthesis is almost always in the lower lumbar spine but is not always painful: it may be discovered quite by chance during X-ray investigations for non-spinal prob-lems.

DIAGNOSIS AND ASSESSMENT

On the basis that scoliosis is by far the most common spinal deformity, the remainder of this chapter is devoted largely to it.

Scoliosis is a problem not just because of the abnor-mal body shape but also because it tends to be progres-sive. The greater problem is that advanced scoliosis is very much more difficult to treat well than is mild or moderate scoliosis, but there is no certain way of know-ing which curve will progress nor how far it will progress. The partial solution to this problem is a com-bination of early diagnosis and continued vigilance: in other words, a long-term programme of regular visits to the clinic for examination and repeat imaging, at least until bone maturity is achieved, sometime between the ages of 16 and 19 years. Once progression is confirmed a scheme of treatment, possibly including surgery, can be planned for the patient.

Early detection was only partially successful when left to parents and teachers—it is difficult to notice subtle changes in posture in someone who is seen casually on a daily basis. A formal programme of clinical examination at school (school screening) was expected to solve this prob-lem but proved to be too expensive for the small number of cases discovered. Most school nurses and doctors are now quite capable of detecting early scoliosis during rou-tine health checks in schools.

The clinical examination is extremely simple and requires merely the inspection of the back of a child bend-ing forward, looking for a tell-tale rib hump (see Figure 13.3). Other asymmetries of the trunk which can be seen quite easily in the erect posture are waist creases, shoulder heights and a prominence of one shoulder blade. General awareness of scoliosis has increased in recent years, but the ideal of consistent early detection has not yet been achieved, and is probably an unrealistic goal.

Imaging of the spinal curvature is the next step, once the consultant staff are satisfied that the deformity war-rants an accurate baseline measurement against which to judge future developments. For the majority of scol-iosis clinics, this imaging will be in the form of X-rays, at least for the first examination. Thereafter, many clin-ics will repeat the imaging in the form of one of the new

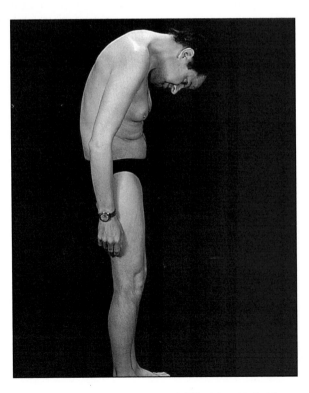

Figure 13.12 Ankylosing spondylitis (rheumatoid spondylitis) causing a fixed kyphosis and loss of forward gaze.

computerised trunk-shape measurements which can quantify the asymmetry of the deformity without the risk of exposure to radiation (see Quantec imaging, page 184 and Figure 13.22). On the erect standing anteroposterior X-ray film view, a standard measurement of the side-to-side bend (Cobb, 1948) and the rotation (Perdriolle & Vidal, 1985) allows comparison with similar measurements made at intervals of months or years. The Cobb method uses an ordinary protractor to measure the curves in degrees, and the Perdriolle method uses a specially designed protractor to measure the rotation. On this view one can also measure the extent to which the spine is out of balance, i.e. by how many centimetres the cervicothoracic junction is shifted off to one side of the lumbosacral junction (Figure 13.13). This information is of particular importance when considering the possibility of surgery.

These X-ray films should also show the iliac crests so that a rough assessment can be made of the patient's skeletal maturity (Risser, 1958): in general, idiopathic spinal curvatures will cease or slow in their progression as skeletal maturity is reached (Figure 13.14). The lateral (side) standing view is used to assess the extent of lordosis or kyphosis.

THE RIB HUMP

The rib hump is measured by one of a number of devices available for this purpose—either directly on the patient's back or by one of the photographic imaging techniques (Isis, Quantec). A very simple but useful measure is that produced by a spirit level (inclinometer) placed transversely across the rib hump with the patient in the forward-bending position. However, the Quantec technology can provide a volumetric measure of the rib hump, reflecting more accurately that part of the deformity which most distresses the patient.

FURTHER EXAMINATIONS

Further examinations depend on the circumstances. For example, if the patient with idiopathic scoliosis is being considered for surgical treatment, anteroposterior X-ray film views will be needed, with the patient bending to each side as far as possible to assess curve stiffness. In congenital scoliosis, there is always the suspicion that there may be other abnormalities in the spinal canal (e.g. split cord or diastematomyelia), kidneys and heart. Computerised tomography, magnetic resonance scanning, myelography, intravenous pyelography, and cardiac and lung function tests are necessary (in varying combinations) in preparation for surgery.

TREATMENT

CONSERVATIVE

For many years there was a widely accepted rule of thumb whereby idiopathic scoliosis was left untreated if the Cobb angle was less than 20°, treated conservatively in a brace (Milwaukee or Boston) if it was between 20° and 40°, and treated by spinal fusion if it was beyond 40°. This rule remains in many centres but variations to it are appearing: bracing has been abandoned, not only because it is unacceptable to self-conscious teenagers but also because studies

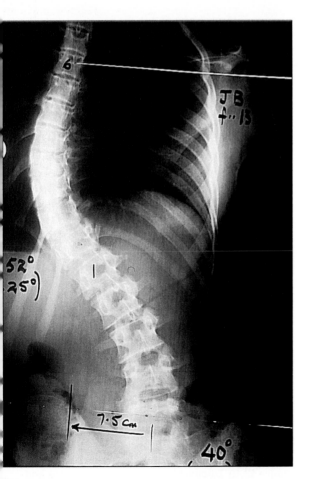

Figure 13.13 Scoliosis with out-of-balance curve in a 13-year-old girl (unusually convex to left side).

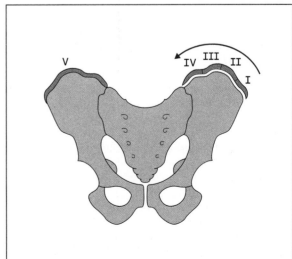

Figure 13.14 Risser measurement of skeletal maturity, graded I-IV. Grade V is when the iliac apophysis fuses with the iliac blade.

have raised serious doubts about its efficacy (Dickson *et al.*, 1980); and there is a trend to recommend surgery for curves reaching 35°.

The controversy over bracing is far from settled. The non-bracing philosophy relies on the scoliosis halting its progression spontaneously or proving its need for surgical treatment by showing progression to 35° and beyond.

There was a time when it was thought that certain exercises had some influence on the deformity, but this has been disproved: the only exercises now prescribed for scoliosis are as part of a bracing regimen.

Electrical stimulation of the muscles on the convexity of the curved spine through the night, has been used as a substitute for bracing mild curves. This is because it is more acceptable to patients and because it was seen to counteract some muscular imbalance thought to have produced the scoliosis in the first place. This treatment also remains controversial but has certainly declined in popularity.

SURGICAL

The decision to opt for surgery is based on three factors: curve severity, curve dynamics and the skeletal maturity of the patient. Severity relates to the degrees of bend (Cobb angle) and rotation with a rib hump. Dynamics consist of the rate of curve progression, curve stiffness and spinal balance. Skeletal maturity describes the level of development of the whole patient as well as of the bone of the spine, irrespective of the patient's chronological age.

A decision in favour of surgical treatment is likely to be made:
- For a patient with a progressive curve which corrects but little on side bending and shows a definite list to one side.
- Where the curve is greater than 35° and there is an unsightly rib hump.
- Where the patient has a Risser sign of III or less and has not yet reached the menarche (Figure 13.15).

The purpose of surgery is not only to halt progression of the curve but also to achieve some correction of the curve and its rib hump. All the operations involve a spinal fusion (bone graft) of some sort, to slow the growth of the spine and to stabilise it in the grafted position. All modern operations involve the insertion of some system of metal fixation to stabilise the spine until fusion is complete: all these systems provide some correction as well.

In congenital scoliosis, the purpose of surgery is to set the stage for future growth to halt the progression of the deformity, and possibly to reverse it. Striving too much to achieve correction during the operation, however, can be dangerous for the spinal cord.

The operations most commonly performed (together with bone grafting) are the:
- Harrington posterior instrumentation (Harrington, 1960): a rod supports hooks at either end of the spine so as to spread open the concavity of the curve (distraction); this is sometimes combined with a compression system on the convex side.

- Harrington–Luque technique: as above, but sublaminar wire-loops along the concavity are used to help pull the curved spine towards the straight rod—thus most closely resembling Andry's deformed tree (Figure 13.16A and B).
- Zielke method (Zielke, 1982): an anterior instrumentation through the chest (and through the diaphragm, into the abdomen, if necessary) which places screws transversely through the vertebral bodies, supporting a rod passing through the screw heads. This technique is ideal for curves with an apex at the thoracolumbar junction. It is capable of an impressive degree of derotation of the spine. The Webb–Morley system is a British version of this German system which in turn was based on the pioneering design of Dwyer in Australia.
- Cotrel–Dubousset (CD) (Cotrel & Dubousset, 1985): this system is applied posteriorly and is a major advance on the Harrington system, using rods on both sides of the spine and multiple hooks or screws. It is also capable of impressive derotation (Figure 13.17A and B).

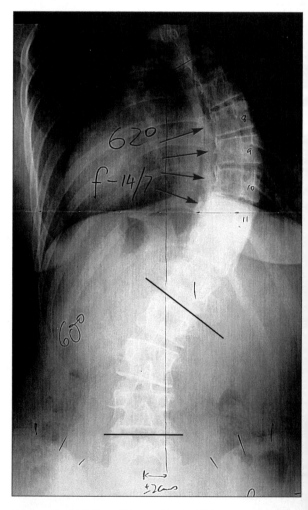

Figure 13.15 Idiopathic scoliosis 62°, severe and rigid, in a girl aged 14 with a Risser sign of only II.

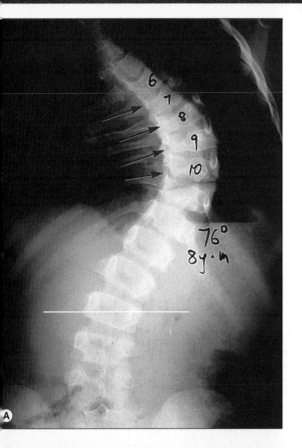

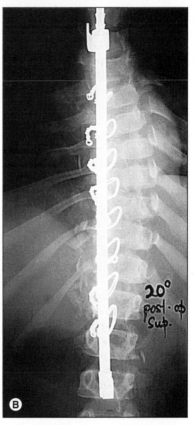

Figure 13.16
Idiopathic
scoliosis before
(A) and after
(B) the
Harrington-
Luque surgical
technique.

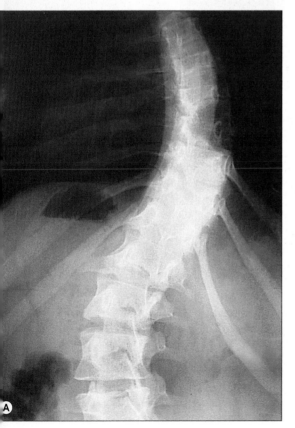

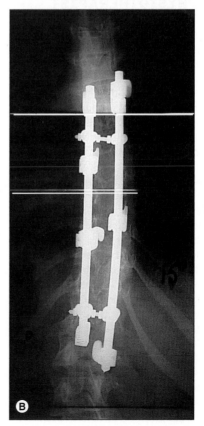

Figure 13.17
Scoliosis
before (A) and
after (B) the
more modern
type of
instrument-
ation such as
the Cotrel-
Dubousset.

• Luque segmental sublaminar system (Luque, 1982): a posterior procedure, ideal for neuromuscular (paralytic) scoliosis, where most of the thoracic and lumbar spine has to be fused in one operation. Double rods are secured to the spine by wires looped around the laminae (Figure 13.18).

Two other procedures are frequently used in conjunction with the above operations, usually under the same anaesthetic: anterior discectomy, at several levels, most often through a thoracotomy, to loosen a particularly stiff curve, and excision of part of several ribs in the rib hump (costoplasty) to improve the appearance of the distorted chest wall (Barrett *et al.*, 1993).

In congenital scoliosis, it is sometimes necessary to remove all of a 'wedge' vertebra, by a combined anterior and posterior approach; in other patients, it is necessary to destroy the vertebral body endplates along the convexity of a curve (epiphyseodesis) to slow down the deforming growth on that side.

In the presence of a stiff, severe kyphosis, such as in juvenile osteochondrosis (Scheuermann's disease), it is necessary to perform an anterior release and posterior compression with fusion. In ankylosing spondylitis, it is too dangerous to operate on the thoracic spine directly, for fear of producing paralysis. A combination of osteotomies (cutting across vertebrae) in the lumbar spine and at the cervicothoracic junction will produce gratifying improvements in posture and forward gaze.

ROLE OF THE PHYSIOTHERAPIST

Until the recent disillusionment with bracing, physiotherapists were intimately involved in scoliosis bracing programmes. With the reduction in bracing, and the realisation that exercises alone could not alter the course of scoliosis, it was thought that there would be little part for physiotherapists to play in the management of spinal deformities. However, physiotherapists are more intensely involved than ever before because of the greater complexity and hazard of the newer operations for spinal deformity.

Since many of these operations require entry into the chest and through the diaphragm, the physiotherapist is required to prepare the patient for surgery and to perform a thorough pre-operative assessment. This includes recording the patient's posture in sitting and standing, and supervising basic lung function tests (Figure 13.19). Breathing exercises are of the utmost importance, especially in those conditions such as the muscular dystrophies, where lung function is severely diminished even before surgery. Intensive pre-operative training will ensure a safer and shorter postoperative recovery period. The physiotherapist has a further important role as confidant, giving reassurance and encouragement. The physiotherapist is the most appropriate communication link between the patient and all members of the treatment team.

During the immediate postoperative recovery period, the physiotherapist helps to restore a clear airway, encourage deep breathing in spite of pain, supervise the function

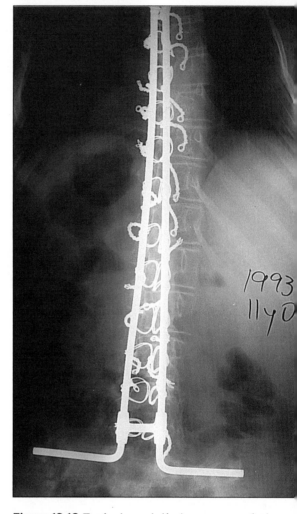

Figure 13.18 Typical paralytic (neuromuscular) scoliosis after surgery with the Luque segmental sublaminar system.

and safety of the chest drain, and help the return of joint movement in all limbs. Chest drains pass from the pleural cavity, between two ribs, into a sealed bottle. They are necessary for the removal of air and blood left over from the operation and generally stay in place for 2–3 days. The chest wall incision and the chest drain together cause significant postoperative pain. The pain will tend to restrict the patient's breathing and this is where the role of the physiotherapist is vital (Figure 13.20).

The role of the physiotherapist continues uninterrupted throughout the rest of the rehabilitation, encouraging an early resumption of sitting, standing and walking. Although most modern internal fixation systems are meant to do away with the need for postoperative bracing, many centres advise bracing for some weeks or months, as added protection for the developing fusion. A plaster of Paris or fibreglass cast is applied before discharge, with the physiotherapist assisting and supervising (Figure 13.21). On the return visit 6 weeks later, when postoperative swelling has settled and the

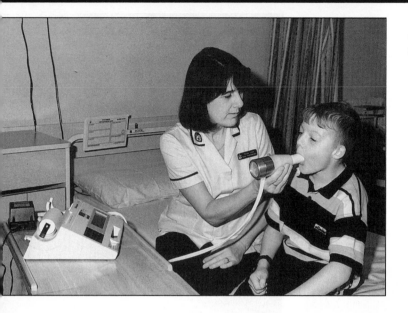

Figure 13.19 Physiotherapist conducting pre-operative respiratory function tests.

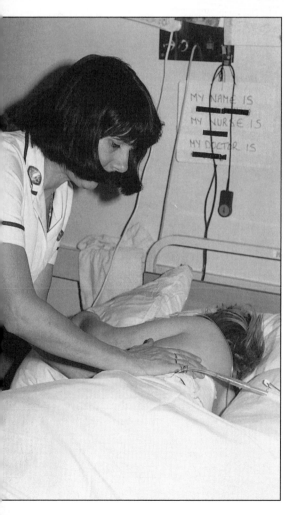

Figure 13.20 Physiotherapist helping post-thoracotomy scoliosis patient with postoperative breathing exercises.

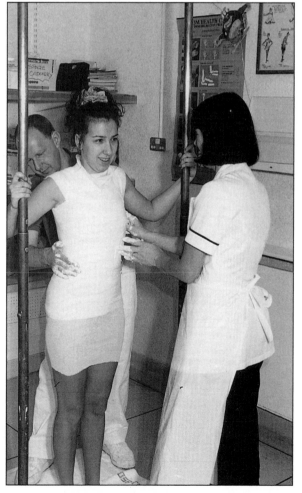

Figure 13.21 Physiotherapist and technician applying postoperative cast.

wound is quite healed, a lightweight removable polythene jacket is applied, to be worn for 4 months during school and daytime activities. Again, it is the physiotherapist who should supervise the fitting of the brace and the teaching of its use in such a way as to ensure that the patient will happily comply for the required period. The physiotherapist is the patient's best adviser on a programme of gradually increasing activity in the first weeks after surgery.

In the months and years after surgery, it is necessary to continue measurements of the chest wall deformity to be able to quantify the success or failure of surgery in that area which most concerns the patient. This is a concept much neglected until recently, because of the surgeon's obsession with the deformity of the spine alone. There is an opportunity here for an expanded role for the physiotherapist in the management and control of modern computerised image capture and processing technique. Quantec imaging produces a computer-generated digitised image of the patient's chest wall, captured in one fiftieth of a second, without any exposure to radiation and sufficiently accurate for the purposes of comparison with previous and later images (Figure 13.22A and B). From the information obtained it is also possible to make a number of useful calculations, including angles of lordosis and kyphosis, the Cobb angle and the difference in volume of the two sides of the asymmetrical posterior chest wall. Not only is this type of information far more useful than standard X-ray image, it should also result in a much reduced use of X-rays and the associated exposure to radiation.

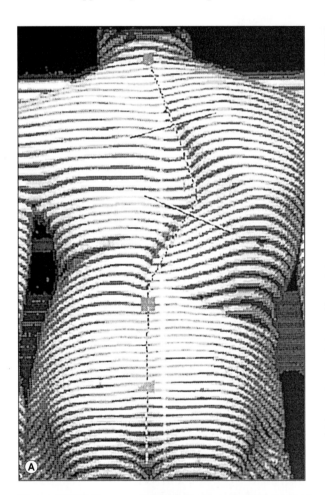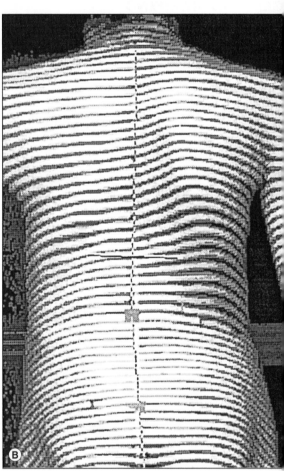

Figure 13.22 Measurement of chest wall asymmetry by the 'Quantec' system. Computer-generated images before **(A)** and after **(B)** surgery. This technology can measure the volume of the rib hump.

REFERENCES

Andry N. *Orthopaedia*. 1743. Facsimile reproduction of the 1st ed in English. Philadelphia: JB Lippincott; 1961.

Barrett DS, MacLean JG, Bettany J, Ransford AO, Edgar M. Costoplasty in adolescent idiopathic scoliosis. Objective results in 55 patients. *J Bone Joint Surg* 1993, **75B**:881-885.

Cobb J. *Outline for the study of scoliosis. Instructional course lectures*, vol V. American Academy of Orthopaedic Surgery: JW Edwards; 1948.

Cotrel Y, Dubousset J. New segmental posterior instrumentation of the spine. *Orthop Trans* 1985, **9**:118.

Goldberg CJ, Fogarty EE, Moore DP, Dowling FE. Scoliosis and developmental theory. Adolescent idiopathic scoliosis. *Spine* 1997, **22**:2228-2238.

Harrington PR. Surgical instrumentation for management of scoliosis. *J Bone Joint Surg* 1960, **42A**:1448.

Luque ER. Segmental spinal instrumentation for correction of scoliosis. *Clin Orthop* 1982, **163**:192-198.

Mehta MH. Infantile idiopathic scoliosis. In: Dickson RA, Bradford DS, eds. *Management of spinal deformities*. Boston: Butterworth; 1984, 101-120.

Mehdian H, Shimizu N, Draycott V, Evans G, Eisenstein S. Spinal stabilization for scoliosis in Duchenne muscular dystrophy. Experience with various sublaminar instrumentation systems. *Neuro-Orthopedics* 1989, **7**:74-82.

Perdriolle R, Vidal J. Thoracic idiopathic scoliosis curve evaluation and prognosis. *Spine* 1985, **10**:785-791.

Risser JC. The iliac apophysis: an invaluable sign in the management of scoliosis. *Clin Orthop* 1958, **11**:113.

Scheuermann HW. Kyfosis dorsalis juvenilis. *Ugeskr Laeger* 1920, **82**:385.

Zielke K. Ventral derotation spondylodesis: results of treatment of idiopathic lumbar scoliosis. *Zentral Orthop* 1982, **120**:320-329.

GENERAL READING

Dickson RA, Stamper P, Sharp AM, Harker P. School screening for scoliosis: cohort study of clinical course. *BMJ* 1980, **281**:265-267.

Leatherman KD, Dickson RA. *The management of spinal deformities*. London: Wright; 1988.

Lonstein J, Bradford DS, Winter RB, Ogilvie JW, eds. *Moe's textbook of scoliosis and other spinal deformities*, 3rd ed. Philadelphia: WB Saunders; 1994.

Scheuermann HW. The classic: kyphosis dorsalis juvenilis. *Clin Orthop* 1977, **128**:5-7.

Stagnara P. *Spinal deformity*. (English translation: John Dove). London: Butterworths; 1988.

SECTION 4

TREATMENT OPTIONS

orthopaedics (orthopaedix). That part of
surgery which deals with the
abnormalities, diseases and injuries of
the locomotor system

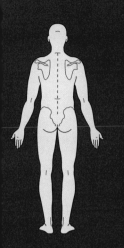

14

K L Haywood & B J Hollins

EXAMINATION OF A MUSCULOSKELETAL CONDITION

CHAPTER OUTLINE

- **Examination process**
- **Initial examination**

- **Objective examination**
- **Subjective examination**

INTRODUCTION

Over the past decade, the treatment of musculoskeletal conditions has progressed and diversified. It is no longer acceptable to consider a musculoskeletal examination as purely the assessment of muscles and joints of a particular functional area. When treating a patient in an outpatient department, physiotherapists are now expected to assess and to treat a whole range of clinical problems. These include neurodynamics, muscle imbalance, connective tissue tension, postural or ergonomic awareness, repetitive strain injuries, stress and social problems, and even metabolic or systemic syndromes. All of these features, and many more, need to be under consideration when a patient presents with a seemingly straightforward musculoskeletal problem. This eclectic approach to a patient's localised mechanical problem may present great difficulties to the physiotherapy student. A question which is often difficult for the newcomer to address is when to deviate from the highly structured examination format presented to students in their early days of training. Making assumptions too early and elaborating on a specific aspect of a patient's condition could result in inappropriate treatment being chosen. Conversely, accepting a clinical concept and performing a modality without careful, thoughtful and precise examination appropriate to that modality, may still result in only partial success.

The longer one is in practice, the clearer it becomes that the 'normal' state does not exist. All people possess varying degrees of abnormality in the form of asymmetrical structure, deviations of body posture, muscle imbalance, adverse mechanical tension, and malfunctioning metabolic processes and systemic organs. It should also be recognised that many individuals experience varying degrees of social pressure. If excessive, this causes stress which may be reflected through the musculoskeletal system.

When looking for an abnormality, you should ask, 'Just how significant is the patient's abnormality and is it appropriate to prioritise such findings?' One way to address this question during examination of a musculoskeletal condition, is to retain the orderly, systematic approach outlined by Maitland (1986, 1987, 1991) and others (Corrigan & Maitland, 1988; Grieve, 1994). On occasions, certain parts of the examination may require expansion, but this should be achieved without deviating too far from the logical sequence. These examination formats have been developed over a significant time, and condense a wealth of experience into practice which should be respected by the novice.

New physiotherapists should strive to become reflective practitioners, aiming to develop skills which enable them to perform a detailed analysis of the patient's findings before treatment. This analysis may well show that further examination of the patient in specific areas is necessary and appropriate to the chosen course of action. Careful analysis of patients as complete entities often reveals not only more appropriate courses of action, but also that they are knowledgeable informants of their own condition—patients live with their condition for 24 hours a day and must be given credit for this accumulated experience (Gadow, 1980).

In this chapter, the basic subjective and objective examination of a musculoskeletal condition will be explored, incorporating points from the authors' clinical experience. Making sense of a clinical examination of the patient is like solving the crime in a detective novel; the greater the number of clues pointing to a particular structure being at fault, the more reason the clinician has for considering the finding significant to the patient's problem and for prioritising treatment to this part of the patient's condition.

EXAMINATION PROCESS

The physiotherapist must continually analyse and reflect on the information gained from the examination. As outlined by Maitland (1986, 1987), Grieve (1994) and other eminent authorities in the field, examination is an ongoing process.

For a musculoskeletal problem, the examination can be divided into the:
- Initial examination.
- Assessment during treatment.
- Assessment between treatments.
- Retrospective assessment.
- Assessment before discharge.

INITIAL EXAMINATION
The initial examination consists of:
- Database collection.
- Subjective examination.
- Objective examination.
- Case history analysis.

On concluding the first consultation, the physiotherapist should have gained sufficient information from the case history analysis to know the characteristics of the patient, their presenting signs and symptoms, the severity and irritability of the disorder, the instability of the segment, any contraindications and precautions, and the progression of the disorder. This information should also assist in deciding whether a clinical diagnosis is possible or appropriate, identification of the stage of the disorder and the formulation of a plan for management.

ASSESSMENT DURING TREATMENT
Assessment during treatment consists of testing the subjective and objective markers before, during and after treatment. This assists in establishing the relevant success or failure of a particular treatment.

When implementing treatment, the physiotherapist should consider a wide range of factors, including the:
- Patient as a whole.
- Patient's attitude.
- Age of the patient.
- Irritability of the condition.
- Severity of the pain.
- Instability.
- Objectivity.
- Assessment of change in the condition.

ASSESSMENT BETWEEN TREATMENTS
The efficacy of a treatment modality and clinical diagnostic assumptions can only be assessed against the change achieved between treatment sessions (Maitland, 1986). The physiotherapist's and the patient's expectations of change are important. These expectations should be discussed, with both parties being fully aware of factors which influence the situation, e.g. social circumstances, ergonomics, home exercise, avoidance of certain activities.

RETROSPECTIVE ASSESSMENT
The physiotherapist should continually note changes or patterns of improvement in both subjective and objective outcome measures. Re-examination of salient clinical features and the physiotherapist's own clinical assumptions should take place every three or four treatment sessions. Reflection, or a second opinion, may totally change the course of action.

ASSESSMENT BEFORE DISCHARGE
This decision must be made against evaluation of the patient's prognosis and response to physiotherapy. The aim is to make the patient independent of medical care.

INITIAL EXAMINATION

Treatment can only be effective when linked with regular efficient examination and assessment, and this starts with the initial examination. The initial examination of the patient consists of collection of data from medical notes, subjective patient information, objective findings and, most importantly, non-verbal information.

The initial visit is often a new experience for the patient, who may appear rather apprehensive and require reassurance by the physiotherapist. At this point the patient should be told that many questions will be asked during the examination. Some of the questions may seem strange, some may have been asked many times before or some may seem of little immediate relevance. Confidence can be inspired by reassurance that the answers to such questions can be of great assistance to the physiotherapist.

During the examination, although patients should be kept to the point kindly and firmly, they must feel they have time to answer the questions and recognise that their view of the problem is considered informative. The physiotherapist must listen to the patient. The patient, in turn, should not be made to feel subordinate or given the impression that they are complaining unnecessarily, otherwise they will be selective when providing information, and this can be misleading. The questions asked or instructions given need to be simple and delivered singly. The answer to one question should be established before moving on to the next and, similarly, the result of one physical test needs to be determined before proceeding to another. The physiotherapist needs to clarify information as it is gathered. Some questions or physical tests may cause the patient confusion and the physiotherapist should be sensitive to this situation and reconstruct questions or instructions if required.

To comprehend the situation fully, the physiotherapist should aim to identify mentally with the patient. This entails a commitment to develop an equal patient–physiotherapist relationship; it is a therapeutic relationship which is most rewarding to both parties (Stimson & Webb, 1975; Strong, 1979; Tucket et al., 1985; Thornquist, 1990).

DATABASE COLLECTION

To obtain a comprehensive database, information should include the:

Name and address of the patient.

Unit number.

Date of examination. This is important for future reference, e.g. in establishing the duration of the problem before presentation to the medical service, or the duration of the course of treatment.

Date of birth. This allows consideration of whether the condition is expected or may have arisen as a result of other factors associated with a particular 'time of life', e.g. osteoporosis in a postmenopausal woman (Dixon, 1995).

Occupation and hobbies. A physiotherapist needs to understand the biomechanical factors associated with an individual's occupation and hobbies. The relation between these factors and the current problem can be established during the subjective examination.

Social history. What are the social circumstances of the patient, and is the individual able to cope? Are there factors arising in the social history that may relate directly to the physical problem? For example, is the low back pain aggravated by the patient caring for small children? Sensitivity is required when enquiring about an individual's social situation.

Compensation. Is industrial compensation being sought by the patient? If so, the physiotherapist must be sensitive when enquiring about this and also when determining the progress of the claim at the time of examination. This is an added burden for the patient and may complicate the picture. However, there is no evidence to suggest that a relation between compensation and a victim's continuing complaint of physical disability exists (Croft, 1995a,b).

SUBJECTIVE EXAMINATION

The subjective examination can be divided into four parts. These are:

Part 1. The type of disorder and the site of symptoms.

Part 2. The behaviour of clinical features.

Part 3. Special questions.

Part 4. History of the present complaint.

Part 1: Type of Disorder and Site of Symptoms

To open the questions and to establish the type of disorder the patient is experiencing, two suggestions by Maitland (1986, 1991) are appropriate: 'Would you like to show me where your main problem is located?' and 'As far as you are concerned, what is your main problem at this present time?'

Such questions appear to be more effective than simply asking the patient 'Where is your pain?' The approach aims to emphasise that the physiotherapist is interested in the patient's view of the situation and how it affects them now, not how others in the medical profession perceive the problem. The physiotherapist needs to have an understanding of the factors causing the greatest concern to the patient. For example, is pain the major concern, or reduction in the range of movement of associated joints?

Clinical features discovered during the examination are recorded accurately on a body chart, which enables the physiotherapist to have an overview of all the information gained.

Body Chart

A body chart is a pictorial representation of the patient's complaint (Figure 14.1A and B).

It is helpful to introduce the body chart at this early stage of the examination as it is difficult to obtain an accurate subjective examination in a logical chronological order without a clear understanding and visual record of the patient's clinical features. The physiotherapist needs to understand fully what the patient is referring to when the problem is described as 'it'. With this knowledge, the physiotherapist will be able to place the patient's responses to questions in their correct context. However, the patient's spontaneous answers may not reflect clinical priorities. Obtaining an accurate and precise description will indicate the distribution of symptoms and may even indicate a possible cause. Clinical reasoning may direct the examination process to an area of the body which in the patient's opinion is of less importance. At the appropriate time, full justification of the physiotherapist's actions must be given to the patient, otherwise misunderstandings may occur and any placebo effect achieved by the thorough examination may be lost.

Obtaining an accurate and precise description of the distribution of the symptoms helps to indicate whether a problem is local or referred, and what structure may be causing its production. A patient who has a clear understanding of the exact area of the problem is often found to be both physically and psychologically stable.

Interpreting a patient's story with conviction of where the problem lies requires caution at times. For example, nerve root pain is usually worse distally. This distal distribution of pain may be deep within a peripheral structure. In this way, a spinal problem could well mimic a peripheral joint syndrome, with local soft tissue tenderness and movement signs. From clinical experience, however, the depth of the pain may help to locate the structure at fault; for example, the more distal a joint is from the spine, the more likely a pain will be located deep within that joint if it is that joint at fault. Conversely, not all superficial pain is referred pain. Such pain could have many causes, not the least a localised inflammatory reaction, a skin condition or even an emotional component.

If a clinical feature is intermittent or variable, it is fair to say there could be a mechanical origin to the problem. All mechanical problems should be described as having a variation in their intensity as the parts move mechanically.

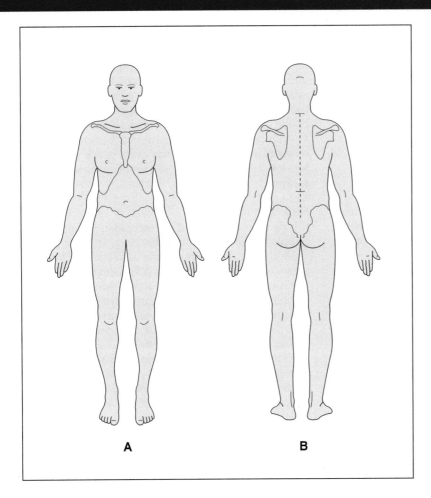

14

Figure 14.1 Body chart. (A)
Anterior and **(B)** posterior view.

A   B

However, patients occasionally have difficulty in expressing the varying nature of their symptoms, so a careful analysis and rephrasing of questions is essential to pursue the assessment further. The physiotherapist should assume that a problem which is described as 'constant' is actually variable until proved otherwise. Also, if symptoms are intermittent, is the patient ever completely free of pain? If so, when?

If after interrogation it seems that symptoms do not vary, this suggests the condition is non-mechanical in origin, which may indicate that physiotherapy intervention for a mechanical problem is inappropriate.

To clarify whether two or more symptoms are related or separate, such questions as 'Do the symptoms always occur together?' or 'Do you feel that the two problems are related?' can often be quite helpful. Patients may be quite clear about their perceived relation between two or more pains, and their feelings about this relation can assist the physiotherapist greatly. If related, the physiotherapist needs to identify structures which could influence the symptoms, while at the same time keeping an open mind.

Valuable information about the nature of the symptoms can be obtained by elucidating what the problem feels like to the patient. An answer can direct the clinical thought processes. For example, a 'sharp' or 'catch' pain probably indicates that a mechanical structure is catching on a pain-sensitive area. The more frequently this 'catch' occurs, the more likely a localised inflammatory response can be expected; often described as a 'dull background ache'. A severe nerve root irritation is often described like a 'gnawing toothache'. In contrast, a severe irritation of a peripheral nerve may be described as a 'burning pain'.

Rather than identifying the sensory components of pain, some patients express the emotional experience of their pain, ranging from 'intolerable' or 'unbearable' to 'devastating' or 'diabolic'. Patients may express that they can no longer cope with the pain when, in fact, they can no longer cope with the current situation. The more severe the emotional distress, the more descriptive the expression (Craig, 1984). The physiotherapist needs to be aware of such descriptors of pain. A consideration of both emotional and biomedical support needs to be made in the final analysis.

Disturbances of the nervous, circulatory and autonomic systems can frequently be associated with musculoskeletal problems. Any evidence of anaesthesia, tingling, pins and needles, or swelling should be documented accurately on the body chart. Further investigation of the relevant system should be pursued in the objective examination.

Before proceeding to the next step, it is vital to mark with a tick on the body chart any areas of the body which the patient indicates are totally free from clinical symptoms on the day of the first assessment. Apart from documenting accurately the patient's condition and increasing the accuracy of the body chart, it can sometimes stimulate a patient to mention odd symptoms which were felt to be irrelevant to the present condition. Without ascertaining these areas at the first session, a later change in the patient's presentation may be difficult to identify.

Once the body chart is complete, it is essential to identify which anatomical structures could give rise to the clinical features presented by the patient; also, to consider the questions that need to be asked about the behaviour of symptoms so as to prove or disprove the physiotherapist's assumptions. Questions must be formulated skilfully to pursue relevant information quickly and efficiently, without prompting the patient. The inexperienced clinician may find it helpful to make a list of questions for each suspect joint. For example, if a patient complains of both shoulder and cervical spine pain, the clinician may want to investigate further, to ascertain if one area is predominantly at fault. To assess the cervical spine further, it may be helpful to enquire about the effect of activities such as reading, reversing the car and looking up at the ceiling, or prolonged flexion. Involvement of the shoulder may require further information about the ability to fasten brassieres, zips, and aprons, to tuck shirts into trousers and to wash and dry oneself.

Having planned the questions, the physiotherapist is ready to move on to the next stage of the subjective assessment.

Part 2: Behaviour of Clinical Features

The purpose of this stage is to determine specifically which structures are at fault and to ascertain the appropriate objective examination; also, to establish the complexity of forces which bring on the symptoms, whether the problem curtails activity, and how the patient manages to reduce or cope with symptoms. It is helpful to divide the behaviour of the clinical features into:

Aggravating and easing factors.
Morning, day and night variation in pain.
Coughing and sneezing.

Aggravating and Easing Factors

There are five good reasons for a very careful analysis of the factors that may aggravate or ease the patient's condition. Firstly, assumptions made about the nature of the condition can be proved or disproved . By assessing the biomechanical implications determined from the patient's explanation, the physiotherapist should be able to ascertain the structures that are being affected, e.g. compressed, stretched, contracted, and therefore to identify the possible

sources of pain. If a clear biomechanical analysis is difficult, the physiotherapist must be open-minded to decide whether the problem is mechanically based.

Secondly, the irritability of the condition must be determined. The physiotherapist should think in terms of sustained and quick activities for each functional area. Irritability concerns: the factors that aggravate symptoms and how soon these symptoms are provoked by the activity; the severity of the symptoms; the time the individual can tolerate the activity; the factors that ease the symptoms; and the length of time it takes for the problem to settle. The answers will result in safer manual handling of the patient. A patient's condition may be described as reflecting a highly irritable state if, for example, severe pain is caused by minimal activity and takes a long time to ease. In such situations the objective examination would be both minimal and specific, needing to highlight key elements and avoid aggravating factors. A physiotherapist should be conscious of the fact that a patient should not leave the department in a worse state than on arrival. A consideration of irritability will help to reduce this complication.

Thirdly, the severity of the condition should be established. It is not the same as irritability. The severity of a complaint is the intensity and spread of a symptom, established from the body chart, which will affect the amount of activity possible. The intensity and extent of the symptom, and their variation, are assessed by the patient, not the physiotherapist. A visual analogue scale (VAS) may be useful in grading the level of severity. This is a scale from 0 to 10, where 0 represents no symptom present and 10 is the worst imaginable manifestation of a symptom (Dixon & Bird, 1981). For example, a patient who complains of a pain in the lumbar region of 5/10 on a VAS scale when standing, which increases to 9/10 and also produces pins and needles in the foot, can be considered of high severity. This condition is both intense and extensive and will limit how much lifting the patient will be able to do.

Fourthly, the presence of instability of a segment should be suspected when the patient is inconsistent in identifying those activities that aggravate or ease the problem. This is especially the case when the inconsistency is coupled with reports of feelings of heaviness, latency, 'giving way', catch pains or locking.

Finally, patients often indicate the most effective treatment modality by describing their own home-management programme or experiences that have been of positive benefit. For example, if rest eases the symptoms, the physiotherapist needs to know the position in which this occurs, how readily the symptoms ease and the length of time it takes for them to settle. Suggested easing factors may help guide the physiotherapist in the choice of treatment modality. For example, a patient with neck pain may experience pain relief on holding and lifting the head, indicating that manual cervical traction could be of benefit to the patient. Choosing a treatment modality which enhances positive experiences is more likely to motivate patients to take control of their own care. During the explanation of aggravating and easing factors, a patient often reveals poor postural and ergonomic awareness. Hence, treatment can be directed at empowering the patient towards responsibility for this aspect of self-care.

Morning, Day and Night Variation in Pain

From clinical experience it has been found that mechanical problems should settle with overnight rest, most musculoskeletal problems usually taking no longer than 1 hour of rest to ease. If sleep is disturbed and the patient is unable to achieve beneficial rest, the physiotherapist needs to identify possible reasons for this. Many factors need to be considered when evaluating a patient's diurnal variation of pain:

Type of Bed and Pillows

The ideal bed is that on which the patient is comfortable and relatively pain free. A hard bed is not necessarily the most suitable, but the patient may benefit from a hard base with a softer mattress on top. The softness of the mattress may be adjusted to suit the patient's needs.

Feather pillows adapt readily to the shape of the head and neck and therefore will support the underlying area well when the muscles relax. Foam pillows often 'bounce' and therefore provide limited support. Butterfly pillows may be helpful, particularly in patients with cervical spine problems. Having too many pillows may force the neck into an uncomfortable flexed or side-flexed position. As a guide, the neck should be supported in mid-range, but the precise position of comfort is very individual and patients should be advised to experiment with different pillows.

The physiotherapist must consider that activities during the day may have aggravated the condition to an extent that sleep is disturbed, for example, the latent onset of nerve root pain. If this latency is not taken into consideration, it may lead to inappropriate treatment when the pain is reduced.

Night Pain

After considering the type and number of pillows and the suitability of the bed, increased pain overnight may alert the clinician to an inflammatory component or to a serious pathology. In such cases, the pain may be constant and non-fluctuating, and is often not relieved by rest: the patient may need to get up and move around during the night to try to ease symptoms—even so, the pain may not be relieved. Pain not relieved by rest should put physiotherapists on their guard. This may not, however, be the whole story, as the dark quiet atmosphere of a bedroom may be the ideal fermenting ground for the patient's emotional or marital problems. For the clinician new to examination, it may be a daunting prospect to take on board this aspect of a patient's problems.

Morning Pain

If pain is not reduced by the morning after a night's rest, the physiotherapist needs to determine why. If the pain is not present on waking, this suggests it has been eased by rest, but if the pain is present on rising, this suggests it is aggravated by climbing out of bed—possibly implying a mechanical basis to the problem, with a low threshold of activity. Severity and irritability levels must be established to guide the analysis of the examination findings.

Increased pain and stiffness in the morning which does not settle within 1 hour should alert the clinician to the presence of an inflammatory condition or the possibility of an autonomic, systemic or emotional component. In certain inflammatory musculoskeletal conditions, stiffness may be the main complaint on waking. The length of time required for the stiffness to ease indicates the possible pathoanatomy of the condition. For example, if stiffness lasts for less than 30 minutes, this implies normal degenerative symptoms with a slight localised inflammatory component, but if the stiffness lasts for more than 30 minutes a more generalised inflammatory condition should be suspected, e.g. ankylosing spondylitis, rheumatoid arthritis.

Day Pain

The physiotherapist needs to understand how a patient's symptoms vary over 24 hours. For example, how do the symptoms experienced at the end of the day compare with those throughout the day? This will involve identification of the problem as having time-dependent, activity-dependent or latent qualities. Analysis will assist in determining the structures at fault and a possible diagnosis. For example, a degenerative mechanical condition with no inflammatory component is most likely to be activity dependent.

Coughing and Sneezing

During a cough or sneeze, there is an increase in intra-abdominal pressure. The pain during coughing or sneezing has therefore often been reported as discogenic in origin (Nachemson & Morris, 1964); however, the thoracic spine or accessory muscles may also be implicated. Also, quadratus lumborum strain and subsequent shortening is an under rated syndrome that often produces pain on coughing or sneezing. To aid in the differential diagnosis, the patient's posture when the pain occurs should be considered.

Part 3: Special Questions

A detailed analysis of the answers to 'special' questions should take place before the patient's history of the present complaint is ascertained. By placing the onset of clinical features in chronological order, it may well be discovered that the systemic and musculoskeletal symptoms are related: for example, a hip problem in a female may have manifested after the onset of a gynaecological problem, or a middle-aged business executive with an arm pain worse on exertion may have noticed the onset of the pain during a period of high blood pressure, increased stress and a tightening feeling in his chest indicating a possible cardiac component.

Certain questions to identify specific precautions and contraindications to treatment are mandatory. Questions to rule out contraindications to tough manual techniques should never be rushed, regardless of the treatment being considered as these questions act as pointers towards more serious pathology, and also provide an overall picture of the patient's general state of health and subsequent healing potential.

Radiological Reports

Always ask patients if they have had a recent radiological examination, and aim to view the X-ray films. The films will have been seen by a radiologist or an orthopaedic surgeon, and a report written. This report should be read, as the professional judgement of these experts is essential. However, caution is necessary in the analysis of findings from an X-ray examination. Some patients can experience severe pain with significant limitation in movement which is not reflected in the findings, while other patients with gross findings may well present with a good range of movement and very little pain. Patients may be distressed if their X-ray films show no evidence of abnormality, but they should be assured that this can be quite normal and does not imply the problem is 'all in the mind'. Investigations such as radiography, magnetic resonance imaging (MRI) scanning and computerised tomography (CT) scanning have been described as 'Telling the truth, but not the whole truth, and nothing but the truth' (Lord, 1995).

General Health

If the patient is receiving treatment for any other condition, it is important to identify the problem and the treatment. This information may influence the physiotherapist's decisions about the prognosis of the presenting condition and potential treatment regimens. Poor general health in itself may be very informative because of its influence on the prognosis. It can be caused by emotional, metabolic or systemic factors, and may cause the patient to lose weight. If weight loss is sudden or unexpected, it should be identified with caution, as it may suggest carcinoma.

A physiotherapist should read a patient's hospital report before or soon after the first assessment. These notes will provide important information about the current status of the patient's general health, concurrent investigations and the referring consultant's opinion of the condition. If it seems, however, that a patient's condition has deteriorated significantly since the last review by the consultant, the physiotherapist may decide to seek further advice from the referring consultant.

If a patient is overweight and this is considered to have a negative effect on the condition, the physiotherapist may need to address weight loss as part of the treatment regimen. Obesity is a particular problem for weight-bearing joints. The physiotherapist should be sensitive to the patient, but it may be necessary to refer the patient to a specialist for weight control.

Severe pain may show in the patient's face. Often, when sleep is disturbed by pain, the patient seems to be very tired both physically and mentally.

Operations

Abdominal operations are of particular importance, especially if they involve the intestines. Such operations may reduce the efficiency of vitamin D absorption, increasing the patient's chance of developing osteoporosis (Dixon, 1995).

Drug History

If the patient is taking medication regularly at the time of assessment, it is beneficial to know which drug, why and how often it is taken, and the length of time it has been taken. Such questioning may reveal a condition not mentioned by the patient under 'general health'. If the patient takes analgesics, the physiotherapist needs to ask certain questions: 'How many painkillers are you taking daily?' 'Are the analgesics taken for the pain, because of your apprehension about the pain, or as an habitual response to the problem?' 'How many analgesics have you taken today [on the day of the examination] and when was the last one taken?'

Recent analgesia may mask any pain produced during the objective examination. Answers to the questions above will assist physiotherapists in developing their understanding of the nature, severity and irritability of the condition, and in their consequent planning of any objective examination.

If the patient admits to having taken corticosteroids, it is important to identify the condition for which these were taken and whether high doses were required over a prolonged period. In time, high-dose corticosteroids affect the quality of bone and soft tissue and predispose to osteoporosis (Dixon, 1995). Therefore, caution is required when planning an objective examination and potential treatment regimens for such patients.

Patients may be given anticoagulants after surgery—for example, following an open reduction with internal fixation of a fractured ankle. As anticoagulants make patients more susceptible to bleeding, forceful treatment techniques should be avoided.

Rheumatoid Arthritis

Rheumatoid arthritis is a systemic, multisystem inflammatory disorder (Walker, 1995). The inflammatory process may lead to a reduction in the quality of soft tissue and bone. Osteoporosis and weakness of the ligaments supporting the involved joints are potential consequences of the disease process. The physiotherapist needs to establish if there is a family history of rheumatoid arthritis or any other inflammatory disorder, e.g. ankylosing spondylitis.

Spinal Cord Involvement

A patient may report difficulties with, or alterations in, the normal walking pattern, or be aware of tripping for no apparent reason. Such findings can indicate an abnormal increased tone, and, if coupled with bilateral tingling in the hands or feet, a physiotherapist should suspect the possibility of an upper motor neurone lesion. Such findings indicate caution and a possible return to the referring consultant for further investigations.

When a patient presents with problems associated with abnormal bladder control and sensation, e.g. a reduced awareness of the need to pass urine, the physiotherapist should be alerted to the possibility of irritation of the nerve roots supplying the area. The prevalence of localised lesions of the pelvic region should not be underestimated and the physiotherapist should attempt to distinguish between a pelvic problem and one due to actual nerve irritation or damage. The physiotherapist needs to keep an open mind about the implications of such symptoms until the examination is completed.

Complaints of headaches, drop attacks and dizziness have many potential causes, including vertebral artery insufficiency, middle ear problems, hypotension, disturbances of the cervical proprioceptive mechanism or autonomic involvement, psychological implications, cord ischaemia, migraines, ligamentous laxity, and musculoskeletal or skeletal problems from the thoracic spine.

Diabetes

Diabetes may adversely affect soft tissue repair and can be associated with osteoporosis and diabetic neuropathies. As a consequence, the diagnosis of diabetes may influence the patient's prognosis and treatment. It would be wise for the physiotherapist treating a patient with diabetes to enquire about the stability of the condition, medication taken and disposition to diabetic comas.

Part 4: History of the Presenting Complaint

The therapist must be prepared to investigate fully the history of the patient's presenting complaint. A detailed history should come last, especially when considering peripheral joint problems, but this is not to imply that it is of least importance. Valuable time can be saved during the analysis stage of a patient's examination by establishing and understanding the chronological order of presentation of the patient's symptoms. The physiotherapist may include information about the onset, progression and relation of relevant aspects of the musculoskeletal condition, as well as relevant systemic problems, trauma, surgery, stress and social difficulties experienced by the patient. This approach will provide an holistic view of the patient and their problems.

An accurate history enables the patient to be classified into one of three possible pathological stages:
- Inflammation.
- Tissue repair.
- Tissue degeneration.

The history can also indicate the short- and long-term goals of treatment, prognosis and outcome. Such predictions come with practice and are often demanded in the documentation of local trust hospitals.

Present History

The present history of the patient's presenting complaint can be divided into its onset and its progression.

Onset

When investigating the onset of the presenting complaint, three main points need to be established:
- When did the problem start?
- How did the problem start—gradually or of sudden onset?
- Did the onset involve some form of injury or was it spontaneous?

All responses to these questions need to be expanded to obtain sufficient relevant information.

If the problem developed after physical injury, the physiotherapist must establish the exact sequence of events. An understanding of the mechanism of injury and subsequent biomechanical or kinesiological implications of the forces involved is required. This analysis assists in the recognition of the damaged structures, the potential for successful healing and the most beneficial treatment modalities. The following checklist may help an inexperienced physiotherapist to progress through this stage of the examination.
- Was the patient able to walk away from the incident? The answer indicates the severity of the initial trauma and the extent of underlying tissue damage. If the patient could not leave the incident unaided, the clinician should ascertain the extent of the assistance required; for example, was the individual able to take full weight on the injured limb?
- Did the patient notice any immediate joint or tissue swelling? Swelling noticed within minutes of the injury implies that bleeding has occurred in the tissues, for example, due to the tearing of a ligament. However, although swelling is frequently noticed immediately, it should be remembered that an haemarthrosis may have a gradual onset.
- What has been the patient's progress since the trauma? Has the pain increased, decreased or remained static? If swelling was present at the time of trauma, has it subsided? If any self-care was instituted, what was it and was it effective? Answers to these questions will help the physiotherapist to assess the progression and prognosis of the condition. Information about the events between the time of the trauma and the patient's presentation to the physiotherapist are important. If the intensity of the pain or the distribution of symptoms has increased, the physiotherapist should seek to identify why this has happened. If the problem is improving spontaneously, the prognosis should be good.

If the problem had a spontaneous onset with no known injury, the physiotherapist should delve deeper into the patient's history to ascertain any predisposing incidents. For example, patients may recollect unusual, unguarded or sustained movements or activities, particularly occurring when they were tired, cold or wet.

When enquiring about the patient's occupation, it may be informative to determine if the job requirements have recently changed. If there has been change, the physiotherapist should establish the reasons for the change and the demands of the new work. If the alteration in work activity coincides with the onset of the problem, it would be worthwhile to pursue this area of enquiry. Any alteration in the patient's activities of daily life may provide a clue to the onset of the condition. For example, a patient who spends long periods sitting may react adversely to their usual desk or chair being changed. Any infection or high temperature coinciding with the time of onset may have significance to musculoskeletal pain of spontaneous onset, and this should be noted.

Clinicians should attempt to analyse the meaning of the patient's descriptions of their problems and avoid making judgements based on their own preconceptions. For example, to avoid prompting a patient, skilful questioning is needed to assess if a 'sudden onset' occurred over minutes, hours or days. Spontaneous comments should not be undervalued, as they often provide keywords or phrases that can give valuable information on follow-up. Throughout the taking of the history, the physiotherapist attempts to rationalise the pathogenesis and prognosis of the disorder. It is essential that the physiotherapist listens to the patient and shows a concern for their problem: to quote GD Maitland, 'Acceptance of the patient and his story is essential if trust between the patient and the clinician is to be established.'

Progression

After investigating the onset of the presenting complaint, the physiotherapist establishes a detailed history of its progression, covering the period from the onset of the problem to the day of the examination. The physiotherapist needs to identify the order of occurrence of each clinical feature, as this provides the chronological progression of the condition. To categorise this progression, the patient may be asked to choose from the terms:

- 'Better'. In this case the prognosis is good, and the physiotherapist must be sure not to make it worse.
- 'Worse'. In this case both the physiotherapist and the patient need to be aware of the prognosis. It may be possible only to halt the progressively deteriorating condition. The response is slow and patience is required.
- 'About the same'. In this case the condition is fairly static, and treatment could be fairly vigorous, depending upon the condition's severity and irritability.

Any treatment for the condition before the patient presented to the department should be noted. Information based on this treatment, e.g. the type of treatment, by whom it was administered and its relative success, may assist the physiotherapist in choosing a suitable treatment modality.

Past History of the Complaint

Here, the physiotherapist attempts to identify the particular stage and progression of the pathology. A 'progressive pathology' is indicated by a patient who experiences repeated bouts of symptoms which are of increasing severity and brought on by progressively less severe incidents. The severity of the exacerbating incident should always be assessed against the degree of disability produced.

Questioning is an investigative procedure and is directed to the start of the patient's condition, e.g. the initial injury, an aggravating occupation or hobby, any falls or road traffic accidents, pregnancy. Having established this part of the history, the physiotherapist needs to understand the frequency, intensity and distribution of the clinical features, by ascertaining:

- Details of the first onset of the original problem.

- The history between the first onset of the problem and its current presentation.
- The number of incidents between the initial and current onset of the condition.
- The time between incidents, and whether these intervals are regular or irregular.
- The patient's status between incidents, e.g. was full fitness achieved between the periods of pain?
- Whether the patient has noticed exacerbation of the problem related to certain activities.
- How the current incidence of pain for which the patient is seeking treatment compares with the first incidence of pain.

The subjective assessment should continue until the physiotherapist has identified those structures which require attention during the objective examination, and until it is known how far the objective examination can be taken without aggravating the disorder, to establish the most important and useful information at the first appointment (Butler, 1991).

OBJECTIVE EXAMINATION

After completing the subjective examination, the next step is to reflect upon the information and to consider the most appropriate examination with which to proceed. This reflection should identify several important aspects of the patient's condition; for example, the nature of the problem and its irritability, the severity of pain and the instability of the segment. Before proceeding with any manual handling, the precautions and contraindications evident from the patient's history should determine the type of examination. The physiotherapist should decide whether the objective examination is to be aimed at the spine, merely checking for peripheral joint involvement, or the reverse.

While it is essential to determine the examination with which to proceed, the aim should be to perform as many tests as possible to prove or disprove clinical judgements. In this respect it is not wise for the inexperienced physiotherapist to deviate too far from the detailed examination of a patient (Maitland, 1986, 1991; Corrigan & Maitland, 1988; Grieve, 1994). Without the clinical experience to make sound decisions about what to omit from an examination, fundamental errors of judgement can be made. To pay attention to detail at the expense of a wide-ranging holistic view of the patient's condition requires a sound and accurate subjective examination, which can only be acquired with practice. A novice physiotherapist should aim to be thorough in the objective examination, performing routine tests even if these are not expected to provide further information, e.g. performing neurological tests in the patient with no peripheral pain. The results of such tests contribute to the overall picture and will assist the physiotherapist in maintaining an open mind until the examination is complete.

Finally, the physiotherapist should reflect on the information gained from the examination for the same length of time as it took to acquire it. This reflection follows two pathways. Firstly, the physiotherapist must determine the relevance of the information gathered and decide if the information is appropriate to the patient's presenting problem. Secondly, the physiotherapist should evaluate the efficiency of the testing procedures. Could the tests be improved, and were they sufficiently refined to give valid results? This type of reflection and attention to detail will ensure that the physiotherapist learns from each patient. In the long term it will save the physiotherapist time, and make the clinical diagnosis more reliable (Egan *et al.*, 1996).

The basic tests performed on the musculoskeletal system can be found in any good text (Hoppenfeld, 1976; Maitland, 1986, 1991; Corrigan & Maitland, 1988; Magee, 1992; Grieve, 1994; Bogduk & Mercer, 1995). The tests fall into several broad categories and the reader is referred to the above texts for specific details on their performance. Each category will be discussed in the light of clinical experience.

Observation

Spending time looking at the patient as a whole and at the specific area affected is not time wasted. Although abnormalities of shape and form are 'normal' in a patient, it can be very informative to note the degree to which the abnormalities exist and the relation to the affected area. While asymmetry may not be relevant at the time, it may indicate predisposing factors which, if not handled appropriately, could lead to a recurrence of the patient's condition. Deviations of the musculoskeletal alignment in one area so often set up compensatory effects in different areas of the body. For example, over-supination of the foot has an effect on tibial rotation and hence knee extension. This in turn determines the position of the patella, the degree of hip extension and the position of the femur. Femoral position and the length of the femur in turn affect pelvic rotation and position. Changes in pelvic position can change lumbar lordosis quite profoundly. Other areas that can also be affected include the thoracic kyphosis, the position of the shoulder girdle, the cervical spine and even the temporomandibular joint alignment. Hence, observation of the patient as a whole is essential.

Areas to be observed are the skin, soft tissues, joints, muscles and the structural symmetry. Skin colour, texture and condition can indicate circulatory, inflammatory, autonomic or neurological conditions which may not otherwise be suspected; for example, brown or black pigment in the skin is common with venous and cardiac insufficiency. Arterial insufficiency is also detected by the rubor colour of the limb which slowly develops with postural changes. Inflammatory or irritative conditions will appear red, although inflammation deep within the tissues will not be obvious on visual inspection. New skin grafts or scars also appear red in their early stages, but gradually change to a bluish tone and then eventually fade to white. Such skin markings indicate past surgery or trauma, both of which must be investigated. Bruising indicates trauma to the tissues and should alert the physiotherapist to the presence of tissue healing. Dry scaly skin can follow conditions with reduced nerve conduction, whereas dry skin with excessive wrinkling occurs in dehydration or after sudden, excessive weight loss. Increased sweating can be indicative of increased autonomic activity. The changes outlined above illustrate a few examples of the trophic skin changes that may be noticed during observation of the patient and which may indicate an underlying pathology.

Soft tissue contours, abnormal humps or bumps may indicate a benign collection of adipose or fibrous tissue, mild effusion, knotted muscle fibres or even a more sinister overgrowth of tissue which requires further investigation.

Joints within the functional area can be observed by noting the crease lines lying over the joint area. Asymmetry of joint range can be predicted when there is an observed change in these crease lines. The losses of joint range may be small and are not always apparent when performing passive or accessory movements. Altered contour or asymmetry in the size of the joint may be indicative of bony enlargement, the presence of joint effusion or asymmetrical congruency of the joint.

Observation of the muscle tone, bulk and contour can be informative about muscle lesions, wasting or imbalance. Muscle imbalance occurs not only in sedentary individuals but also in active people who train using selective patterns of movement without considering total body conditioning or contralateral equality of movement. It is therefore possible for a very active or athletic person to have quite profound muscle imbalance and selective weakness of particular muscle groups. Certain viral conditions can also present with selected muscle wasting.

Finally, a variety of antalgic postures may be adopted to relieve pain or as a protective deformity. Deviations in posture may also occur to compensate for bony asymmetry or decreased range of movement. This can be detected by relating specific points of the body to an imaginary plumb-line lying in the sagittal and frontal planes.

Functional Activities

Functional activities such as walking or undressing are informative not only in the biomechanical analysis of the patient's problem but also in the functional disability it created for the patient. However, observing the patient undressing or asking the patient to walk in a normal manner is not always helpful. The complex combination of movements needs to be slowed down by means of video for analysis by the inexperienced clinician. When this is not possible, provided that the irritability of the patient's condition allows, tasks can be repeated in such a way as to reinforce certain biomechanical components. For example, walking on the toes or heels, in inversion or eversion of the foot, will stress different joints and should aid in the differential diagnosis. If weightbearing activities such as walking are performed with very little difficulty by the patient, the physiotherapist may request that the patient performs more demanding tasks, such as squatting or step-ups or even standing and squatting on one foot. The type of functional activity requested should be geared to the patient's ability. It will depend upon the patient's pathology, irritability, severity, instability and age and whether or not they normally uses walking aids. It should not be forgotten that the upper limbs have weight-bearing functions in addition to their prehensile tasks.

Other Related Joints

Those joints which lie deep to the area of pain or those which could refer clinical features to the functional area being examined, should be tested briefly. This includes the spine. The purpose of this examination is twofold: firstly, to exclude these joints as the source of the patient's problem; secondly, to determine whether any local pain or loss of range predisposes to problems elsewhere. These screening or clearing tests usually consist of active movements either in one plane of movement or in a combined movement. Further stress may be applied at the end of range in the form of overpressure. The aim of these tests is to establish a differential diagnosis and to exclude any contribution to the presenting problem by the joint being tested. Any findings must be carefully considered together with the patient's total subjective and objective presentation.

The extent of spinal dysfunction must never be underestimated. It is therefore good practice for all physiotherapists new to clinical examination to examine the spine, even if the patient has already been diagnosed as having a local problem such as carpal tunnel syndrome or tennis elbow. Quite often patients have primary causes or secondary associated lesions within the appropriate area of the spine. While spinal movements, compression and quadrant testing can all provide important information, the most useful examination is palpation of the spine. This may produce a significant sign at an appropriate level; it may not, however, reproduce the patient's distal pain or clinical features. This does not exclude the spine as a cause of the patient's complaint. If the findings are of sufficient significance, the spine should be considered as a component of the patient's presenting problem.

Neurological Testing

Neurological tests performed as part of a musculoskeletal examination involve testing the conduction of a spinal nerve and nerve root, the spinal cord and the cauda equina. To test the integrity of the spinal nerve and the nerve root, the dermatomes, myotomes and reflexes are tested (Maitland, 1986). In clinical practice it is generally accepted that these tests are performed when spinal pain or sensory changes radiate past the shoulder or buttock. However, for the novice physiotherapist, neurological testing should always form a part of the routine examination of spinal conditions. Inexperienced physiotherapists can not rely on their subjective examination alone to rule out the presence of neurological signs.

When performing neurological tests for sensory change, muscle strength and reflexes, the reliability and validity of the findings depend on the quality of the examination.

Sensitive, appropriate and efficient measuring procedures are essential. Neurological tests should be carried out before performing neurodynamic tests.

Neurodynamic Tests

Tension tests have long been part of the routine spinal examination performed by physiotherapists (Maitland, 1986), and involve a combination of tension placed on neuromeningeal structures and joint movement. The physiotherapist is looking for reproduction of the patient's pain and a decreased range of movement in neural tissue. If such findings are present, they must be included with all other examination findings to form part of the total picture. Tension tests have a high sensitivity and the neural stretching may lead to an increase in the patient's clinical features. From clinical experience, this flare-up of symptoms frequently has a latent onset. Therefore, on the patient's first attendance, tension testing should be restricted to a minimum. The aim should be to investigate the condition using a gentle stretch, never forcing the structures.

Specific tension tests used in examination include the straight leg raise (SLR), the passive neck flexion (PNF) and the prone knee flexion (PKF). Recently, upper and lower limb neurodynamic tests and the slump test, have been included as a routine part of the peripheral joint musculoskeletal examination (Butler, 1991). These tests look for movement as well as tension.

Neurodynamic tests also have a low specificity, and the novice physiotherapist may be confused by the many structures which are being moved during the performance of the tests. If the neurodynamic tests prove to reproduce the most prominent clinical feature and the physiotherapist wishes to use them as a form of treatment, then careful and sensitive differential testing of the neuromusculoskeleton should be carried out before treatment (Butler, 1991).

Swelling

The examination of swelling has both a subjective and objective component. During subjective questioning, the physiotherapist should ascertain and draw on the body chart the position of any swelling felt by the patient—although this is not always visible—if the swelling varies and if there is any visible colour change of the skin. Also, it is necessary to ascertain what activities aggravate the swelling and to determine if it is activity or gravity dependent. Answers to these questions may indicate the type of swelling and its cause. Finally, if the patient reveals that the swelling was a result of a traumatic insult, the time of onset of the swelling should be ascertained. Immediate swelling indicates there may have been a tear of the soft tissues, whereas a slow onset indicates an inflammatory reaction.

Examination of swelling includes palpation of its position, size, shape, colour, temperature, tenderness, movement, consistency, surface texture, ulceration, margins and associated swellings. Systematic attention to detail and consideration of underlying anatomy will help to uncover its possible cause. Measurements are essential so that changes occurring later can be recognised. In contrast, vague statements about size and inaccurate and misleading objective measurements should be avoided.

Soft Tissue Palpation

Palpation of the soft tissues, as outlined by Hoppenfeld (1976), is often an underused diagnostic tool in clinical practice. A sound anatomical knowledge is required to interpret and understand the information gained by palpation of the soft tissues. Although referred tenderness, secondary soft tissue lesions and congenital malformations may be misleading to the clinician, the value of sensitive palpation as part of the diagnostic tool, particularly of the periphery, should not be underestimated. Palpation provides information about the state of the tissues with regards to temperature, sweating, soft tissue thickening, tightness, swelling, joint lines, bony anomalies, state of the tendons and their sheaths, muscle belly fibres and even the superficial sites of nerves. These tissues and the relevant information that palpation provides, act as an adjunct to clinical diagnosis. Raised local temperature and sweating indicate an area of increased activity, provided that the room temperature and the state of anxiety of the patient have been taken into consideration.

Soft tissues should be palpated sensitively but firmly, noting any undue dysfunction. This is only significant if palpation reproduces the patient's symptoms and the structure palpated is easily accessible. Tenderness may be referred from a distant site, possibly in the spine. These secondary findings in distal structures often require a localised treatment together with treatment of their proximal source to rehabilitate the patient fully.

Muscle Testing

Muscle groups which lie within the functional area being examined should be tested by isometric contraction. A static hold with a slow build-up of manual resistance followed by a slow release is adequate for the initial test. This will reproduce the pain or indicate the gross loss of strength. However, the test is not very sensitive and as a result it is necessary to investigate further any pain produced during a muscle contraction, to determine its true cause. For example, pain produced during a muscle contraction may be caused by joint compression. Likewise, any muscle weakness identified by testing may be due to disuse, trauma, disease, neurological deficit or pain inhibition, and further testing is necessary to isolate the specific cause. The decision to investigate further is taken after analysis of all the examination findings, and will be carried out at a subsequent attendance.

In cases of peripheral nerve injuries, muscle tears or hand injuries, it may be necessary to perform graded tests for muscle strength, e.g. the Oxford grading (Daniels *et al.*, 1995). The reader is referred to standard texts (Cole *et al.*, 1988; Kendall *et al.*, 1993) for the starting positions for each muscle to be investigated and the directions of manually applied force.

Manual testing of muscle groups is relatively unspecific and is difficult to interpret if muscle weakness is present. If, however, no weakness of muscle groups is observed, the test can be considered to produce strong evidence that all muscles are clinically normal.

Normal muscle length is an anatomical feature that should be tested clinically, although the results should be interpreted with care. Muscles which pass over two joints produce more reliable tests when movement of one joint is restricted to permit free movement of the other joint over which the muscle acts.

If, after final analysis of the patient's examination findings, it is believed that the patient's problem is an imbalance of muscle length, strength and functional working, then further testing procedures (Jull & Janda, 1987; Norris, 1993) should be carried out in a subsequent attendance, before treatment of the muscle imbalance.

Gaining accurate measurements of a muscle bulk is almost impossible, and care must be taken to avoid demotivating patients by the use of unreliable methods of measurement. Also, it should be acknowledged that muscle bulk measurements do not necessarily equate to muscle strength.

Palpation of the muscle belly is a very under-rated examination. Following trauma or acute pain, muscle fibres frequently become 'knotted', a finding which is only detected on deep palpation. If this procedure is omitted, the use of massage or related stretching techniques may not be considered as part of the treatment regimen, to the detriment of the patient's recovery. For example, fibres of the calf musculature are often affected in the patient with a fractured ankle complex or fractured calcaneum.

Active Movements

Testing active movements within the unrestricted joint range of a functional area before the examination of passive or accessory movements, makes any subsequent manual handling safer and more informative. Active movements test the integrity of the soft tissues, especially joints and muscles, and inform the physiotherapist about the quality and range of movement possible. It is important that the patient is in full control of the movement at all times.

There are several considerations regarding the examination of the active range of movement.

Firstly, transference of knowledge gained during the subjective examination and observations of tests performed so far, is required.

During the subjective examination, an assessment should have been made of the pathology, irritability, severity and instability in the affected area, and the patient's response to pain. This knowledge should be utilised when examining active range of movement. For example, if a patient's condition has been assessed as very irritable, the instructions given to the patient before any movement should be adapted accordingly. Instructions may include asking the patient to move until they first feel an increase in pain, and then to stop and return to the position of comfort. The physiotherapist should enquire about the patient's pain and other clinical features only after the patient has returned to the neutral position. Active movements should not be hurried in a patient with an irritable condition. It is important to wait until any aggravated clinical features have settled before continuing the examination. It may only be possible to examine one or two movements on the first visit, and further investigations may have to be deferred.

In contrast, patients whose condition is not irritable can tolerate more investigation at the first visit. They are asked to move the body part as far as possible into the available range of movement and then to return to the neutral position. If the pain or clinical features were minimal and subside quickly, the movement may be repeated and gentle overpressure applied if the end of range was pain free. Overpressure should be released gently and the patient returned to the neutral position. The purpose of applying overpressure is to allow the clinician to perceive the end-feel of the joint.

Secondly, if all active movements have failed to reproduce the patient's clinical features, rapid repeated movements or combined movements within a functional activity can be tested and analysed.

A comparison needs to be made between the various activities which aggravated the condition during the subjective examination and the active movements performed in the department (Edwards, 1988).

Functional movements of the body rarely occur in one plane of movement but are usually a combination of movements in several planes. Therefore, when examining active ranges of movement it is sometimes necessary to combine several movements into functional patterns.

Finally, the quality of the movement and the patient's non-verbal response should be observed. The purpose of observing active movements is not only to note the range of movement and the point at which the patient's symptoms are provoked, but also to give the physiotherapist the opportunity to note the quality of the movement produced and the patient's non-verbal response to such activity.

Passive Movements

Careful, precise passive movements are performed in anatomical or functional planes of movement. These are performed when active movements do not reach the end of the normal range. The physiotherapist performs them for two reasons: firstly, to determine if the passive range differs from the active range, and secondly, to calculate the end-feel of the movement. The end-feel informs the physiotherapist about the restricting or inhibiting factors that prevent any further movement. This could be pain or muscle dysfunction, in which case the end-feel is open-ended and 'empty'; or it could be due to soft tissue restriction, when the end-feel is 'tighter'. The feel of the soft tissues will guide the clinician

when judging the pathological state and subsequent treatment regimens. If the soft tissues are tight, it is essential to perform combined end-of-range passive movements. The number of passive movements performed will depend upon the pathology, irritability, severity and instability of the patient's condition, and the patient's response. It may only be possible to perform minimal passive movements if the factors mentioned above are intrusive.

Accessory Movements

Accessory movements give the most information to the physiotherapist conducting the examination, especially if the patient has some joint involvement. However, they must be performed accurately and require the most skill, acquired by painstaking practice. Expertise in this area improves a physiotherapist's knowledge of the musculoskeletal system. Several authors have suggested that the skilful application of accessory movements is diagnostically reliable in the examination of the spine (Jull *et al.*, 1988; Phillips & Twomey, 1996).

Depending on the irritability, severity and instability of the patient's condition, the maximum number of accessory movements are performed to assess the integrity of the joint complex and soft tissues. Kaltenborn (1980), Maitland (1991) and Grieve (1994) outline specific accessory movements for each functional area. During the performance of these accessory movements, the physiotherapist is looking for several features, one of which is pain. The point in the range where pain occurs, together with its site and distribution, are important. The more information the physiotherapist is able to elicit about the nature and characteristics of the pain during the performance of the movement, the greater the usefulness of the tests.

The clinician is also looking for the relation between pain and resistance. Resistance is detected in the absence of friction-free movement, and information is required concerning its intensity throughout the joint range. It is also necessary to note any muscle spasm, end-feel and limitation of joint range. All these relations are recorded on a movement diagram (Maitland, 1986; Grieve, 1994), which is used to communicate what is felt by the physiotherapist and patient throughout the range of accessory movement of the joint.

If the therapeutic results of the movements described above are to be used as a form of treatment, this information is vital to help the practitioner decide upon the grade, force, amplitude, direction, duration and frequency of the technique applied.

Finally, the most important part of the examination of a musculoskeletal condition is to reflect upon and analyse the findings. Reflection, analysis and clinical decision making form the topic for the next chapter.

REFERENCES

Bogduk N, Mercer S. Selection and application of treatment. In: Refshauge K, Gass E, eds. *Musculoskeletal physiotherapy: clinical science and practice*. Oxford: Butterworth Heinemann; 1995.

Butler DS. *Mobilisation of the nervous system*. Melbourne: Churchill Livingstone; 1991.

Cole JH, Furness AL, Twomey LT. *Muscles in action: an approach to manual muscle testing*. Oxford: Churchill Livingstone; 1988.

Corrigan B, Maitland GD. *Practical orthopaedic medicine*. Cambridge: Butterworths; 1988.

Craig KD. Emotional aspects of pain. In: Wall PD, Melzack R, eds. *Textbook of pain*. London: Churchill Livingstone; 1984.

Croft AC. Biomechanics. In: Foreman SM, Croft AC, eds. *Whiplash injuries: the cervical acceleration/deceleration syndrome*, 2nd ed. Baltimore: Williams and Wilkins; 1995a.

Croft AC. Soft tissue injuries. In: Foreman SM, Croft AC, eds. *Whiplash injuries: the cervical acceleration/deceleration syndrome*, 2nd ed. Baltimore: Williams and Wilkins; 1995b.

Daniels L, Worthing K, Hislop HJ. *Muscle testing*, 6th ed. London: WB Saunders; 1995.

Dixon AJ. Osteoporosis and the family doctor. In: Butler RC, Jayson MIV, eds. *Collected reports on the rheumatic diseases*. Tunbridge Wells: Arthritis and Rheumatism Council; 1995.

Dixon JS, Bird HA. Reproducibility along a 10 cm vertical visual analogue scale. *Ann Rheum Dis* 1981, **40**:87-89.

Edwards BC. Clinical assessment: the use of combined movements in assessment and treatment. In: Twomey LT, Taylor JR, eds. *Physical therapy of the low back: clinics in physical therapy*. Churchill Livingstone; 1987.

Egan D, Cole C, Twomey LT. The standing forward flexion test: an inaccurate determinate of sacroiliac dysfunction. *Physiotherapy* 1996, **82**:235-242.

Gadow S. Existential advocacy: philosophical foundation of nursing. In: Spicker SF, Gadow S, eds. *Nursing images and ideals: opening dialogue with humanities*. New York: Springer; 1980.

Grieve G. Mobilisation of the spine. *Notes on examination, assessment and clinical method*, 6th ed. Edinburgh: Churchill Livingstone; 1994.

Hoppenfeld S. *Physical examination of the spine and extremities*. Appleton-Century-Crofts; 1976.

Jull GA, Bogduk N, Marsland A. The accuracy of manual diagnosis for cervical zygapophyseal joints pain syndrome. *Med J Australia* 1988, **148**:233-236.

Jull GA, Janda V. Muscles and motor control in low back pain: assessment and management. In: Twomey LT, Taylor JR, eds. *Physical therapy of the low back: clinics in physical therapy*. Edinburgh: Churchill Livingstone; 1987.

Kaltenborn KM. *Mobilisation of extremity joints*. OLAF Norlis Bokhandel, Universitetsgaten Oslo; 1980.

Kendal FP, McCreary EK, Provance PG. *Muscles, testing and function*, 6th ed. Baltimore: Williams and Wilkins; 1993.

Lord S. Clinical indicators of headache referred from the upper synovial joints. *Proceedings from the physical medicine research foundation's 8th international symposium on musculoskeletal pain emanating from the head and neck. Current concepts in diagnosis, management and cost containment'*. Banff, Canada. October 13-15, 1995.

Magee DJ. *Orthopaedic physical assessment*, 2nd ed. London: WB Saunders; 1992.

Maitland GD. *Vertebral manipulation*, 5th ed. London: Butterworths; 1986.

Maitland GD. The Maitland concept: assessment, examination and treatment by passive movement. In: Twomey LT, Taylor JR, eds. *Physical therapy of the low back: clinics in physical therapy*. Churchill Livingstone; 1987.

Maitland GD. *Peripheral manipulation*, 3rd ed. London: Butterworths; 1991.

Nachemson A, Morris JM. In vivo measurements of intradiscal pressure. *J Bone Joint Surg* 1964, **46A**:1077.

Norris CM. *Sports injuries. Diagnosis and management for physiotherapists*. Oxford: Butterworth Heinemann; 1993.

Phillips PR, Twomey LT. A comparison of manual diagnosis with a diagnosis established by unilevel lumbar spinal block procedure. *Man Ther* 1996, **2**:82-87.

Stimson G, Webb B. *Going to see the doctor: the consultation process in general practice*. London: Routledge Kegan Paul; 1975.

Strong PM. *The ceremonial order of the clinic: parents, doctors, medical bureaucracies*. London: Routledge Kegan Paul; 1979.

Thornquist E. Communication—what happened during the first encounter. *Scand J Primary Health Care* 1990, **8**:133-138.

Tucket D, Boulton M, Olson C, Williams. <11> *Meeting between experts. An approach to sharing ideas in medical consultations*. London: Tavistock; 1985.

Walker DJ. Rheumatoid arthritis. In: Butler RC, Jayson MIV, eds. *Collected reports on the rheumatic diseases*. Tunbridge Wells: Arthritis and Rheumatism Council; 1995.

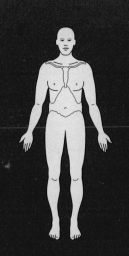

15 B J Hollins

MUSCULOSKELETAL PATIENT CASE HISTORY ANALYSIS

CHAPTER OUTLINE

- Case history analysis
- Case history analysis format
- Analysis of the subjective examination
- Subjective and objective asterisk

- Analysis of the objective examination
- Setting objectives
- Formulating a management plan
- Long-term goals

INTRODUCTION

Analysing the case history of a patient with a musculoskeletal problem consists of interpreting and reflecting on the data obtained at the initial examination. Ideally, it should take place immediately after completing the subjective and objective examination (see Chapter 14). The value of immediate analysis of every detail of the patient and their environment cannot be overemphasised; with both the patient's story and the patient's emphasis on certain points so recently implanted in the physiotherapist's mind, the clinical analysis is likely to be patient oriented.

Analysing a patient in this way, however, is only part of the clinical decision-making process. Clinical reasoning, or decision-making, is a highly complex phenomenon, which begins with a patient's referral and should continue on, in the form of reflection, after a patient has been discharged. Higgs & Jones (1995) define clinical reasoning as 'the thinking and decision making processes which are integral to clinical practice'. If the reader wishes to explore this subject further, there is a growing body of literature (Mattingly & Fleming, 1994; Dutton, 1995; Higgs & Jones, 1995; Basmajian & Sikhar, 1996). Many of these authors have produced models to provide structure to a physiotherapist's thought processes.

This text is based on the work of Higgs & Jones (1995), and expands on a small portion only of their overall clinical reasoning model; the analysis of the patient's data after an initial examination. It takes the novice physiotherapist through the first stages of analysing a subjective and objective examination, consideration of the stage of pathology, setting and prioritising objectives and planning the initial treatment. The aim is to assist students in their early stages of clinical decision making.

The complexity of a patient's musculoskeletal problem may be a daunting prospect to students. They perceive they have insufficient knowledge and skill to tackle the patient's sometimes numerous problems. Novice physiotherapists should be heartened by the understanding that the most knowledgeable person in the process is the patient. The physiotherapist's objective is to acquire that knowledge and analyse it. Hence, while biomedical knowledge and physiotherapeutic skill are essential in data analysis, they are only part of the picture. During clinical decision making, cognition and metacognition are equally essential. Students are capable of this. The novice simply takes longer to climb up the spiral, which begins with the initial referral and spreads upwards and outwards towards a final outcome. The spiral gets larger as each decision or interaction takes place. The process is one of clarification, where each finding generates further questions to be reflected upon and clarified. For the final outcome to be successful, there must be a growing understanding of the patient and their problems (Higgs & Jones, 1995).

This chapter aims to point out two aspects of clinical decision making: firstly, to give structure to the initial analysis of a patient's data, and secondly, to explain why analysis may follow certain commonplace features. Physiotherapists do not routinely think through a clinical examination and perform predetermined treatment plans. They actively reason, adapting and changing their plans in harmony with the patient's changing clinical features and environment; a process of continual cue gathering, pattern recognition, hypothesis generation, idea testing, reflection and adaptation to outcomes—ideally with the patient and physiotherapist working together. The physiotherapist should be the patient's advocate (Gadow, 1980).

Most of the text is taken from clinical experience, with suggested references for further reading. The student is encouraged to read the literature in this area critically, to evaluate the findings of the research and to scrutinise carefully 'good' practice.

CASE HISTORY ANALYSIS

During the process of reflecting back over the data of a patient's initial case history, quite intuitively the physiotherapist intermingles the three dominant methods of clinical reasoning proposed by Higgs & Jones (1995) in their model. They point out that the physiotherapist reasons in many ways, one being to subconsciously relate the patient's presenting problems to their own perception of normality.

However, does normality exist? As pointed out in Chapter 14, most people after a certain age have a predisposition to neuromusculoskeletal problems. The 'normal' adult can be found to have, for example, social stresses, abnormal joint signs, muscular imbalance, body asymmetry, neurodynamic dysfunction, and autonomic, systemic and metabolic abnormalities; all manifestations of normal bodily degeneration. Instinctively, the more experienced physiotherapist clarifies data as they are being received, by comparing the findings with what is an expected degree of normal abnormality (Maitland, 1996). Novice physiotherapists can achieve this by asking themselves questions such as 'Does this particular sign or symptom fit into an accepted degree of normality or is it a clinical dysfunction?', 'How comparable is this particular sign or symptom with other abnormal features?', 'Does it fit into the patient's story?', 'Can I group any abnormal clinical features?', 'Can I change this clinical feature to produce normalisation of the dysfunction?', 'Will I be able to measure any change I make?' and 'If I make a change towards normalisation will it be a beneficial change or could it be harmful to the patient?'

This type of questioning can follow through every component of the subjective and objective examination as the examination progresses.

The most important part of the analysis is the assessment that takes place at the end of the subjective and objective examination. To assist the novice to structure this process, a format has been suggested on page 205. An explanation of this format is given below.

ANALYSIS OF THE SUBJECTIVE EXAMINATION

The aim of the subjective examination is to collect data on the kind of disorder and the area and behaviour of the symptoms, to ask special questions to rule out clinical precautions and to take a chronological history of the patient's problems. The more thoroughly this is completed, the easier the analysis.

AGE

A patient's age should not be taken for granted. Adolescent patients who present with minor trauma should follow through a normal healing timescale (Evans, 1980). If they do not, the physiotherapist should consider why. Likewise older active males, unlike active females, may not have developed delicate osteoporotic bones. Activity, diet and sex are more accurate indicators of osteoporosis than is age alone (Spector, 1990; Anderson & Francis, 1994; Dixon 1995; Twomey & Taylor, 1994). Consideration of the length of time the patient has been aware of the dysfunction may have more relevance than chronological age.

OCCUPATION AND HOBBIES

Understanding the condition from the patient's perspective should be at the forefront of the physiotherapist's mind while performing the analysis. Attempting to 'live in the patient's shoes' as the patient goes through their daily routines of work and hobbies can be very informative. It can reveal the mechanism of injury or repetitive injury. Understanding the background of neuroplastic changes which have taken place before the patient's visit, enhances the decision-making process.

NATURE OF THE PATIENT
Patient's illness response

There is a growing recognition that pain is a complex experience, involving not only a variety of biological factors such as neural activity, endocrine responses and immune function (Kidd et al., 1996) but also a wide range of psychosocial factors (Melzak & Wall, 1993; Wells et al., 1994 Shacklock, 1995; Adams et al., 1997). The process of analysing how the patient lives with their condition can help to relate specific clinical features to the person as a whole. For example, a patient who complains of a 'hurt' which manifests when digging may be referring to a mechanical low lumbar pain. Alternatively, the patient may be explaining a painful experience, such as a marriage problem, which dominates the patient's thoughts whenever they are digging. In the former case, an ergonomic analysis and advice are necessary (Khalil et al., 1993). In the latter case, the hurtful experience needs analysing

Case History Analysis Format

Assessment of Subjective examination

1. Age _____

   Any significance _____

2. Jobs/Hobbies _____

   Any significance _____

3. Nature of Patient _____

   Patient's illness response _____
   Patient's attitude _____

4. Pain chart
   List structures under pain/symptoms _____
   Structures which can refer pain/symptoms _____
   Other sources of symptoms _____

5. Nature of condition
   Factors supporting hypothesis

Source/Mechanism	Pain	Aggravating factors	Easing factors	Diurnal cycle	History

6. Severity

	Supporting evidence
None	
Mild	
Moderate	
Severe	

7. Irritability

	Supporting evidence
None	
Mild	
Moderate	
Severe	

8. Instability of segment

	Supporting evidence
None	
Mild	
Moderate	
Severe	

9. Stability of condition changing to

	Supporting evidence
Better	
Worse	
Same at present	
Stable	

10. Latency

	Supporting evidence
None	
Mild	
Moderate	
Severe	

11. History

Significant clues	Interpretation

12. Is there any reason for caution? _____

13. Any special tests necessary to rule out contraindications? _____

14. Is a neurological test necessary? _____

15. Any extra physical examination procedures necessary to confirm diagnosis? _____

16. Stage in pathology

Significant clues	Evidence
Inflammatory	
Tissue Repair	
Degeneration	
Purely mechanical	
Non mechanical	

17.
Subjective asterisk* _____

Case History Analysis Format

Assessment of objective examination

1. Objectivity

2. Clinical diagnosis

Clinical Features	Expected abnormalities or positive findings	Unexpected abnormality or positive findings	interpretation

3. Functional Restriction

Abnormal findings or supporting evidence	Other areas needing attention

4. Objective asterix*

5. Are there any extra physical tests which should be performed at a later stage and why? _____
_____

6. Stages of pathology

	Supporting evidence
Inflammatory	
Tissue repair	
Degeneration	
Purely mechanical	
Non mechanical	

7. Working hypothesis _____

8. Prognosis _____

9. Objectives in order of priority _____

10. Management plan _____

11. Long term goals _____

The above Case History Analysis form is expanded upon in greater detail below:-

Pain, hurt, fear and physical disability can often go together in a patient's mind and become confused (Shacklock, 1995). The association of chronic pain and depression should not be forgotten when interpreting a patient's story; masked depression is a common problem and can manifest as musculoskeletal pain (Fishbain et al., 1997).

Further information on the various aspects of the relation of a patient's illness responses and their disability can be found in several texts (Stimson & Webb, 1975; Tuckett et al., 1985; Herlzlich & Pierret, 1987; Seigel, 1990; Melzak & Wall, 1993; Wells et al., 1994; Shacklock, 1995; Adams et al., 1997).

Patient's attitude to the problem

A patient's attitude towards the problem is not necessarily the same as the patients 'illness response', as presented above. The former can stem from beliefs, while the latter can stem from a suffering of some kind. People have varying degrees of endurance (Melzack, 1973). A stoical personality may seem brave due to certain beliefs of the patient, and as a consequence this presents a different picture of a problem than a patient with a seemingly 'overactive personality' (Douglas, 1994). Both scenarios may, however, present with the same objective findings.

When the findings of the subjective examination do not match with those of the objective examination, a patient's musculoskeletal problem needs careful consideration. The patient's over- or underemphasis of a clinical feature such as pain, should be handled with caution. Both situations can be equally as misleading. As described by French (1994), the intensity of the pain experienced and the way in which people respond are not merely a function of the degree of physical damage incurred. There are many factors influencing pain perception, including familial, cultural and situational factors and past experiences. Anthropological and ethnographical studies by the sociologists and anthropologists, for example Strong (1979), Klienmann (1981) and Douglas (1994), showed that a person's pain cannot be fully understood without knowledge of their sociocultural beliefs.

PAIN CHART

The pain chart, completed early in the interview, provides a great deal of information about the possible source of a problem. For example, a complaint of pain deep within the groin and radiating into the upper anterior thigh may stem from abnormalities of the lumbar spine, sacroiliac joint or hip joint; local soft tissues underlying the pain, e.g. skin, fascia, ligaments, contractile structures; neurological or circulatory structures; systemic organs, e.g. gynaecological or abdominal organs; a tumour, infection or other disease process. Further information on the differential diagnosis of the above can be found in several textbooks (Cyriax, 1984; Maitland, 1986, 1991; Grieve, 1989; Goodman & Snyder, 1995; Murtagh and Kenna, 1997).

NATURE OF THE CONDITION

The 'nature' of the condition refers to the fundamental qualities or characteristics which make up the abnormality, i.e. the type of syndrome or pattern. For example, the nature of an inflamed nerve root is made up of the characteristics of a toothache-like pain within a dermatomal distribution, which is worse distally and in conditions which irritate the inflammation, i.e. when closing down the intervertebral foraman or compress or stretch the inflamed nerve (Rydevik & Olmarker, 1992; Olmarker et al., 1997). In contrast, the nature of a mildly degenerative spinal joint problem is made up of the characteristics of a deep local aching-like pain, which is made worse by compression or stretch to the joint. The joint displays a typical capsular pattern (Cyriax, 1984), and on palpation a combination of resistance and pain are evident (Jull & Bogduk, 1986; Kuslich et al., 1991; Murtagh & Kenna, 1997).

Although it may be difficult to isolate the specific structure or soft tissue at fault (Bogduk et al., 1981; Bogduk, 1983; Kuslich et al., 1991; Schwarzer et al., 1995), integration of pain chart with other features of a patient's story can reduce the number of structures or disease processes suspected. Infection, for example, can be ruled out if the other features of inflammation are absent, such as temperature, swelling, tenderness, redness—or rash as in herpes zoster—and possible causative infectious agent (Table 15.1).

This type of interpretation should be followed through with each predominant clinical feature. It helps to make sense of a patient's story and dispel incorrect assumptions. It is important to keep an open mind when interpreting a patient's data, as it is very easy to make assumptions. For example, when an elderly patient with cervical pain complains of dizziness, this could strongly indicate vertebral artery involvement, and should also alert the clinician to treat the neck with care (Grieve, 1989a). Dizziness, however, can have several causes. For example, it can be associated with reduction of proprioceptive input due to reduced joint range (Grieve, 1989; Grant, 1994). Whereas conditions with dizziness require great caution, those of reduced joint range require vigorous joint mobilisation and soft tissue stretches.

As well as looking at each aspect of a patient's story for possible identification of dysfunction patterns, a generalised overview is also essential. This helps to indicate the dosage or type of treatment required, when initially testing out a hypothesis with a treatment regimen. Consideration should be given to the condition's severity, irritability and stability and any contraindications or precautions to the prescribed treatment.

IRRITABILITY OF THE CONDITION

This can be described by how easily and to what extent the condition is aggravated, the length of time the patient can perform a task before it becomes necessary to stop due to an increase in symptoms, the time it takes for the symptoms to settle, and the extent of the settlement of the symptoms (Maitland, 1986). The answers all contribute to describing the irritability of a patient's condition. This information is an essential part of the analysis. The level of irritability should always be considered when deciding on how vigorous the treatment should be within the department, by self-help or at home.

SEVERITY OF THE CONDITION

This describes the intensity of any pain and the extent of its distribution when undertaking a particular activity. This is not the same as irritability. Severity is purely a subjective measure of the feeling and distribution of pain, which may change with activity. It is not related to the aggravating or easing factors of the pathological condition, only to the subjective manifestation, which in itself can inhibit function. For example, a condition which is severe but non-irritable can be handled quite vigorously without affecting the pathology adversely. In contrast, an irritable condition must always be handled with care—it could take a long time to settle a pain or inflammatory reaction.

STABILITY OF THE CONDITION AND INSTABILITY OF THE SEGMENT

Newcomers to case history analysis may become confused by the terms instability of the segment (or tissues) and stability of the condition. In this chapter, instability will refer to a condition where the integrity of the soft tissues has been compromised, for example by such factors as tissue trauma, lengthening or attenuation. The stability of the condition (Maitland, 1986; Grieve, 1994) refers to the progression and stability of the condition as a whole and can be described as either 'better', 'the same' or 'worse'.

The instability of the segment can be estimated by establishing answers to the following: 'How stable is the condition from one day to another?', 'How much do the clinical features fluctuate?' and 'How much does the condition vary for no apparent reason?' Also, analysis of symptoms is required to determine if the same mechanical provocative factor can have a variety of effects. Clinical features such as 'catch' pains, locking, 'giving way' and a feeling of apprehension towards certain movements, together with answers to the above questions, all direct the clinician towards analysing the instability of a segment at both a subjective and an objective level. The patient presenting with a history of instability and unstable objective findings needs to be handled with care until the nature of the instability has been established. Provoking the problem can so easily lead to a loss of the patient's confidence.

The patient with instability can sometimes display the feature of latency. Latency describes the symptom which presents some time after the incident rather than having an immediate onset. It can occur after a movement, holding a position, at the end of the day or even the next day. There can be many causes, one of which is instability of the segment. It is essential to discover latency during the analysis stage because it will affect the strategy for patient management—the vigour of the chosen treatment, the manual handling of the patient, and the time of day treatment is implemented. The physiotherapist should plan to see a patient when the symptom is both better and worse.

To establish the stability or the progression of the condition, the physiotherapist needs to obtain information on:
- Whether or not the condition is improving spontaneously.
- Whether or not the condition is in equilibrium.
- The length of time the condition has been in this state.
- Whether or not the condition is deteriorating and, if so, at what rate.

The answers to these points will assist the physiotherapist in determining the potential prognosis for the condition. For example, if the problem is becoming worse, treatment may be difficult and should be approached with caution. Any further deterioration in a patient's condition may undermine the patient's confidence in the physiotherapist. However, if the condition is improving, treatment should enhance this progress.

In conclusion, stability of the condition, instability of the segment and latency in the onset of symptoms should all be carefully considered in the management of the patient. All three should give reason for concern.

HISTORY OF THE CONDITION

Analysing a patient's history in the correct chronological order is an important step in the differential diagnosis. For example, a 65-year-old male patient complains of pain over his left anterior upper thoracic area. This pain is made worse by any activity which overexerts the patient and forces him to take in deep breaths. False assumptions may be made unless careful notice is taken of the history of this condition. The pain originated from an incident 6 months before presentation, when the patient was forced both to use his left arm and over reach to hold a heavy weight in an awkward position. These clinical features are also characteristic of a heart problem. By analysing the history of the clinical features, the patient's differential diagnosis is clearer.

CONTRAINDICATIONS AND PRECAUTIONS

It is a professional duty not to cause harm to the patient during the course of physiotherapy management. Physiotherapeutic intervention should facilitate a patient's natural healing process. During data analysis, it is essential to consider both a patient's healing potential and the vulnerability of the patient's condition. The healing process may be slowed down by certain diseases, such as diabetes mellitus and those that result in poor circulation. Even a patient with good healing potential may still be vulnerable e.g. the fit healthy teenager who presents with a low lumbar problem. While youth should predispose to good healing properties (Evans, 1980), it is not always consistent. The lumbar intervertebral disc of an adolescent may contain more fluid in the nucleus pulposus (Taylor, 1990; Bernick et al., 1990). As such, these patients may be vulnerable to vigorous handling techniques poorly applied during physiotherapeutic intervention.

It is the duty of the physiotherapist to be fully aware of any contraindications or precautions to the planned treatments (Grieve, 1989; Kitchen & Basin, 1996; Jones & Barker, 1995). Any indications that caution is necessary—identified as a result of answers from the subjective examination or elsewhere—must be taken seriously. It is far better to be overcautious, especially if mistakes or oversights could harm the patient or have legal implications. Every time a patient attends the physiotherapy department, the suspected clinical feature should be checked and documented.

STAGE IN PATHOLOGY

To assist the novice physiotherapist in interpreting the many aspects of a patient's story, a patient's pathology can be divided into several possible stages (see Table 15.1). The three stages of inflammation, tissue repair and degeneration have been tabulated in their simplest form, combining the findings from the subjective and objective assessment (see below). While this type of classification may be artificial, it can often clarify a complex problem.

Interpretation is all about listening, believing, being open-minded, not allowing theoretical knowledge to obscure a view, and yet being thorough, logical and methodical in the decision-making process.

SUBJECTIVE AND OBJECTIVE ASTERISK

By selecting and using an asterisk (*), a subjective and/or objective clinical feature can be used as an outcome measure that is a future indicator of a treatment's success or failure (Maitland, 1986). This practice assists in making each treatment more scientifically measurable and outcomes more objective. If the reliability of the measurement is unknown, it becomes difficult to interpret the results (Riddle, 1992). There are many factors which may affect the reliability of a clinical measurement, including the clinician, the instrument and the patient (Gass, 1995; Sackett et al., 1991). When recording measurements, it is important to also document any factors which could be contributing to the errors. This makes the recording more trustworthy, and judgements based on the measurements more scientific.

If one aspect of a patient's condition is changing at a different rate from the other, then the physiotherapist's

Clinical features relating to stages in pathology			
Clinical feature	**Stage of inflammation**	**Stage of tissue repair**	**Stage of degenerative process**
Pain	**Background, throbbing ache**	Intermittent pain, with nagging ache if irritated	Intermittent
Irritability	**Irritable**	Depends on structure	None
Aggravating activity	**All movements**	Movements in line with tissue stress	Activities involving end-of-range movements and sustained rest
Instability of segment	**Stable**	May be unstable, depends on trauma	Stable
Night pain	**Rest causes increased 'stiffness'**	Likes to rest in position away from tissue tension	Often cannot lie still for too long
Morning	**Stiff for at least 30 minutes**	Stiff for short time	Stiff for few minutes only
Day	**Pain–time dependent**	Pain–time and activity dependent	Pain–activity dependent
X-Rays	**Normal**	Possible visualisation of tissue repair	Loss of joint space, sclerosis or bone osteophytes
History	**Possible infection, irritation, trauma**	Previous trauma or operation	Long insidious onset, predisposing factors
Observation	**Redness? Swelling?**	Possible scar? Operation? Thickening? Deformity?	Loss of joint range in capsular pattern, muscle imbalance
Joint range	**All ranges restricted by pain and swelling**	Pain when move in line of injury	Pain end of range with restriction in capsular pattern
Muscle	**Pain inhibition**	Depends on damage	Muscle imbalance
Palpation	**Heat, swelling, tenderness**	Tenderness and thickening over healing tissue	Bony enlargement, soft tissue thickening, tenderness

Table 15.1 Clinical features relating to stages in pathology.

objectives are only partially being met. The patient is not a machine. Mechanical dysfunction may be only part of a patient's problem. The subjective change should match the changes in the objective signs, and, to be meaningful, all findings should be measured critically and sensitively. The careful usage of asterisks or outcome measures can assist in this process.

ANALYSIS OF THE OBJECTIVE EXAMINATION

OBJECTIVITY OF THE CONDITION

This refers to the number of significant findings from the objective examination, i.e. the soft tissue changes, joint signs, muscle changes, bony anomalies, neuromeningeal involvement, and so on. The mere task of calculating the number of positive objective findings or functional restrictions, relating them to the level of tissue damage, clinical response to change and length of time the patient has suffered the damage, and using this information to produce an objective score (1–10), can be very helpful to the new clinician. These considerations can help in the realistic setting of both short-term and long-term goals. Expectations can be based upon the degree and extent of the tissue damage which needs to be rehabilitated. To enhance this part of clinical reasoning, the reader should be familiar with the healing potential of different structures, and the healing process (Evans, 1980; Peacock, 1984; Woo *et al.*, 1990; Barlow & Willoughby, 1992).

FORMULATING A CLINICAL DIAGNOSIS FROM THE OBJECTIVE FINDINGS

Although all patients should be considered in a holistic manner, taking into account the impact of the mind, body and soul (Stalker & Glymour, 1989), it is often useful to consider a clinical diagnosis. This is a working hypothesis based upon clinical findings, and helps to direct treatment at a particular aspect of the patient's problem. The clinical diagnosis may be the same as, only part of, or even different from, the pathological diagnosis. It is the clinically oriented part of the patient's presentation, believed to be the focus of the problems.

There are many ways of arriving at a clinical diagnosis (Gass, 1995). All methods should incorporate a holistic overview coupled with a sympathetic systematic attention to detail, equating anatomy, physiology, biomechanics and normal function with possible dysfunction. Initially, every part of a patient's story and each positive objective finding should carry equal weighting. Later, to make sense of the vast amount of information and to simplify the process of clinical reasoning, the student needs to focus on a particular aspect of the patient's problem. This focus could take two forms, either to formulate a clinical pattern or syndrome or to work through a functional movement analysis.

Clinical Syndromes

While reflecting back over the patient's case history, the physiotherapist should attempt to relate clinical features to each other. It may be possible to group some findings and to formulate a clinical syndrome. For example, ligamentous problems have local pain, made worse by palpation and stretch. Muscular problems also have local pain, made worse by palpation, stretch and contraction of the relevant muscle. Joint problems not only have local pain, but the pain may also be referred distally at the segmental level. This pain is made worse by palpating and stretching the local soft tissue structures, together with compression of the joint surfaces. The practice of grouping clinical features to produce clinical syndromes is expanded upon elsewhere (Stoddard, 1983; Cyriax, 1984; Grieve, 1989; Corrigan & Maitland, 1994; Goodman & Snyder, 1995; Murtagh & Kenna, 1997).

To establish the source of the problem, it may be necessary to investigate differential tests further (Maitland, 1986, 1991; Grieve, 1994; Hoppenfeld, 1996; Magee, 1997). A lot can be gained from analysing blood tests, X-ray films, electromyograms, computerised tomograms and magnetic resonance imaging scans. For further reading at a basic level the reader is referred to Rowley & Dent (1997).

To assist the novice when looking specifically for mechanical damage to the musculoskeletal system, a plan for the differential diagnosis of musculoskeletal pain is outlined in Figure 15.1. Pain is the clinical feature chosen to help facilitate the process of formulating a clinical syndrome. Syndromes are presented in their simplest forms. This artificial and dogmatic approach is designed to help the new student: it is not intended to be exhaustive. As the clinician progresses, the model will outlive its usefulness; indeed, the oversimplification will become a hindrance to understanding the complexity of the patient's problems. Figure 15.1 has been constructed from clinical experience. This type of approach is, however, controversial; Grant (1988) suggests that diagnostic skill is best improved by not imposing diagnostic models. The reader is therefore encouraged to become an evidence-based practitioner. To achieve this, clinical experience must go hand-in-hand with good scientific research.

To complicate the story, most patients present with more than one syndrome. One way of streamlining the analysis is: firstly, to consider the patient's worse sign or symptom and develop the thinking process from this focus; secondly, to consider only those clinical features which are comparable in their expression, i.e. that can be related to a specific mechanical anomaly; thirdly, to consider the syndromes in their purest form; finally, to instigate treatment aimed at the most prominent clinical feature or syndrome. The results of the intervention form the beginning of the analysis. For example, if the patient is made worse, at least treatment was affecting the problem. Reassessing the intervention will further enlighten the physiotherapist.

The trial and error of looking for pure syndromes, treating them according to the clinical guidelines, and assessing the results at the next attendance, is questionably one of the best ways of gaining clinical expertise. It is questionable because of the lack of scientific evidence evaluating the effectiveness of physiotherapeutic techniques (Waddell *et al.*, 1996; Bogduk & Mercer, 1995).

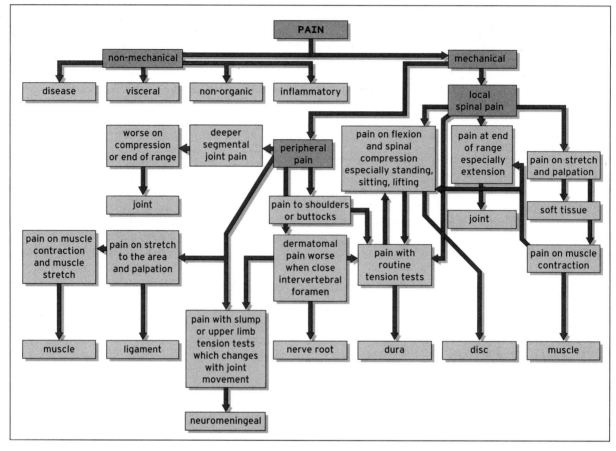

15

Figure 15.1 Differential diagnosis model for musculoskeletal pain.

FUNCTIONAL MOVEMENT ANALYSIS OR RESTRICTION

Often it is not practical to aim for a clinical syndrome or diagnosis. The patient's diagnosis is perceived by the patient as a functional restriction, not a disease process (Lewit, 1991). This functional inability may consist of several different tissue changes which all contribute to some degree. By noting the quality of each component of a particular functional movement, instigating changes to any abnormalities found, and re-evaluating the movement, it may be possible to simplify the cause of the patient's musculoskeletal problem.

Analysing every component of a functional movement carefully should help to establish the specific tissues needing attention—as Nordin & Frankel (1989) point out, the orientation of collagen fibres in soft tissue reflects the tissue's function. For example, a patient may be unable to raise their arm above their head in the scapular plane. Several concurrent causes may be at fault. Lack of cervical side flexion or extension can be caused by cervical joint restriction or soft tissue tightness. Thoracic spine extension, rotation and side flexion have been implicated in arm movement. Costovertebral and costotransverse joint accessory glide could be abnormal. Sternoclavicular and acromioclavicular joint glide also occurs during arm elevation, as well as clavicular rotation. Any restrictions of these movements will result in reduced arm range. The active and accessory ranges of the glenohumeral joint will have a profound effect on the patient's ability to attain elevation. Joint movement is dependent on muscle action, and a detailed assessment of upper limb and scapular thoracic muscle strength, balance and length is essential. Finally, irritability or tension of neuromeningeal tissue must be ruled out (Cyriax, 1984; Palastanga *et al.*, 1994; Schneider & Pardoe, 1985; Grieve, 1989; Maitland, 1986, 1991, 1994; Butler, 1991; Janda, 1994; Norkin & Levangie 1992). The above is a simple analysis, and is by no means exhaustive as there are many other reasons for inability to raise the arm. The quality of each component of the functional movement should be considered and, if necessary, manual techniques, specific exercise or patient education provided (McKenzie, 1981; Kaltenborn, 1989; Hunter, 1994; Maitland, 1986, 1991, 1994; Butler, 1991; Mulligan, 1995; Edwards, 1992; Baurdillon *et al.*, 1992).

Using the patient's functional restriction as a measurable factor for change, as described above, takes the problem from the patient's perspective. This must motivate the patient to comply with treatment.

Two methods are presented to assist the data analysis part of clinical reasoning: formulation of a clinical diagnosis and functional analysis. There are many other ways of approaching a problem. The student is advised to be critical of their own reasoning process. Indeed, it has been suggested that many diagnostic errors are caused by an inability to think things through, not the result of inadequate medical knowledge (Bordage & Alan, 1982; Bordage & Zacks, 1984; Bordage *et al.*, 1990; Bordage & Lemieux, 1991). As the clinician's expertise develops, it becomes feasible not only to view the patient as a whole but to challenge diagnostic paradigms—Faucault (1973) explains that diagnosis is only a construction based on a diagnostician's knowledge and beliefs. The patient's problem has many causes and as many answers, all of which will help clarify the situation.

Clinical Features Related to Stages in Pathology

Reaching a conclusion on clinical diagnosis alone provides insufficient information from which to determine treatment. Using the 'brick wall' concept, Maitland (1986) points out that a clinician does not treat the pathology but the stage in the pathology presenting at the time of treatment. To help the newcomer interpret this concept, Table 15.1 has divided pathology into three different stages—inflammation, tissue repair and degeneration. Although the word degeneration has been used, it must be considered a process rather than a static phase. Once again, the reader is asked to consider these stages in their simplest form. The table works through clinical features obtained during the initial subjective and objective examination. Its purpose is to organise the mechanical musculoskeletal part of the patient's problem. The table is clinically based not evidence based and should be used as a guideline only.

Establishing the stage in pathology assists the clinical decision-making process. However, it must be remembered that this is a dynamic process and the clinician's thinking should change in accordance with the patient's condition. To summarise this point: in the clinical decision-making process, the clinician has analysed the findings of the initial subjective and objective examination; the findings are used to formulate a clinical diagnosis or working hypothesis and to decide on a stage in the pathology of the musculoskeletal system. The next step is to set objectives.

SETTING OBJECTIVES

Objectives should be both holistic and realistic, and should include both short-term and long-term goals. Their production should be a dual process, incorporating both the patient's and the physiotherapist's ideals. Gadow (1980) suggests that if patients become part of the objective-setting process, they will take on more responsibility for achievement of the objectives. Having too many objectives confuses both the patient and the physiotherapist. Examination is an ongoing process—as a patient's condition changes, so do the objectives. Once objectives have been set, they should be prioritised.

Prioritising objectives

As previously mentioned, at times it may be difficult to isolate just one clinical diagnosis. A condition may seem very complex, with many aspects which could all equally be regarded as a priority for treatment. In this case, the physiotherapist may benefit from some guidelines to assist in making the initial steps in the planning of treatment. For example, if a patient has a swollen joint and is experiencing a lot of pain and muscle weakness, the physiotherapist may assess that it is appropriate to address the inflammatory process first. By reducing the swelling, the patient's pain may ease and any painful inhibition of muscle action will hopefully reduce, resulting in improved muscular contraction (Janda, 1993).

Often the patient presents with both spinal and peripheral joint signs. In such cases, the spinal component of the problem should be treated first (Maitland, 1986). Later assessment of the peripheral component may well reveal an improvement. Some quite interesting changes can occur to the periphery after spinal treatment. To treat the causative component first is still the case with such concepts as 'neurodynamic dysfunction' (Butler, 1991). If neurological tissue tension is present, it is necessary to find the cause of nerve tension, which may well be a central spinal joint problem or an inflammatory process elsewhere. Once the cause has been considered, it may or may not be necessary to stretch the neuromeningeal structures. The novice physiotherapist must be cautious. If there is a lack of knowledge and relevant examination of the pathodynamics of neurological tissue tension, its treatment can so easily irritate the patient's condition (Butler, 1991).

A traumatic incident often presents with several conflicting clinical features. It must not be forgotten that if the patient has received sufficient force to stretch, break or tear a particular structure, e.g. a fracture of the distal end of the radius, the same force will also have reached other vulnerable areas of the body, including the spine (Foreman & Croft, 1995). The immediate soft tissue injury and inflammation should be treated first. However, other structures which could also be damaged should be investigated as soon as possible, especially if pain does not subside. It is very useful to remember that spinal pain can be complex and radiating (Jinkins, 1997).

The management of a degenerative condition should be aimed at reducing the intensity of clinical features in the functional area. However, at the earliest opportunity, the physiotherapist needs to take into consideration predisposing factors which may be facilitating the degenerative process, e.g. tight tissues, muscle imbalance, work ergonomics, posture, back care. These, together with many other considerations, should be placed into a package of education and home regimens. The patient should assume responsibility for alleviating degeneration of the system. The patient needs to be involved in the rehabilitation programme for it to be realistic and to achieve long-term success (Gadow, 1980).

Once objectives have been set and prioritised, the clinician is ready to formulate a management plan, should this be necessary.

FORMULATING A MANAGEMENT PLAN

The aim of treatment should be to make the patient independent of the physiotherapist as soon as possible. Treatment may need to involve several stages—for example, passive and assisted treatment followed by home treatment—before the patient obtains long-lasting independence. Passive treatment is that which can be applied only in the department by a qualified physiotherapist. Assisted treatment requires a great deal of active participation by the patient, with some assistance and education by the physiotherapist. Self-help treatment implies that it is the patient's sole responsibility for examination, treatment and evaluation. This treatment is self-administered at home. Finally, independence requires patients to have a great deal of self-awareness and understanding of how to care for themselves.

Passive treatment

If passive treatment is necessary, its choice will depend upon many factors, probably most predominantly the stage in the pathology of the condition. Table 15.2 outlines three stages in pathology—inflammation, tissue repair and degeneration. For each stage there is a recommended set of treatment modalities, together with the manner in which they should be applied. The list is fairly general and contains modalities which most physiotherapists should be able to administer early in their careers. Treatment modalities should be directed at the clinical feature of a pathology. The pathological diagnosis will remain the same, but the patient's clinical features are expected to change as the modalities are applied.

Assisted treatment

Assisted treatment requires the expertise of a qualified physiotherapist as the treatments can only be administered in the physiotherapy department. At the same time there is much that the patient can achieve independently. A self-help attitude is to be encouraged. For the patient to be fully motivated into this aspect of treatment it is vital that suboptimal or inappropriate treatments are not administered. Regular supervision of activities taking place in the department is essential. To suit the patient's individual needs, management should include spending quality time with the patient, regularly completing a subjective and objective evaluation of progress, and adapting and modifying the treatment regimens accordingly. This is an essential component of assisted treatments. The patient can be easily demotivated by suboptimal treatment. If the patient has travelled from afar for treatment in the department only to receive modalities which could have been carried out at home, the value of such physiotherapy is questioned.

Modalities for musculoskeletal conditions			
Stage in musculoskeletal condition	**Inflammation**	**Tissue repair**	**Degenerative process**
Aim	To reduce inflammation	To facilitate natural repair and restore optimal function, to increase tensile strength, to maintain tissue length	To reduce pain, to improve function, to reduce factors predisposing to degeneration
Modalities	Electrotherapy to decrease the inflammation Ice to reduce heat	Electrotherapy to facilitate natural tissue repair Ice? Heat?	Electrotherapy for pain or inappropriate Heat for relaxation
	Massage in elevation for swelling, taking care not to increase scar formation	Massage to facilitate tissue reorganisation	Massage to stretch and mobilise soft tissues
	Support and compression	Support to facilitate healing and reduce deformity; plan when to remove	Support to facilitate movement; support may be inappropriate
	Muscle work for protection; muscle work may be inappropriate unless gentle	Muscle work to restore optimal function and encourage good-quality repair	Muscle work to reduce dysfunction and achieve optimal balanced function
	Passive movements to maintain range if appropriate	Active, passive, accessory, physiological movements to restore optimal function and increase tensile strength, all tissues gently extended to maximum length	Active, passive, accessory and physiological movements in isolation or combined to mobilise and stretch for optimal joint, soft tissue and neurological range

Table 15.2 Modalities for musculoskeletal conditions.

Treatment administered in the department should be of a nature which cannot be administered at home. Unsupervised treatments should always be accompanied by education so that patients are fully aware of the purpose of the treatment, of how to be effective, and of how to progress and pace themselves. Either the physiotherapist or the patient should be measuring the outcome.

Self-help

There are many advocates of self-help treatment regimens (McKenzie, 1981; Evjenth & Hamberg, 1989; Key, 1991). However, it must be stressed that this is not an easy option for the physiotherapist. To be effective, physiotherapists must administer, through continual assessment, an appropriate treatment regimen which has been carefully monitored and adjusted to the patient's needs. There should be an open channel of discussion with the patient, either by follow-up sessions or by telephone calls, to be sure that the patient is in control of their condition and has sufficient knowledge to eventually take full responsibility.

LONG-TERM GOALS

Decisions regarding the appropriate long-term management of the patient are always difficult. In an ideal situation, not constrained by cost, it is a decision which should be monitored by seeing the patient regularly. From the outset, the plan should be discussed with the patient. This reduces disappointment and unrealistic promises or patient expectations. The inexperienced physiotherapist must not expect to cure all ills and not be disappointed when patients have not reached, cannot reach, will not reach, or do not even want to reach, professional goals of recovery.

Clinical decision-making challenges many assumptions. For example, young sporty clinicians may assume that their younger patients need vigorous home exercise regimens to maintain joint range and to keep muscles or nerves fully stretched, or that they require advice on healthy eating habits, back care, ergonomics, and so on. However, it must not be forgotten that if the patient wishes to remain a 'couch potato' and enjoys smoking, being overweight and sleeping on a soft bed, then that is their choice. As soon as the patient's ideal is reached, discharge should be arranged, with no guilt on the part of the physiotherapist. The physiotherapist's job is to give information to patients, not to change beliefs (Coward, 1989). In contrast, it is not the remit of overstretched physiotherapy resources to continually repair the damaged tissues of the patient who persists in activities known to be harmful to the neuromusculoskeletal system. If the patient insists on indulging in such activities for self-gratification, then it is a free choice. The patient should be warned, however, that physiotherapy resources are scarce. Adequate advice should be provided on the safety aspects, ergonomics and home treatments of the chosen activity.

CONCLUSION

Analysing the case history of the patient with a musculoskeletal problem, consists of interpreting and reflecting on data obtained from the initial subjective and objective examination. Taking each part of the examination and performing both a specific and a mere generalised analysis, as well as producing a working hypothesis and testing out the hypothesis in the form of a treatment (specific for the patient's stage of pathology), are all important aspects of the clinical reasoning process. However, reflecting on the results of the initial treatment trial is where the student will perhaps gain most of the knowledge specific to the patient.

This chapter has attempted to give advice to the inexperienced musculoskeletal clinician, and is based on personal clinical experience in this field. Health care is now directed towards evidence-based practice. Clinicians are advised to read critically about the process of examination, to develop skills in performing both the subjective and objective examination, to question the accuracy and usefulness of the tests performed, to interpret carefully assumptions regarding functional disability and clinical diagnosis, but, most importantly, to reflect upon their own practice. Recognition of weaknesses or even mistakes may help to develop a more sensitive practitioner and this can only be of benefit to the patient.

REFERENCES

Adams N, Taylor DW, Rose MJ. *The psycho-physiology of low back pain.* Edinburgh: Churchill Livingstone; 1997.

Anderson FM, Francis RM. Osteoporosis in men. *Hospital Update* August, 1994:399-400.

Barlow Y, Willoughby J. Pathophysiology of soft tissue repair. *Br Med Bull* 1992, **48**:698-711.

Basmajian JV, Sikhar WB. Clinical decision making in rehabilitation. Edinburgh: Churchill Livingstone; 1996.

Baurdillon JF, Day ER, Bookout MR. Examination of muscle imbalance. In: (ed. Baurdillon JF, et al.) *Spinal manipulation.* Oxford: Butterworth Heinemann; 1992.

Bogduk N, Mercer S. Selection and application of treatment. In: Refshauge K, Gass E, eds. *Musculoskeletal physiotherapy: clinical science and practice.* Oxford: Butterworth Heinemann; 1995.

Bordage G, Grant I, Marsden P. Quantitative assessment of diagnostic ability. *Med Educ* 1990, **24**:413-425.

Bordage G, Lemieux R. Semantic structures and diagnostic thinking of experts and novices. *Acad Med* 1991, **66**:570-572.

Bordage C, Zacks R. The structure of medical knowledge in the memories of medical students and general practitioners, categories and prototypes. *Med Educ* 1984, **18**:406-416.

Butler DS. *Mobilisation of the nervous system.* Melbourne: Churchill Livingstone, 1991.

Corrigan B, Maitland GD. *Muskoskeletal and sports injuries.* Oxford: Butterworth Heinemann; 1994.

Dixon AJ. Osteoporosis and the family doctor. In: Buyler RC, Jayson MIV, eds. *Collected reports on the rheumatic diseases.* Tunbridge Wells: Arthritis and Rheumatism Council; 1995.

Douglas M. *Risk and blame: essays in cultural theory.* London: Routledge; 1994.

Dutton R. *Clinical reasoning in physical disabilities.* Baltimore: Williams and Wilkins; 1995.

Edwards BC. *Manual of combined movements: their use in the examination and treatment of mechanical vertebral column disorders.* Edinburgh: Churchill Livingstone; 1992.

Evans P. The healing process at cellular level: a review. *Physiotherapy* 1980, **66**:256-259.

Fishbain DA, Cutler R, Rosomorff HL, Rosomoff RS. Chronic pain–associated depression: a review. *Clin J Pain* 1997, **13**:116-137.

Foreman SM, Croft A C. *Whiplash injuries.* Baltimore: Williams and Wilkins; 1995.

French S. The psychology and sociology of pain. In: Wells PE, Frampton V, Bowsher D, eds. *Pain management by physiotherapy,* 2nd ed. London: Butterworth Heinmann; 1994.

Gass EM. Principles of examination and measurement. In: Refshauge K, Gass E, eds. *Musculoskeletal physiotherapy: clinical science and practice.* Oxford: Butterworth Heinemann; 1995.

Goodman CC, Snyder TEK. *Differential diagnosis in physical therapy.* Philadelphia: WB Saunders; 1995.

Grant R. Vertebral artery concerns: premanipulative testing of the cervical spine. In: Grant R, ed. *Physical therapy and the cervical and thoracic spine.* Edinburgh: Churchill Livingstone; 1994.

Grieve GP. *Mobilisation of the spine. Notes on examination, assessment and clinical method,* 6th ed. Edinburgh: Churchill Livingstone; 1994.

Higgs J, Jones M. *Clinical reasoning in the health professions.* Oxford: Butterworth Heinemann; 1995.

Hoppenfeld S. *Physical examination of the spine and extremities.* New York: Appleton Century Crofts; 1996.

Hunter G. Specific soft tissue mobilisation in the treatment of soft tissue lesions. *Physiotherapy* 1994, **80**:15-21.

Janda V. Muscle strength in relation to muscle length, pain and muscle imbalance. In: Harms-Ringdahl K, ed. *Muscle strength.* Singapore: Churchill Livingstone; 1993.

Janda V. Muscles and motor control in cervicogenic disorders: assessment and management. In: Grant R, ed. *Physical therapy of the cervical and thoracic spine.* Edinburgh: Churchill Livingstone; 1994.

Jones K, Barker K. *Human movement explained.* Oxford: Butterworth Heinemann; 1995.

Jull G, Richardson CA. Rehabilitation of the active stabilisation in low back pain assessment and management. In: Twomey LT, Taylor JR, eds. *Physical therapy of the low back.* New York: Churchill Livingstone; 1994.

Key S. *Back in action.* London: Vermillion; 1991.

Khalil MT, Abdel-Moty ME, Rosomoff RS, Rosomoff HL. *Ergonomics in back pain.* New York: Van Nostrand Reinhold; 1993.

Kidd BL, Morris VH, Urban L. Pathophysiology of joint pain. *Ann Rheum Dis* 1996, **55**:276-283.

Kitchen S, Basin S. *Claytons electrotherapy.* London: WB Saunders; 1996.

Kuslich SD, Ulstrom CL, Nicheol A. Tissue origin of low back pain and sciatica. *Orthop Clin North Am* 1991, **22**:181-187.

Lewit K. *Manipulative therapy in rehabilitation of the locomotor system.* Oxford: Butterworth Heinemann; 1991.

Magee DI. *Orthopedic physical assessment.* Philadelphia: WB Saunders; 1997.

Maitland GD. *Peripheral manipulation,* 3rd ed. London: Butterworths; 1991.

Mattingly C, Fleming MH. *Clinical reasoning forms and inquiry in the therapeutic practice.* Philadelphia: FA Davies; 1994.

Melzack R, Wall PD. *Textbook of pain.* Edinburgh: Churchill Livingstone; 1993.

Mulligan BR. *Manual therapy 'Nags', 'Snags', 'MWMS', etc,* 3rd ed. New Zealand: Plane View Services; 1995.

Murtagh J, Kenna C. *Back pain and spinal manipulation.* Oxford: Butterworth Heinemann; 1997.

Norkin CC, Levangie PK. *Joint structure and function.* Philadelphia: FA Davies; 1992.

Olmarker K, Kikuchi S, Rydevik B. Anatomy and physiology of spinal nerve roots and the results of compression and irritation. In: Giles LBF, Singer KP, eds. *Clinical anatomy and management of low back pain.* Oxford: Butterworth Heinemann; 1997.

Palastanga N. Soft tissue manipulative techniques. In: Boyling JD, Palastanga N, eds. *Modern manual therapy.* London: Churchill Livingstone; 1994.

Palastanga N, Field D, Soames R. *Anatomy and human movement structure and function* (student edition). Oxford: Butterworth Heinemann; 1994.

Riddle DL. Measurement of accessory motion. Critical issues and related concepts. *Phys Ther* 1992, **72**:865-873.

Rydevik B, Olmarker K. In: Jayson MIV, ed. *The lumbar spine and back pain.* Edinburgh: Churchill Livingstone; 1992.

Sackett DI, Haynes RB, Guyalt GH, Tugwell P. *Clinical epidemiology. A basic science for clinical medicine,* 2nd ed. Boston: Little Brown; 1991.

Schwarzer AC, April CN, Bogduk N. The sacroiliac joint in chronic low back pain. *Spine* 1995, **20**:31-37.

Shacklock MO. *Moving in on pain.* Oxford: Butterworth-Heinmann; 1995.

Spector TD. Trends for admissions for hip fractures in England and Wales. *BMJ* 1990, **300**:1173-1174.

Stoddard A. *Manual of orthopaedic practice.* London: Hutchinson; 1993.

Taylor JR. Development and structure of lumbar intervertebral discs. *Man Med* 1990, **5**:43-47.

Twomey LT, Taylor JR. Bone loss and osteoporosis of the spine. In: Boyling JD, Palastanga N. *Modern manual therapy.* London: Churchill Livingstone; 1994.

Waddell D, Feder G, McIntosh A, Lewis M, Hutchinson A. *Low back pain evidence review.* London: Royal College of General Practitioners; 1996.

Wells PE, Frampton V, Bowsher D. *Pain management by physiotherapy.* Oxford: Butterworth Heinemann; 1994.

Woo SLY, Horibe S, Ohland KJ. The response of ligaments to injury healing of the collateral ligaments. In: Daniel D, et al., eds. *The ligaments structure function injury and repair.* New York: Raven Press; 1990.

GENERAL READING

Burnick S, Walker JM, Paule WJ. Age changes in the annulus fibrosus in human intervertebral discs. *Spine* 1990, **16:5**:520-524.

Corrigan B, Maitland GD. *Practical orthopaedic medicine.* Cambridge: Butterworths; 1991.

Low J, Reed A. *Electrotherapy explained: principles and practice.* Oxford: Butterworth Heinemann; 1990.

Pritchard P. In: Frankenberg R, ed. *Time health and medicine.* London: Sage; 1992.

Siegal B. *Peace, love and healing.* London: Rider; 1990, chpt 3.

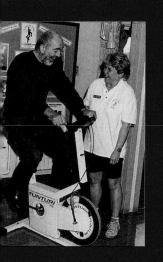

16 E Mellor

FUNCTIONAL RESTORATION PROGRAMME

CHAPTER OUTLINE

- Functional restoration programmes
- Setting up a functional restoration programme

- A model of a functional restoration programme
- Discharge

INTRODUCTION

The patient with chronic low back problems is frequently referred to the physiotherapist when previous surgery has failed or surgery is not possible. Alternatively, patients may be referred by their general practitioner as a last resort for pain relief.

Physiotherapy offers such patients a variety of treatments, which may be either 'hands on' or 'hands off', combined with exercise, education and advice. Physiotherapists know that for management to be effective they must gain the patient's compliance and confidence. When referral for treatment is early, patients usually accept that they have a very important part to play in their understanding and control of pain. For example, there is no future in treating a patient who encourages the recurrence of pain by sitting incorrectly for a week, only to return for further treatment a week later. In the long run this type of patient becomes poorer financially, physically and psychologically.

Functional restoration has evolved a physical and psychological approach (Mayer & Gatchel, 1988) to the management of the patient's problems, where specific diagnosis is not necessarily all important. Experience from the implementation of functional restoration programmes demonstrates that socioeconomic factors often play the most important part in determining a positive or negative effect of treatment on the patient recovering from a spinal condition, whatever the pathology.

When patients are at the stage when they can no longer cope, they are usually referred for functional restoration programme treatment as an end of line 'treatment'. This is often too late for achieving full recovery as they are likely to have been on state benefits for years, are physically unfit and are not motivated sufficiently to perform the basic activities of daily living. Such patients become introverted and dissatisfied with life, have family problems and are often unemployable. They may also be unwell due to the side effects of drugs.

These patients may now feel that they have medical, psychological and socioeconomic problems from which there seems no escape. This downward trend needs to be stopped, by referral to a rehabilitation programme while the person is still employable, if at all possible. Referral should be within the first 6–12 months, so that chronic pain has not been established.

FUNCTIONAL RESTORATION PROGRAMMES

HISTORICAL DEVELOPMENT

It could be said that low back pain is an epidemic, as it affects the majority of people at some time in their life. It causes an increase in the number of lost working days, which causes a reduction in national production and leads to greater demands on state benefits. There does not seem to be an increase in the number of precipitating injuries or in back pathology. In the UK, return to work is not always a viable option for people with chronic back problems because of the work ethic, unemployment levels, the benefits' system and the impact of litigation on a patient's rate of recovery.

In the UK there are many functional rehabilitation courses, e.g. back schools and out-patient and in-patient programmes. These are of varying length—many up to 4 weeks, some even longer. There are also pain clinics which primarily offer alternative methods of pain relief and combine these with functional rehabilitation.

At a meeting in 1995 organised by the Society for Back Pain Research, the results from several established programmes in Scandinavia and Britain were discussed. This showed that out-patient courses produced the same results as in-patient courses. Some physiotherapists have found that one-to-one advice and treatment are more effective than group courses, hence a variety of programmes has been developed to respond to this demand. These programmes take into account the local requirements which are governed by the environment, economics, the content and available staffing levels.

MEASURING OUTCOMES OF FUNCTIONAL REHABILITATION

In the USA, the Commission on Accreditation of Rehabilitation Facilities (Pope *et al.*, 1991) has produced specific guidelines for work-hardening programmes for patients with long-term back pain problems. The outcomes are evaluated by performance on the programme, after which the patient may have:

• Returned to work.
• Met the programme's goals.
• Declined further services.
• Not complied with organisational policies.
• Demonstrated limited potential to benefit.
• Required further healthcare intervention.

ASSESSMENT

There are different systems for the self-assessment of pain, disability and psychological state available to professionals in this field. There is also a comprehensive guide to the most commonly used questionnaires (Pynsent *et al.*, 1993). Objectives determined as a result of assessment should be measurable and repeatable and should cover the patient's ability to perform activities of daily living and specific ranges of movement and stamina for the performance of exercises.

Any tests and questionnaires should be explained to the patients to make them aware that their responses should relate to the exact time of the assessment. When answering the questions, the patients must mark the correct comment relating to their physical status at the precise time of completing the assessment form. Patients have a tendency to complete forms while reflecting on a previous state— usually when the condition was at its worst—not realising that improvement has been gained.

Although the assessor should not change any of the patient's responses, it is essential to note whether the patient has not scored the sections correctly to reflect his or her present ability. Patients tend to dislike filling in forms, and some may have difficulty with reading and writing. The more simple the questionnaire, the better for cost and time effectiveness.

Questionnaires may be completed at the time of the initial assessment, on the first or last day of the programme, at follow-up assessment or at any further follow-up by post. Strength and stamina may be regularly tested throughout the programme and these results often encourage the patient to continue improving.

SETTING UP A FUNCTIONAL RESTORATION PROGRAMME

A high level of co-operation between the providers and the purchasers of the service is required to set up a functional restoration programme. The facilities and staff have to be chosen specifically for the type of programme. The programme leader is nominated early in the planning process, and may be an anaesthetist, a clinical psychologist, an orthopaedic consultant, a physiotherapist or any other person with sufficient specific knowledge and experience in this specialist field. The facilities should be carefully planned, the proximity of the patients' accommodation to areas where theory and practical sessions are held is of obvious importance.

FACILITIES

It must be decided whether the programme will be residential or non-residential; in both cases, the level of support within the patients' accommodation must be determined.

Patients' Accommodation

If the course is residential, accommodation must be available on site. Ideally, all the patients should have their own room. If dormitory accommodation is provided, this must cater for both sexes if the courses are mixed, and the patient must have an acceptable level of privacy. There must be adequate provision of baths, showers and laundry facilities. Both residential and non-residential courses require designated areas where the patients can relax in the evenings, at lunchtime and during breaks in the course programme.

Accommodation Requirements for the Course

Accommodation needed for the successful implementation of the course is listed below:

Interview/Assessment Room
This should comprise a small room where one-to-one interviews can be held in privacy.

Teaching Area
A room large enough to accommodate the patients in comfort, with chairs and teaching facilities, should be available. Useful equipment includes a model of the articulated spine, a skeleton, slide projector and video recorder.

Gymnasium

A full-sized and well-equipped gymnasium is required for activity sessions in the programme. It is also useful to have additional recreational activities available, such as table tennis and badminton.

Swimming Pool

Many hospitals have hydrotherapy pools but these are not appropriate for use in a functional restoration programme as they are usually too small to accommodate all the patients on the course. If the hospital does not have a swimming pool on site, arrangements should be made to use a public facility so that the patients can benefit from group exercise in a large pool.

Workshops

Not all hospitals have workshops where work activities can be simulated. If these are not available, the occupational therapy department should develop functional activities with equipment that simulates those movements required of patients attempting to return to employment after the programme.

This type of structured environment is also suitable for encouraging patients to resume practical hobbies, e.g. woodwork or metalwork, they may have given up because of their back pain. It is also an environment in which patients may experiment, developing new hobbies and leisure activities they may pursue at home after the programme or at weekends while on the programme.

Office Facilities

Staff require office space for planning activities, documentation of the course, recording patients' progress, audit and storage of records. This area should be out of bounds to patients and should be securely locked when unoccupied.

Changing Facilities

Both the staff and the patients will require adequate changing facilities as they will be participating in several activities requiring different clothing.

Leisure/Sports Facilities

The provision of leisure facilities is obviously of importance when patients are attending residential rather than non-residential courses. When developing a programme, course planners should investigate the availability of leisure activities such as golf and tennis. If there are suitable walks within easy access of the course location, these should be mapped out.

Meals/Refreshments

The patients are encouraged to have a balanced diet of nourishing food, and dietary advice may be required by some of the participants. Special dietary requirements on the grounds of preference, religious conviction or medical need must be catered for. Both residential and non-residential courses should have restaurant facilities on site where patients can buy meals. If food is provided, there will be control over the quantity and quality consumed during the course, and the meals can also be timed to fit in with programmed activities. If this is not possible, self-catering facilities should be provided.

Course organisers should also consider the provision of refreshments. Are these to be provided in the working areas or are the patients to go elsewhere?

STAFF DEDICATED TO THE PROGRAMME

The programme leader should be identified early in the planning stage as he or she will determine the content of the programme and identify the personnel required to implement the courses successfully. The number and type of staff recruited will depend on the professional orientation of the course leader, the proposed length of the course, whether the course is to be residential or non-residential and its proposed content.

Professional support will be required from the physiotherapists, occupational therapists, clinical psychologists, dieticians and secretarial staff.

REFERRAL

The course leader should determine the source of referral that will be accepted on the programme. This could include referral by an orthopaedic surgeon, neurosurgeon or general practitioner. Other referral sources may be determined, but care must be taken to ensure that the objectives of the programme continue to be met from the larger recruitment base.

Referral Criteria

The inclusion and exclusion criteria for course participants should be agreed and adhered to as far as possible. It is very easy to have good admission criteria and then be persuaded to relax these to allow particular patients onto a programme. In hindsight, these patients seldom do as well as those for whom the criteria applied.

COURSE CONTENT

This will be determined by the:
- Physical and personnel resources allocated to the programme.
- Philosophy of the programme.
- Expertise available.
- Size of the group.
- Length of the programme.
- Residential or non-residential nature of the programme.
- Inclusion and exclusion criteria.
- Outcome requirements.

These factors have been discussed above and must be considered by the course leader when constructing the programme.

ASSESSMENT AND EVALUATION

Assessment and evaluation tools to be used on the programme must be identified before the course starts.

The programme should be subject to continuous audit and be responsive to any changes proposed.

COSTING THE COURSE

Determination of the costs of all the items mentioned on page 218, is required so that a business plan can be constructed to enable the host unit to decide on the size of groups, the length of each course and the number of courses that can be run annually. Within the constraints of the resources available, there is an economic break-even point which will show the size and number of courses that can be run effectively. This is a resource-intensive project. In the long term, it is more beneficial to patients to run fewer courses effectively than to spread the available resources so thinly that the courses are inadequately resourced.

A MODEL OF A FUNCTIONAL RESTORATION PROGRAMME

The functional restoration programme described below is based at a hospital specialising in the orthopaedic management of patients. The hospital is situated in the country, 3 miles from the nearest population centre. Public transport connections to the rest of the county are poor and so the course is residential, lasting for 3 weeks.

There are several subspecialty units within the hospital, one of which is the centre for spinal disorders. The programme was developed by the surgeons and physiotherapy staff of this centre.

Over the 3 years of operation of the functional restoration programme at this centre, it has been found that there is a correlation between chronicity of pain, i.e. time since the original onset of low back pain, and non-return to work. In this geographical area, the problem is compounded by lack of employment prospects, the rural environment and lack of accessibility of appropriate back care. It is generally known that early intervention facilitates resolution of symptoms, with the possibility of a rapid return to work. If there is a court claim pending, early intervention again will facilitate return to work, especially if there is an interium payment, but there is evidence from research in other centres that has proved patients do not return to their pre-accident or -incident 'normal' once their claim is settled 4 or 5 years later with a lump sum. Functional restoration programmes are therefore suitable methods of approach either during the early stages of litigation or when the claim has been settled, as the patient is then psychologically compliant.

PROGRAMME LEADER

The team is led by a senior 1 physiotherapist, whose line management is through the physiotherapy manager to the chief executive of the Trust. The contracts department of the Trust helps with marketing issues and referrals from out of the area. For referral of patients, there is close liaison with orthopaedic consultants specialising in spinal disorders.

STAFF DEDICATED TO THE PROGRAMME

The staffing of the programme includes:
- Two whole time equivalent (WTE) chartered physiotherapists, one senior 1 physiotherapist, who is also the programme leader, and one senior 2 physiotherapist.
- One WTE occupational therapist, senior 2.
- One WTE clinical assistant, a physiotherapy assistant.
- A part-time visiting clinical psychologist.
- A sessional pharmacist who gives a 1-hour lecture in each programme.
- A sessional dietician who gives a 1-hour lecture/demonstration in each programme, but is available to take specific referrals for individual advice and guidance.
- A sessional disability employment advisor who gives a 1-hour talk in each programme, from the local Job Centre.

Social workers are available for consultation should their services be required.

As patients are resident in the hospital for the duration of the course, support from other hospital staff is essential, for example, kitchen, laundry, domestic and maintenance staff.

COURSE PHILOSOPHY

A functional restoration programme aims to encourage patients with back pain to improve their lifestyle by improving function and fitness and by increasing their self-esteem. The emphasis is on education, self-help and empowerment.

COURSE AIMS

The aims of the course are:
- To improve function both physically and psychologically.
- To accept and learn to cope with existing levels of pain.
- To improve the quality of life within the constraints imposed by back pain.

COURSE OBJECTIVES

By the end of the programme, the patient should have:
- An increased knowledge and awareness of spinal anatomy, pathology and biomechanics.
- An increased level of fitness and flexibility through exercise.
- Increased self-confidence.
- Decreased levels of anxiety and depression.

REFERRAL CRITERIA

Referral to the programme is accepted from either an orthopaedic consultant or general practitioner. It is important to have information concerning the patient's medical or surgical history, any psychiatric illness, and any treatment given.

After 1 year of operation of the functional restoration programme, the following inclusion and exclusion criteria were agreed at an audit of the patients' results:

Inclusion Criteria

To be accepted onto the programme, the patient should:
- Be motivated to improve functionally.

- Be realistic about potential improvement through the setting of short-term and long-term goals.
- Be functionally independent and medically fit.
- Not expect a cure or great pain relief.

Exclusion Criteria

The patient will be excluded from the programme if he or she has:

- Any history of heart disease or cardiac surgery.
- A previous or ongoing psychiatric history.
- Evidence of current drug or alcohol misuse.
- Equipment in situ at home, e.g. stair lift or wheelchair.
- A pending compensation claim.
- Above threshold scores for anxiety and depression on completion of psychology questionnaires.
- Type 1 diabetes—such patients would be considered for a less physical programme.
- Been unable to complete a quarter of a mile corridor walking test within 5 minutes—these patients would also be considered for a less physical programme.
- Should not be a surgical candidate.

ASSESSMENT

Assessment is usually conducted by the same member of the team so that there is continuity of measurement, although at times it may have to be done by someone else,

for example, an occupational therapist substituting for a physiotherapist or vice versa.

Assessment Tools and Methods

The information needed for assessment will cover socio-economic factors, difficulties encountered in the activities of daily living, how leisure time is spent, past medical history, assessment of pain, present ranges of spinal movement, peripheral joint movement and neurology.

Assessment of Pain

Many different methods of pain assessment have been developed over the years (Huskisson, 1974), and three different sytems are used on the programme described.

Drawing a Pain Pattern on a Physiotherapy Assessment Body Chart

On the physiotherapy assessment body chart (Figure 16.1A), areas of pain are marked by the patient (Figure 16.1B). Normally, the charts comprise outlines of the body on both anterior and posterior views, but only the latter is reproduced here. The level of pain intensity is indicated by the proximity of the hatching lines drawn by the patient: close hatching—high intensity of pain, light hatching—lower intensity of pain.

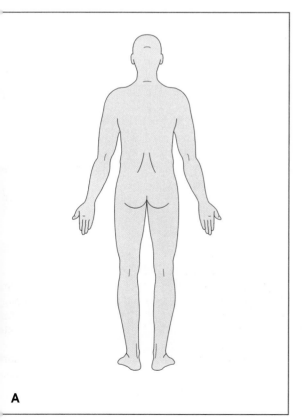
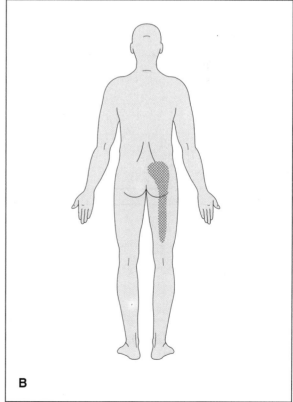

A **B**

Figure 16.1 Body chart outline. (A) Posterior view before completion.
(B) Completed by patient. Areas of hatching denote areas of pain.

Marking an Analogue Scale with the Level of Pain Experienced at the Time

The analogue scale is a straight line, 10 cm long, on which 'no pain' is marked at one end and 'maximum pain' at the other (Figure 16.2A). The line may be marked off in numbered segments to facilitate interpretation of the scale. Patients mark the point along the line that indicates their current level of pain (Figure 16.2B). A comparison of several of these completed scales enables improvement or deterioration to be assessed according to the movement of the patient's marks towards one or other of the line's extremities.

In addition, a comment from the patient on their perceived quality of the day can be a valuable indicator to determine the effectiveness or otherwise of the management programme. A patient may record the same point along the scale, indicating that the level of pain is unchanged. However, if the comment made on three successive assessments was 'bad day', 'average day' and 'good day', respectively, this would indicate improvement in the patient's general condition, and if the comments went from 'good day' to bad day', it would indicate that the condition was worsening and the patient's ability to cope with the level of pain was deteriorating .

Assessing the Amount and Type of Medication Taken

By comparing the amount and type of drugs the patient was taking before entering functional restoration with the amount required during the programme, a direct assessment of medication can be made. Patients should,

however, be warned at the initial assessment that they may have more pain while undergoing the programme because of the level and number of physical activities involved. If a patient feels unable to tolerate any increase of pain, that patient would not be suitable for most functional restoration programmes and may gain more benefit from attending a pain clinic. Patients on the programme should understand why their pain or stiffness is likely to be increased and be made aware that the ethos of the programme is to learn to control pain while improving physical abilities within a structured programme that is designed to be supportive.

Assessment of Range of Spinal Movement

Range of spinal movement is measured using the modified-modified Schober method (Figure 16.3) (Williams *et al.*, 1993).

The distance between the spine of the 12th thoracic vertebra and the lumbosacral junction is measured first with the patient standing, spine erect, and then on flexion of the spine to the point where it is limited by the intensity of pain experienced. The more the flexion of the lumbar spine, the greater the discrepancy between the two measurements.

Assessment of Disability

The Oswestry Disability Index is used in the programme to assess the level of disability identified by the patient (Fairbank *et al.*, 1980). In addition, the programme leader has developed a lifestyle index to be used in the programme

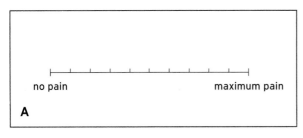

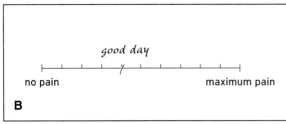

Figure 16.2 Analogue scale. (A) Before completion. **(B)** Completed by patient.

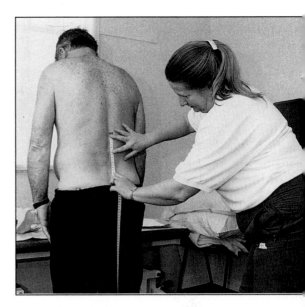

Figure 16.3 Modified-modified Schober method of measuring spinal range of movement by the physiotherapist. At each assessment, spinal range is re-measured as well as the patient's disability and psychology questionnaires, pain level and timed walking test.

This has been developed from the Oswestry Disability Index and is specific to the needs of the programme.

Psychological Assessment

Use of the General Health Questionnaire (Goldberg, 1978) and assessment on the Hospital Anxiety and Depression Scale (Zigmund & Snaith, 1983) provide a comprehensive assessment of the patient's psychological state, which is taken into account when assessing the patient's response to the programme.

Following the initial patient assessment, aims for the programme are agreed. There are normally no more than four or five of these, all of which must be short term, achievable and realistic. Patients will become depressed if aims are unachievable and goals unrealistic. Goals should be changed early in the programme if they are found to be wrong.

The patient accepted for the programme is notified within a fortnight of the initial assessment, and a suitable date arranged for admission. If there are any medical problems, the general practitioner is requested to see the patient before admission, to certify fitness for a reasonably physically demanding programme. This provides protection for the staff of the programme as there are no routine visits from medical staff as in other areas of the hospital. For this reason also, patients bring in any drugs that are likely to be needed and take them as they would at home.

If a patient is found not suitable for the programme at assessment, then the team will give appropriate advice for further management of the problem.

For those who are less physically fit but still independent, e.g. after spinal surgery or if the condition is too widespread to guarantee improvement with surgery, a less physically demanding programme can be set up. This can also be arranged for patients with higher scores than the team expected in the psychological assessment. Experience in running the programme has demonstrated that this type of patient improves more significantly if the physical intervention is associated with a greater input from the clinical psychologist. Although patients recovering from surgery or with high psychological assessment scores are more difficult to rehabilitate, they can be included in functional restoration programmes provided numbers are reduced. By being in a smaller group, such patients can have the additional support required and it allows them to participate by realising their limitations, learning to pace themselves, and not feeling physically or mentally pressurised by the more active groups.

COMPLIANCE AND GOAL SETTING

On initial assessment, the patient must want to be included on a programme and be able to set realistic goals. There should be regular feedback on a daily or weekly basis, because although patients may be included in a group, they also need individual attention. The programmes will work only if they are patient led. To help the patient achieve on the course, the tasks covered must relate to their individual goals. This involvement in shaping the course will lead to improved patient compliance. The flexibility built into each group allows for essential differences in each programme implemented. No two programmes will include the same personalities nor the same problems.

COURSE CONTENT

The course should be reasonably flexible because of the variety of patient problems presented. In the first week there must be more theory, advice on activities of daily living and practical sessions. The last week may contain more sessions encouraging strength and stamina but with the warning that patients must not be overzealous with their new-found fitness. Muscles that have been misused and abused over a period of time do not return to normal after a week's exercise programme.

The content will vary according to the staff teaching the programme and the individual needs of the patient.

Education

Anatomy

The teaching of basic spinal anatomy and pathology are important so that patients can relate to good biomechanical principles. They are made aware of normal body reactions to movement of bone, disc, joint, nerve, muscle and other tissues in the spinal column (Figure 16.4). They learn to appreciate what is or is not comfortable, how to decrease painful postures and why this is so relevant to their condition.

Ergonomics

Instruction in ergonomic principles is very important, relating to the patient's activities of daily living and occupation, hobbies and interests (Figure 16.5). Much thought can be put into daily activities, for example, instruction and advice on:

- Mobilising exercises in bed to reduce stiffness.
- The correct methods of getting out of bed.
- The use of correct body mechanics to suit the individual for completing morning toilet procedures and dressing.
- Achieving good seating for meals.
- Good posture while working.
- The importance of regularly changing activity and position.
- Using good handling techniques in work.
- Some form of appropriate exercise/sport.
- Relaxation techniques or a social activity to ensure the patient is able to 'wind down' in the evening.
- Being able to retire to a comfortable bed feeling, in a healthy manner, physically and mentally tired.

Coping Strategies

Coping strategies for living with back pain are individual to each patient. Every person has a different perception of pain, influenced by different factors, and therefore every patient will have a different way of dealing with it. Discussion is often wide ranging, extending from how to deal with chronic or acute pain to understanding the patient's basic back condition and the treatment techniques to which specific joints,

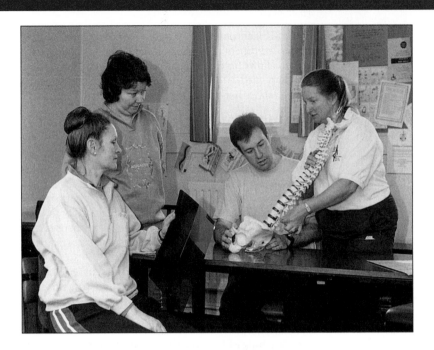

Figure 16.4 Discussion on the ward in the day room with the physiotherapist. Basic anatomy is described, relating to everyday body postures and activities. X-Ray films are discussed, and a video is shown of the patients performing in the gymnasium and workshops, and while walking.

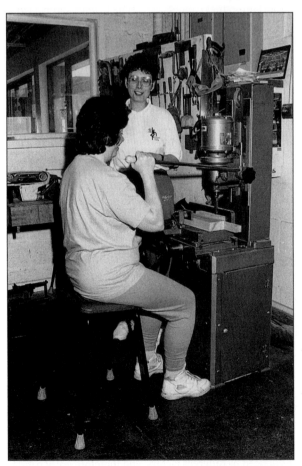

Figure 16.5 Workshop session with the occupational therapist. Posture, body mechanics and ergonomics are practised, either to encourage a hobby or to instruct for return to work.

discs or soft tissues will respond. Although pain is discussed, the emphasis should be on the activity or posture that is causing the patient difficulties in achieving specific activities, rather than concentrating on the fact that because activity is painful it cannot therefore be achieved.

Stress Management

Stress management is closely linked with strategies for coping with pain. Throughout the programme, all the multidisciplinary staff continuously encourage and help to instill patients with confidence during all their activities. Positive thinking, and the importance of keeping an open mind and being prepared to try alternative methods, are dealt with at all sessions, including those with a clinical psychologist.

Relaxation

Relaxation techniques are taught in lying and sitting, and are practised by the patient in the position that gives most comfort. If the patient finds relaxation sessions very beneficial, then audiotapes can be purchased for continued use. Group games are a good method of dropping inhibitions and allowing sociability. Staff try to make opportunities for patients to talk about their general problems on an individual basis while out of the hospital environment on short outings. This means that the patient does not feel singled out and, being in a relaxed environment, they are able to discuss their problems.

Psychological Rehabilitation

Psychological rehabilitation assesses the patient's attitudes towards their problems in both group and individual sessions. Emphasis is on the individual having a more flexible attitude in their thoughts and general approach to the management of back pain. Any specific problem will be dealt with in individual sessions and the clinical psychologist will refer the patient for more specialised help if necessary through the patient's general practitioner. The patient is also able to 'self-refer' to help groups that may be suggested by the clinical psychologist.

Diet

The patient is advised that a healthy, well-balanced diet is essential for an active life. An incorrect balance of foods may cause obesity or lethargy, or a medical problem may result in calcium and minerals not being absorbed and causing referred spinal pain. A condition such as diabetes would need careful observation, as increased daily activities may necessitate a change in diet and drugs.

Drugs

Drugs and their side effects are discussed with the pharmacist. Patients are asked to bring to the hospital all the drugs that may be needed during their stay. They take their own medication as they would at home. Patients are warned that they may have more aches and pains while on the course because of alterations in their lifestyle. They may need to take more medication, but, more importantly, they should learn how to pace themselves so that the increased activity is not necessarily synonymous with increased pain. It is hoped that, in time, by using better body mechanics, altered postures, pain coping strategies and relaxation, and by understanding more about their backs and not being afraid of the pain, the patients will be taking fewer analgesics, thinking about their pain in a different way, coping with it and charting that it has decreased. During the programme, patients may need to take non-steroidal anti-inflammatory drugs or occasionally analgesics, but hopefully they will stop taking any antidepressants. Any alteration in medication must always be agreed with the patient's general practitioner.

Exercise

Restoring function is initially by mobilisation of stiff spinal or peripheral joints, then by gentle stretching of soft tissues that have become shortened, and finally by strengthening muscles to protect the body as a whole. The patient is given an illustrated guide on the exercises to be performed which includes instruction on how to progress the programme as strength and mobility improve.

Although a programme of exercises may be taught in a group session, it should be individually tailored for each patient. All patients will not have the same range, stamina or pain threshold, and will therefore perform differently.

Work in the gymnasium aims to increase fitness, flexibility, strength and stamina while encouraging group participation in activities (Figure 16.6). Apparatus is also used. This will encourage patients to join a gymnasium or leisure centre on completion of the hospital programme and will help them to continue with a fitness improvement programme. In this way, the problem of reduced motivation after the programme is overcome and the patient finds they no longer need to be led by staff or have the set daily routine of the programme. It helps them to learn to be independently active and to fill their days in a worthwhile manner.

Team games are a good way to encourage patients to acquire some competitive spirit. These must, however, be carefully controlled as the patient is more likely to be less aware of their physical restrictions and may suffer soft tissue injury. At all times the physiotherapist must be vigilant to ensure that patients who are generally unfit and susceptible to injury do not push themselves too far. If all warnings are ignored and injury results, the situation may be used to teach pain coping strategies in the acute situation.

Hydrotherapy

Hydrotherapy is a very beneficial treatment modality (Figure 16.7). The warmth of the water facilitates movement and relaxation, soothes aches and provides a medium in which general stamina and fitness can be improved. A programme of specific pool exercises is used, and changed frequently to ensure that interest is retained and boredom avoided.

In the long term, many patients have reported increased symptoms following swimming. This may be due to using the breast or crawl stroke only, as both involve spinal extension. Ideally, the patient should perform warm-up exercises by the poolside before swimming, and should use several swimming strokes, before finishing with cooling-down exercises in a comfortable depth of water (Figure 16.8).

Work Simulation

Work simulation is covered in the theory sessions, when teaching the principles of good posture, body mechanics

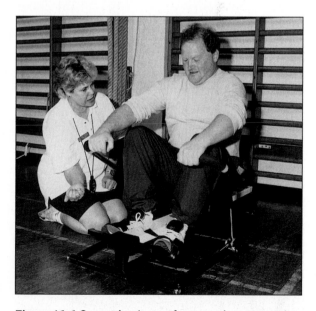

Figure 16.6 Supervised use of gymnasium apparatus with the programme assistant. After learning basic exercises for mobilising, stretching and strengthening, patients learn to use apparatus safely and to do circuits to increase their fitness and stamina.

and ergonomics. These principles are then put into practice in a workshop involving heavy or light activities. The patient learns by trial and error on attempting different tasks and by having them corrected. The task is thus made easier to perform and is more comfortable. Feedback by video recording is an excellent tool to show how postures may be changed and corrected, although the patient may feel self-conscious. The video recording should also be used to show the progression in gait re-education and in exercise sessions where range and rhythm or speed of movement are most noticeably improved.

Tasks taught may relate to activities of daily living, for example, perched on a high stool to brush teeth in the morning. Several methods can help the patient to cope with activities of daily living: adopting a certain position to put socks on, correct transfers with suitable back supports for the car, techniques to make housework less of a strain

on the spine, the availability and use of long-handled gardening tools, and seating assessments related to a hobby or work station. Many patients will need similar advice, but, as no two people have the same problems, individual sessions have to be planned into the programmes for specific assessments for seating or job simulations.

Activity Re-education

Outdoor activities are an essential part of the course, and help to change attitudes to a variety of situations. For example, the patient who knows that shopping in the supermarket is always a painful experience, will avoid going. As the patient usually undertakes this activity by car, it is not long before other journeys by car are also avoided. Next, appetite may deteriorate and the patient loses interest in food as the foods they prefer may not have been bought by the person doing the shopping. As a result, the

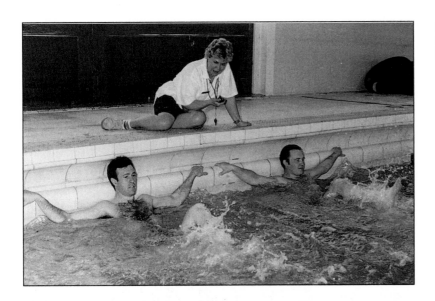

Figure 16.7 Timed kick and swim with the programme assistant to improve stamina.

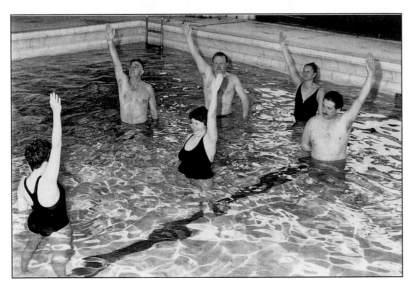

Figure 16.8 Warm-up and stretching exercises with the occupational therapist. A varied daily routine of exercise leads into strengthening and general fitness exercises, completed by team games and relaxation.

patient may gain weight by eating unhealthy 'comfort food' and also because of a greater levels of inactivity. The patient may now not want to be seen socially because of the lack of self-interest they take in their appearance. An increase in anxiety and depression results.

Encouraging outdoor activities in a staged manner helps the patient reverse this trend of deterioration, and increases physical and mental wellbeing. Good physical performances lead to a feeling of achievement. Those patients who have become negative in their thinking or have developed a phobia of the outdoors, may begin to relax and enjoy life again. As a consequence, they become less of a burden to their families, and any strain is reduced.

DISCHARGE

On completion of the programme, goals should be set which can be achieved by the next follow-up attendance. Patients should be encouraged to continue physical activity and to reward themselves for each achievement with a small treat. They must not expect too much of themselves initially, and are encouraged to set realistic goals. Otherwise, if these goals are not achieved, depression may ensue and they may be disinclined to try again; and so starts another downwards spiral.

As fitness improves, the patient's energies should be directed towards outside interests—perhaps retraining for, or returning to, some form of work. Patients who are already in employment are given advice in preparation for their return to work, and those who are on certified sick leave are given an assessment to determine the type of work that may suit them, or are encouraged to enter into a more active lifestyle. If they need to feel useful but are not fit for conventional employment, they may be encouraged to try voluntary work.

If after 6 months patients feel they have better control of their problems, they are discharged to the care of their general practitioner (Figure 16.9). Alternatively, they return to the consultant who referred them. A longer follow-up may be planned to ascertain the success or failure of control of their back problems. Involving the general practitioner in follow-up consultations is also a good way of auditing the availability of continuing healthcare resources.

CONCLUSION

The types of patients discussed in this chapter have, in the majority, been those who have had surgery or who have been unemployed and on state benefits for many years. These are patients who often show a poor response to conventional physiotherapy. There are many simple ways they can help themselves to cope with back pain, but it takes time, by trial and error, to understand the situation and to appreciate what may alleviate their specific pain. Alternatively, it may be that the increased physical fitness and its associated feeling of wellbeing will enable them to be more active and may be sufficient to help them cope better with their pain. If they are also able to continue at this level of activity while taking less medication, they are likely to feel better.

For patients who are less disabled or have fewer physiological problems, programmes can be modified and probably run for less than 3 weeks. In the programme described in this chapter, pathology groups are not mixed. Only those patients whose main complaint is of back pain are included in the programme. This is an individual choice and does not necessarily apply to similar programmes in other parts of the country.

Early results from the programme described show that on completion of the functional restoration programme, the majority of patients have decreased disability scores, are able to be more active, have an increased range of movement and have a feeling of increased physical fitness. Some patients have often found alternative strategies for reducing their pain or use antalgic postures, while others have been able to reduce their medication while on the course.

Psychological scores show there is significant reduction in anxiety and depression levels, confirming that patients are better able to cope both with their back problem and with life in general. Those that return to work are able to adjust ergonomically, improving their working capacity with a decrease in symptoms.

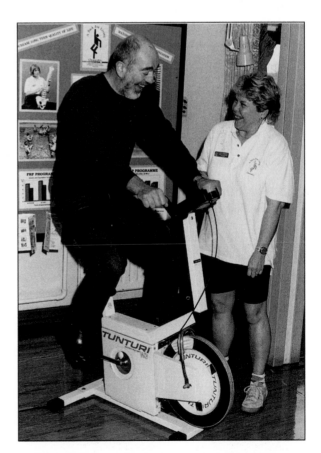

Figure 16.9 Final follow-up 6 months after the programme. This patient is coping much better at work, and has improved range of movement and halved disability scores, and on a normal day is pain free.

REFERENCES

Fairbank JCT, Davies J, Cooper J, O'Brien J. The Oswestry Disability Questionnaire. *Physiotherapy* 1980, **66**:271-273.

Goldberg D. The General Health Questionnaire (GHQ). In: Miller D, ed. *Part of an assessment: a mental health portfolio*. NFER Nelson Publishing; 1978.

Huskisson EC. Measurement of pain. *Lancet* 1974, **ii**:1127-1131.

Mayer TG, Gatchel RJ. *Functional restoration for spinal disorders: the sports medicine approach*. Philadelphia: Lea and Febiger; 1988.

Pope MH, Anderssen GBJ, Frymoyer JW, Chaffin DB. *Occupational low back pain: assessment, treatment and prevention*. St Louis: Mosby Year Book; 1991:202.

Pynsent P, Fairbank J, Carr A. *Outcome measures in orthopaedics*. Oxford: Butterworth Heinemann; 1993.

Williams R, Binkley J, Bloch R, Goldsmith CH, Minuk T. Reliability of the modified-modified Schober and double inclinometer methods for measuring lumbar flexion and extension. *Phys Ther* 1993, **73**:26-36.

Zigmund AS, Snaith RP. The hospital anxiety and depression scale. *Acta Psychiatr Scand* 1983, **7**:478-483.

GENERAL READING

Callaghan MJ. Evaluation of a back rehabilitation group for chronic low back pain in an out-patient setting. *Physiotherapy* 1994, **80**:677.

Harkapaa K, Jarvikoski A, Hakala L, Jarvilehto S. Outcome of rehabilitation programmes for employees with lowered working capacity. *Disab Rehabil* 1996, **18**:143-148.

Main CJ, Wood PLR, Hollis S, Spanswick CC, Waddell G. The distress and risk assessment method: a simple patient classification to identify distress and evaluate the risk of poor outcome. *Spine* 1992, **17**:42-52.

Swift DK. The back rehabilitation programme at Firbeck rehabilitation unit. *Physiotherapy* 1991, **77**:575-580.

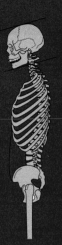

17 J Pitt-Brooke

NEUROMUSCULOSKELETAL ENVIRONMENT INTERACTIONS CONCEPT

CHAPTER OUTLINE

- **Human kinetics: McClurg Anderson's views**
- **Neuromusculoskeletal environmental interactions**
- **Human movement: environmental interactions**

- **Prevention of musculoskeletal injury**
- **Requirement for conditioning in movement habits**
- **Stretching programme**
- **Movement pattern change**

INTRODUCTION

Human movement involves a complex set of interactions, co-ordinated by the central nervous system (CNS), which result in an individual's ability to perform movements within an environment which includes gravity. These complex movements require strength, intricacy and balance. The body's ability to withstand and adapt to the stresses placed upon it as a result of such movements increases its capacity for movement, and yet the physiotherapist is constantly confronted with the effects of failure in the musculoskeletal system. This failure is evident in some of the painful musculoskeletal disorders seen in patients who are often unable to report factors which may have caused the apparent disorder. The resulting painful condition may be due to a number of mechanisms, including mechanical and neurological. A successful approach to the analysis, diagnosis, treatment and re-education of movement therefore needs an understanding of the interaction between body mechanics, muscular and nervous system factors and the environment.

The aim of this chapter is to present the neuromusculoskeletal environmental interactions (NMEI) concept which deals with the causation, prevention and treatment of some

musculoskeletal disorders. The concept embraces human movement interactions within their environment, including gravity, giving consideration to both actions and reactions of the body in movement in terms of its structure and function. It is developed from the work of McClurg Anderson (1951, 1971).

HUMAN KINETICS: MCCLURG ANDERSON'S VIEWS

During the 1940s and 1950s, a particular approach to the diagnosis and treatment of musculoskeletal disorders was developed by a Scottish physiotherapist, Tom McClurg Anderson. This approach was based on a synthesis of knowledge about biomechanical and physiological factors (McClurg Anderson, 1951), and was called 'human kinetics'. McClurg Anderson's ideas were developed at a time when the study of human physiology was in its infancy. With the exception of Sherrington (1947), who analysed the reflex activity of the spinal cord, there had been little study of the complexities of voluntary muscular movement in humans. McClurg Anderson observed the behaviour of the body in movement, and analysed the movement in terms of skeletal mechanics and muscle action. In other words, he observed and analysed the co-ordination of the muscular system by clinical observation alone, and in so doing attempted to unravel the complexity of the neural processes controlling human body movement. He believed, on the basis of certain principles, that it was possible to educate individuals to execute movements with greater efficiency and accuracy. As a result, strain would be diminished, thereby reducing the danger of injury.

The approach developed by McClurg Anderson (1951) was based on the notion that structure and function are subservient to each other. A system of physical analysis was developed to assess the state of muscular and connective tissues in relation to the stresses habitually imposed on them.

McClurg Anderson (1971) identified the need to recognise the basic requirements of normal day-to-day movement habits on muscle function from the perspective of both mobility and postural control, and suggested that such function may materially influence the condition of certain body tissues and therefore the manner in which they fulfil their function. He suggested that, for the same reason, day-to-day movement habits may determine to a considerable extent the injuries or disabilities likely to affect those tissues.

This approach to the analysis of movements advocates consideration of the initial stimulus of each movement and the fundamental character of the movement. The latter entails:

- Lock actions, defined as 'putting a [body] part into a position which will automatically stabilise other parts of the body and lead to more efficient action with the minimum of effort' (McClurg Anderson, 1971). Examples include, the lock action of the neck, involving lower cervical extension with slight upper cervical flexion, i.e. tucking in the chin, which tends to draw the rest of the spine into extension, as well as stimulating retraction of the shoulder girdle. This provides a stable and balanced position from which to move the upper limbs.
- Check actions, defined as 'the proper placing of the feet or body to prevent possible overbalancing while performing a particular movement' (McClurg Anderson, 1971); for example, ensuring that the feet are placed and adjusted so that the base of support is widened in the direction of movement.
- Evasive actions, defined as 'protective limitation of action in a part which leads to alteration in the character of a movement, and to compensatory actions' (McClurg Anderson, 1971). These actions most commonly arise as a result of protective inhibition in response to discomfort. For example, when a person with shoulder weakness or pain tries to reach out to grasp something, instead of flexing/elevating the arm, the person tilts the body forward and to the opposite side, as well as using shoulder elevation excessively. Inhibition of glenohumeral joint movement is the evasive action, while all other movements are compensatory.

If movement is to be harmonious in terms of minimising stresses to the body's structures, there must be a regard for this basic framework. When any part of a movement is altered without regard to its basic framework, compensatory actions are established. This disturbs the harmony of a movement and produces unnecessary muscular tension.

In this context, McClurg Anderson defined movement in terms of efficiency, and his views led him to believe that some patterns of movement were efficient and some were not. Those that were not were the movements which were most likely to cause unnecessary strain to the musculoskeletal system. A definition of good movement according to McClurg Anderson (1971) is; 'a movement which fulfils its function with the minimum of effort and the minimum of strain'.

Minimum effort refers to the type of muscle work involved in producing and regulating movements.

As principal of the Scottish Physiotherapy Hospital and School, McClurg Anderson educated his students in the principles of 'human kinetics'. The essence of the ideas were further developed, particularly in the field of patient handling, by John Vasey, a student of McClurg Anderson, and Lesley Crozier. Vasey and Crozier changed the name of the approach after subsequent developments and published their views under the title 'A neuromuscular approach to human movement' (Vasey & Crozier, 1984).

This chapter draws on some of the original ideas put forward by McClurg Anderson. These have been extended, in the light of more recent scientific findings, as a concept of neuromusculoskeletal environmental interactions, to explain the possible causation of some musculoskeletal disorders and also to suggest an approach to their prevention, treatment and rehabilitation. A preliminary account of this concept can be found elsewhere (Pitt-Brooke, 1995).

NEUROMUSCULOSKELETAL ENVIRONMENTAL INTERACTIONS

CUMULATIVE STRAIN

The term 'cumulative strain' appears in the vocabulary of many orthopaedic practitioners. As a term, it is poorly defined, and has become synonymous with insidious pathogenesis of painful musculoskeletal conditions. These conditions are those in which no obvious accident or direct injury can be identified, but where a series of possible, subliminal insults to the body in terms of 'stresses' and 'strains' can be identified which together may contribute to a subsequent painful condition of the musculoskeletal system. Such painful states probably arise from a structural deterioration in different body tissues as a result of excessive tension being created in them. It is unfortunate that, like many functional parameters associated with human movement, cumulative strain is difficult to quantify and demonstrate scientifically. Few clinicians would question the existence of cumulative strain or its role in the development of many painful musculoskeletal syndromes and 'overuse' injuries. However, it is unsatisfactory to accept anecdotally, the existence of cumulative strain as an entity without trying to define it through some form of analytical and clinical explanation. The inflammatory process specific to overuse injuries is described by Pecina and Bojanic (1993), and may be helpful in other cumulative strain scenarios.

McClurg Anderson's definition of efficient movement suggests that there may be a need to consider movement patterns as contributing to the causation of some painful musculoskeletal disorders. It becomes necessary to consider in more detail how to assess the effects of poor or inefficient movement patterns in individuals, and to analyse how these patterns may lead to pain in those who develop painful musculoskeletal conditions.

A concept of 'muscle imbalance' has gradually gained both popularity and credibility over the past 20 years or so. This concept draws attention to the problems which may be created by muscle shortening (Jull & Richardson, 1994). It seems likely that inefficient movement patterns may contribute to the development of muscle shortening. Contemporary physiotherapy practice has embraced the concept, and both anecdotal and research evidence have helped to develop a range of assessment and treatment techniques to identify and rectify problems of muscle imbalance. Much that is within the concept of muscle imbalance is complementary to the ideas put forward here. Many clinico-anatomical tests have been devised to assess shortening of specific muscles (Janda, 1983; Kendall & McCreary 1994), but assessment needs to focus on both the analysis of movement patterns and specific adaptive muscle shortening, if a complete picture is to emerge of the causation of some musculoskeletal disorders. Without a total picture, treatment and rehabilitation strategies will be incomplete.

Occupational Environment

Indications of the effect of cumulative strain can be demonstrated by considering some typical occupational problems. For example, back pain of epidemic proportions exists in the nursing profession, thought to be associated largely with the cumulative effect of postural strain resulting from the movement requirements of nursing care (Stubbs *et al.*, 1986). Many of the painful problems associated with the upper limbs of patients may result from cumulative strain on structures around the cervical spine and the shoulder complex. A further example may be farmers, many of whom develop strains and sometimes spondylitis at the thoracolumbar junction, from sitting in a bucketed seat. This seat fixes the pelvis as the trunk rotates and bends to enable the farmer to view the ground behind the tractor.

Sporting Environment

In the sporting environment there are many examples of painful conditions associated with repetitive movement patterns. For example, rowers typically complain of painful conditions in the lumbar spine and thoracic and shoulder regions, associated with the need to fix the lower trunk while the upper trunk flexes, extends and rotates, creating, together with the upper limb movement, a powerful pull. The painful conditions of the upper limb associated with racquet sports are familiar to most physiotherapists, as are the various painful conditions suffered by enthusiasts of 'health and fitness gymnasia' in which the predominant form of exercise requires fixing one part of the body, to exercise another more vigorously. Such fixation often results in excessive strain on parts of the body which are poorly adapted for such function.

Part of the difficulty with many of these painful conditions is that their causation is likely to be multifactorial, and the cumulative strain element alone may arise from subliminal strain on a number of different structures, rendering it difficult to examine explicitly and specifically.

EVENTS WHICH MAY LEAD TO CUMULATIVE STRAIN

It is useful to consider hypothetically, the sequence of events which may contribute to cumulative strain. Such a sequence of events was suggested by Pitt-Brooke (1995).

There are predominant functional postures in human movement. Postural fixation is provided for these postures by anticipatory feedforward and feedback mechanisms, from information about movement of the distal part of the limbs. This leads to the need for particular muscles to provide fixation within a specific range. Muscle work specific to range and function has a training effect, and, for fixation, this is isometric muscle work. Specific isometric strength of muscles in an inner to middle range without specific attempts to stretch these muscles may lead to shortening of the musculotendinous unit. This is likely to be associated with adaptive changes in the connective tissues of muscles. An adaptively shortened muscle is less likely to be responsive to the needs of complex movement interactions, and there is some evidence to suggest that such muscles may show altered reactions to excitatory and inhibitory nervous impulses. This may lead to an inability of the affected muscles to respond appropriately to demand, and may result in microtrauma. Microtrauma adds to the adaptive muscle-shortening process, and altered proprioception reinforces these adaptive changes.

It seems likely that cumulative strain conditions are associated with excessive postural holding, which in turn is associated with sustained isometric contraction of certain muscle groups. In this way, the muscles required for postural fixation in movement may be subject to overuse. While this seems a contradiction in terms, there may be a need to recognise abuse of the postural mechanisms to reduce or counteract the effects of such abuse.

It is important, therefore, to review some basic biomechanical, kinesiological and neurophysiological considerations to gain an understanding of how the human body reacts with its environment, including gravity.

BIOMECHANICAL CONSIDERATIONS

To appreciate the different ways in which forces can affect movement and cause stress on the body, it is necessary to consider some basics of biomechanics. Let us start with the centre of gravity and the area of the base of support relative to the movement.

Try the following exercise and consider the difference in body reactions. Stand with your feet wide apart. Keeping your back comfortably straight, flex your hips and knees to lower the body into the base of support created by your feet, maintaining an erect spine. Feel the weight distribution in your feet move from the length of the medial borders of the feet to the lateral borders and the heels. This indicates that the erect spine is tending to displace the centre of gravity of the body towards the back of the base of support. Extend the hips and knees and return to the erect position, and feel the weight distribution return to the length of the medial side of the feet.

Now repeat the exercise, but consciously rotate the pelvis backwards as you do so, inducing flexion in the lumbar spine. Feel the weight distribution more clearly over the medial arches of the feet, nearer the centre of the base of the support.

Repeat the exercise both ways several times, to reinforce the difference in weight distribution in the feet. This reflects the differences in body reactions.

Generally, a movement will be more efficient in terms of reducing the effect of gravitational forces if the centre of gravity of the body is kept low and the line of gravity is kept near the centre of the base of support. This is best achieved in movement by allowing flexion at major joints, including the spine, while maintaining as wide a base of support as possible.

It is important to bear in mind that some people find it very difficult to co-ordinate flexion in the lumbar spine with flexion in the hips and the knees, as a result of years of movement patterns in which hip and knee flexion has been associated with extension in the lumbar spine. This may result in a slightly different reaction.

Essential Point

If biomechanical efficiency during movement of the body is to be maintained, it becomes clear that the base must be mobile, as must all the joints whose movement allows the centre of gravity of the body to be lowered and kept within the base area—equally, normal length of soft tissues, muscles, tendons and their fasciae is important if normal range of movement is to be maintained. Furthermore, if the lowering of the centre of gravity is the first part of every movement, it may reduce the needless control of an unbalanced movement in which the centre of gravity is higher.

SPINAL MOBILITY

At this point, it may be worth considering the mobility of the spine in balance. Since the 1930s, research into the mechanics of the spine has indicated a predominant discogenic factor in the pathogenesis of painful conditions associated with the low back. Numerous studies have been carried out on models and *in vivo*, to discover positions which produce high intradiscal pressure and therefore possible disc damage and pain (Nachemson, 1963; Adams & Hutton, 1985; Adams *et al.*, 1987). In addition, studies have been carried out to measure myoelectric activity in trunk muscles. Evidence from these studies correlates with many model studies (Ortengren & Andersson, 1977).

Measurement of both intradiscal pressure and myoelectric activity in the spine gives a reliable indication of loads in the lumbar spine (Ortengren *et al.*, 1981). The conclusion from most of the research is that to reduce stress in the lumbar spine the load carried should be kept as close to the body as possible. Clearly, the smaller the load, the lower the potential strain on the area. Interestingly, the position of the spine, in particular during lifting, is less important than the relative position of any applied load, and it would seem that this has been the subject of some important misconceptions. Loads on the lumbar spine are applied not just as a result of manual handling but also as a result of some predominant movement patterns. This is an important point.

It may be that a predominant movement pattern in which extension of the spine is maintained while more fundamental biomechanical principles are being ignored, i.e. loads are not being kept close, with inefficient displacement of body parts, causes some of the musculoskeletal disorders which prove so difficult to diagnose and treat using other approaches.

Consider Figure 17.1 and the strain imposed on the lumbar spine and shoulder girdle area as a result of holding this posture. Also consider the number of times this posture is used during a day, often with the trunk being lowered further. Add to this the effect of using outstretched arms, and consider the loading on the lumbar spine. This may be a more subliminal loading and strain on the lumbar spine and shoulder girdle than the obvious strain imposed by handling heavy objects, but the cumulative effect may be as important. If this is the case, reconsideration of how to re-educate this movement pattern is required.

As well as investigations into the positions causing high internal forces in the lumbar spine, research has also tried to ascertain how loads applied to the motion segment are shared between each of the intervertebral discs and facet joints between adjacent vertebrae. Studies carried out on models suggest that facet joints are highly loaded when they have to resist shearing or rotational forces. Furthermore, the amount of loading on facet joints as opposed to the intervertebral disc is significantly affected by the stiffness properties of not only the disc but also the capsules of the facet joints. So, the stiffer the facet joints, the greater the load they take from the intervertebral disc. It is important, therefore, that, wherever possible, this stiffening of the facet joint capsule is prevented, since the intervertebral disc is better designed to absorb stresses than the facet joints. It follows then that movement habits should encourage movement of the facet joints, not stiffening of ligamentous tissues. Facet joint movement will also promote circulation of body fluids through periarticular structures, enabling them to keep healthy.

To summarise, it is important to consider the relation of the body to its base area of support, in terms of both static and dynamic postures. This is important whether or not a load is being carried. To facilitate maximum potential balance in static and dynamic postures, it is necessary to maintain maximal flexibility, particularly in the joints that

For a specific objective movement to occur—for example, lifting a book from a shelf at eye-level—there is co-ordination of many different muscles, all performing these different roles. To summarise, to grasp and lift the book off the shelf, there will be isotonic action of the agonists. This action will be allowed by the reciprocal relaxed lengthening of the antagonists (assuming they have normal muscle length). The bones to which the origins of the agonists are attached will be stabilised by muscles that are also attached to those bones but which also have attachments to bones not required as part of the primary movement. These muscles work isometrically. It is this stabilisation work which is responsible for the majority of energy expenditure due to muscle contraction during the course of a day.

Essential Point

The work of isometric fixator muscles is a requirement for stability. Isotonic muscle work produces mobility, while background postural stability is produced through isometric contraction of muscles acting as fixators. It is the proportion of stabilising muscle work in relation to mobilising muscle work which is at issue in cumulative strain. This proportion is dependent on both bio-mechanical factors, as described on pages 231–232, and neurophysiological factors, as outlined below.

NEUROPHYSIOLOGICAL CONSIDERATIONS

The neurophysiological control of human movement is highly complex and outside the bounds of this chapter. However, it is necessary to appreciate the importance of certain, specific mechanisms in analysing the efficiency of movement patterns in terms of postural stabilisation and cumulative strain. It could be argued that it is the success of the neuromuscular system in controlling unbalanced, inefficient movements that is a major contributor to cumulative strain.

Fundamental to this hypothesis is the role of the CNS in the control of posture, specifically in terms of determining background stabilisation from which active movements can occur. Essentially, the motor control system is influenced by a complicated sensory network which inputs information to the CNS at various levels, both cortical and subcortical. This input helps to generate an output response in the form of muscle activity, to produce either movement or stability. It is the inputs which stimulate large amounts of stabilising output. These inputs need to be minimised if cumulative strain is to be successfully reduced.

Consideration of the control of posture is a prerequisite to understanding the body's response to displacement of its centre of gravity. Such consideration has largely been omitted from traditional biomechanical analysis of movement, and it may be this lack of recognition of the effects of postural mechanisms during movement that has led to the widespread use of what may be considered inefficient movement patterns (Figure 17.2).

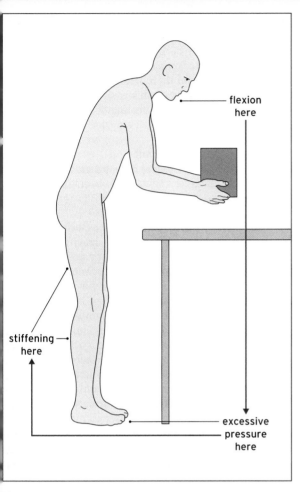

Figure 17.1 Typical posture associated with manual contact of an object.

flexion here

stiffening here

excessive pressure here

are capable of lowering the body into its base, namely, the hips, knees and spine.

KINESIOLOGICAL CONSIDERATIONS

The basic principles of the group action of muscles merits some consideration in developing an understanding of cumulative strain.

For the purpose of clarity, let us recall McClurg Anderson's definition of 'good' (hereafter termed 'efficient') movement: 'a movement which fulfils its function with the minimum of effort and the minimum of strain'.

Minimum effort refers to the type of muscle work involved in producing and regulating movements. This muscle work relies on co-ordination of muscular action. Co-ordination of muscular action relies upon reciprocity between:

- Agonistic and antagonistic muscles/groups.
- Muscles concerned with adjusting and maintaining balance throughout movement.
- Muscles which stabilise the spinal joints and the limb girdles during movement.

BALANCE IN MOVEMENT

The regulation of muscle tone for the maintenance of posture and the preparation for movement is the function of proprioception. To this end, there exists a set of postural reflexes which play an important role in the regulation of the degree and distribution of muscle tone (Sherrington, 1947). When standing upright, the weight of the body is taken largely by the bones and ligaments, with little muscle activity occurring. Sufficient muscle tone is maintained by feedback mechanisms to different parts of the CNS. Any attempt by gravity or any other force to displace the body from this position is actively resisted. This resistance results from the activation of postural reflexes initiated by proprioceptors in the eyes, ears, neck, trunk, limb muscles and feet. These reflexes are part of postural control mechanisms which are integrated in the cerebellum and brainstem to allow sustained muscle activity without fatigue. Isolated postural reflexes can rarely be demonstrated in individuals with intact nervous systems, but their influence can change the degree and distribution of tension in muscles. This is shown in the following exercise (Figure 17.3).

To appreciate those areas of the body that typically sustain the abuse human movement can inflict on some muscle groups, stand up in a space with your feet comfortably apart and your arms down by your sides. Drop your chin to your chest and keep it there. After approximately 30 seconds, and keeping your head down, lift your arms up straight in front of you to the horizontal position

and keep them there. Maintain this position for approximately 30 seconds. Start to become aware of the areas in your body which are becoming uncomfortable, or where you are conscious of tension. Maintain this position for about 30 seconds and then bend forward at the hips by about 30°. Again, maintain this position for about 30 seconds. You will experience a feeling of discomfort or tension in the:

- Feet.
- Lower leg—the gastrocnemii.
- Thighs—the quadriceps and hamstrings.
- Lower back—the erector spinae and quadratus lumborum.
- Shoulders—the trapezii and deltoids.

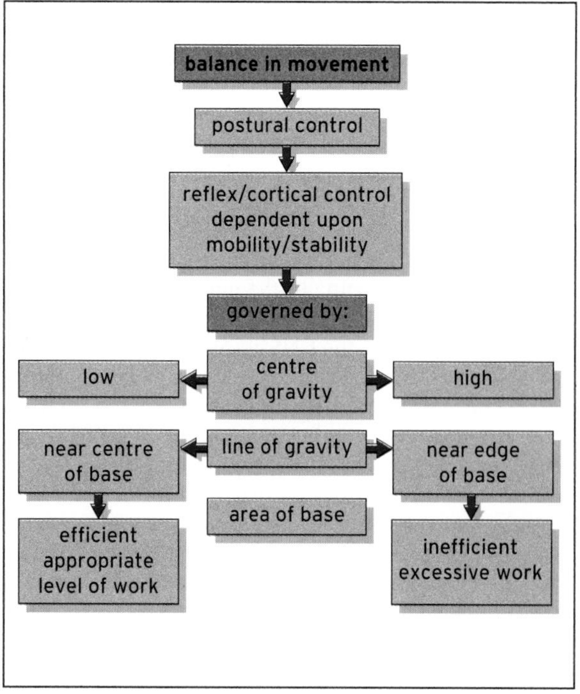

The reason for the tightening feelings experienced during the exercise is that, as the centre of gravity of the body moves forward, there is stimulation of a positive supporting reaction (a postural reflex). The stimulus for this is twofold: firstly, a proprioceptive stimulus is produced by stretch of muscles as a result of dorsiflexion of the toes and ankle; and secondly, an exteroceptive stimulus is evoked by contact of the pads of the feet on the ground. This reaction is characterised by the simultaneous contraction of flexor and extensor muscles. This is a modification of the extensor thrust spinal reflex described by Sherrington (1947). While this reaction produces a rigid limb for support, it also results in a limb that cannot contribute further to any balance reactions. Balance reactions need mobility of joints and fine postural adjustments by the muscles. Attempts at maintaining balance must therefore come from other parts of the body when this supporting reaction of the lower limbs has been stimulated.

This stiffening reaction is stimulated in everyday movements as soon as the weight of the body starts to move forward onto the pads of the toes. When one becomes aware of one's body movements, it is easy to appreciate how many everyday activities result in excessive reflex contraction of muscles. This may lead to adaptive shortening of muscles and reduce mobility of the joints over which they act. Moreover, if the insidious effect of this process extended over a period of years is considered, there may be an explanation in part for the pathogenesis of some painful musculoskeletal syndromes which affect the shoulder complex, thoracic and lumbar spine and pelvic regions.

The reflex stiffening behaviour is a specific reaction to the stimulation produced by the weight of the body moving forward over the toe pads. Similar reactions occur in other regions. The tightening around the shoulder girdle and thoracic region which may have been experienced in the exercise above, results from the stabilisation work in that area, required to maintain the arms in front of the body. The next time you wash up or stand at a sink for any length of time, think back to the exercise and imagine the position.

It may be useful to the reader to consider all the activities and types of movement used during a typical day which stimulate these reflex mechanisms, to appreciate the possible effects on joints, peri-articular structures and soft

Figure 17.2 Balance in movement. (Adapted from Crozier & Cozens, 1995.)

tissues. With this appreciation, it is possible to consider ways in which excessive stimulation of the postural fixation mechanisms can be avoided.

Essential Point

Alterations of balance within movement are essential features of the broad repertoire of complex movements unique to human movement. Reactions to any alteration in balance of the body in movement result from a complex set of interactions between the central and peripheral nervous systems. It could be argued that the effectiveness of the nervous system in allowing an individual to stabilise an unbalanced movement or posture results in a misuse of postural reactions, leading to an excessive requirement for a stability function in muscles. It may be that the excessive requirement for isometric muscle activity, signalled by the CNS in response to poor balance in movement, is incompatible with the maintenance of healthy soft tissue extensibility.

HUMAN MOVEMENT: ENVIRONMENTAL INTERACTIONS

From a synthesis of the points raised in the previous discussion, a model can be developed to explain a possible genesis for many non-specific painful musculoskeletal conditions.

When muscles are subject to excessive tension in resting, postural or active functions, their natural extensibility (contractile element) and elasticity (tendinous element) will be reduced. This is probably due to changes in the structure of fascia and connective tissue within the muscles (McClurg Anderson 1951; Goldspink et al., 1974; Goldspink & Williams, 1981). In addition, sensitivity may be altered, as well as blood and lymphatic circulation.

Over a period of time, deterioration of anatomical structures—for example, connective tissue such as muscle, fascia and ligament—results from excessive tension in different parts of the body. This frequently occurs in a cumulative subliminal manner, leading to cumulative strain in certain structures and tissues. Unfortunately, as already mentioned, cumulative strain is difficult to demonstrate in clinical and laboratory experiments. There is, however, growing evidence that structural deterioration of body tissues can result from progressive injury as a consequence of excessive tension being experienced in different parts of the body (Goldspink et al., 1974; Goldspink & Williams, 1981; Adams & Hutton, 1985; Adams et al., 1987; Pecina & Bojanic, 1993). Such deterioration results in progressive adaptive shortening of structures in response to repeated small-scale inflammatory responses within the tissues, in response to repetitive subliminal strains. Muscle and fascia adapt to their function both in length and structure.

In the context of cumulative strain, the most costly form of muscle work is that which involves sustained contraction, i.e. isometric or static muscle work. It is inefficient in terms of the utilisation of energy because sustained contraction leads to a reduction in blood flow through the muscle. This is the characteristic muscle work of postural control, and is predominant in the trunk and around the

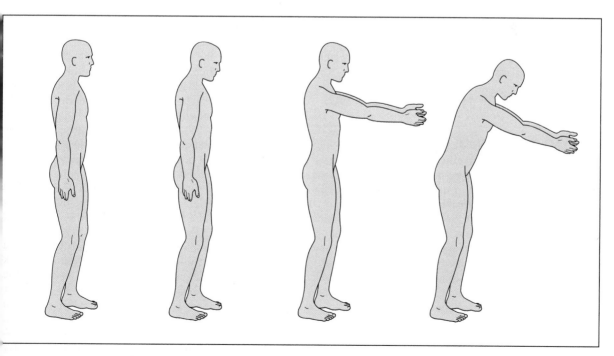

Figure 17.3 Feel the weight distribution in your feet as you progressively move your centre of gravity forward.

limb girdles in most activities of daily living. Think about tasks such as brushing teeth, filling a kettle, reaching to a cupboard, ironing, and pushing a shopping trolley around corners! Some of the muscles may be adapted for their function, i.e. they have a high proportion of slow twitch fibres, but other muscles, although more commonly associated with mobility functions, may be required to act as stabilisers, particularly in the case of top-heavy movements. Alternatively, a threshold beyond which the muscles adapted for postural fixation are prepared, is exceeded.

It seems likely that many problems associated with pain in the musculoskeletal system could be associated with movement patterns which cause cumulative strain on body structures. Painful disorders of the musculoskeletal system which develop insidiously, often with no memorable incident or injury, may result from the gradual deterioration of structures, in particular muscular, ligamentous and connective tissues, which have been subjected to insidious subliminal strain, but which, over a period of time, reach a threshold of intolerance and give rise to pain.

One of the most predominant movement patterns which is likely to be associated with the development of cumulative strain is 'top-heavy bending'. Here, movements begin with the hands, head and upper trunk moving forward. This forward movement of the upper part of the body requires the trunk and leg muscles to stabilise the lower part of the body, rather like an anchor and chain taking the strain of a boat when moored. This top-heavy movement pattern dominates many human actions at work, during recreational activities or at home.

To treat the source of many musculoskeletal problems, it is necessary to change the physical movement habits of those with the painful consequences of strain on soft tissues. It becomes necessary to consider the basic principles of what may be described as 'efficient' movement in terms of minimising the cumulative strain which results from excessive postural stabilisation.

PREVENTION OF MUSCULOSKELETAL INJURY

MINIMISING CUMULATIVE STRAIN

The essential feature of an efficient movement is its segmental nature, in which the various parts of the body come into action progressively, in the proper sequence. This helps to ensure, as far as possible, that the centre of gravity of limb and body parts remain close to the base on which they are moving. In addition, if a movement is efficient, it will facilitate the recruitment of all available forces and reduce the need for reflex postural activity to a minimum. Efficient movements in this context are movements which interact with the environment harmoniously. They are based on the following principles:

The lower the centre of gravity of an object, the greater its stability

In terms of human movement, if the centre of gravity of the body is lowered, reflex postural activity is reduced.

Moreover, the nearer the line of gravity falls to the centre of the base of support, the more balanced the movement will be. The lower the centre of gravity and the wider the base of support, the greater the chance that the line of gravity will fall near the centre of the base. This principle can be applied to movement of all body parts. In the trunk, for example, to lower the body from standing, this principle can be effected by relaxing the knees, hips and low back into flexion.

The greater the area of the base of an object, the greater its stability

Again, in terms of human movement, the base from which movement occurs needs to be wide to ensure maximum stability. This is difficult, as the base is likely to be part of that movement. If a foot is moved in the direction of intended movement, or in the direction to which the body is tending to fall, reflex postural activity will be reduced. Turning of a foot in this manner, is associated with rotation at the hips, and this is likely to reduce or prevent unwanted rotation in the spine. If the two principles mentioned above are combined, this allows the development of a dynamically stable efficient movement. In other words, a moving body requires a mobile base to maintain stability. This is essential. It is the inability to adjust the base as part of a movement which leads to evasive actions elsewhere in the body. Evasive actions are likely to lead to strain or injury.

The closer a load is applied to the fulcrum of the lever, the less effort required to balance it

In human movement, any part of the body or limb which is above, in front or behind its centre of gravity, constitutes a load. In addition, there are external loads (however large or small), which are usually taken by the hands. The fulcrum may be at the wrist or elbow. In either case, if the load is kept as near to the centre of gravity as possible, less effort is needed to balance displacement of the load. In the case of loads taken in the hand, if they are kept in the hand or forearm, as near to the fulcrum as possible, it is likely that the use of gripping actions will be minimised. Intense gripping actions require substantial stabilising muscle work and should be avoided where possible. Reaching beyond the object to be moved with outstretched fingers, applies a stretch to the palmar fascia, which then recoils. The combination of these actions tends to discourage overgripping and encourage the load to fall nearer the palm of the hand rather than the fingers.

A further example of this point lies in analysis of reaching actions. In any reaching action, movement should begin at the shoulder girdle with an initial elevation. This is followed by extension of the elbow and flexion of the shoulder joint, then relaxation of the shoulder girdle. The muscles which would otherwise fix the shoulder girdle become part of the movement, and the action progresses segmentally in a distal direction. Theoretically, this should minimise the need for stabilising muscle activity in the upper trunk and shoulder girdle.

APPLICATION OF PRINCIPLES IN LOWERING AND RAISING THE BODY

All basic actions in human movement requiring a change in body posture, involve an element of lowering and raising the body's mass. To effect a lowering of the body's mass within its base of support, it should be lowered segmentally, starting with the body parts closest to the base. The lowering phase should therefore be initiated by a 'relaxation' of the knees and hips. In continuing this relaxation, gravity would tend to effect a 'relaxation' in the trunk, i.e. flexion in the lumbar spine and increased flexion in the thoracic spine, while the cervical spine increases its lordosis. This is exemplified by the effect of gravity producing a kyphosis over 70–80 years, manifest in many elderly people. This position of 'collapse' is also compatible with fulfilling the requirements of maintained balance on the basis of the principles outlined above.

The 'effort' phase, or raising of the body's mass, should be initiated by gentle movement of the head, so that the cervical, thoracic and lumbar segments become elongated in that order, restoring themselves to their neutral position within the base of support. Raising and lowering the body in this way enhances balance in movement and may help to maintain mobility in the spine (Figure 17.4).

To reinforce these ideas, the following demonstrates the compromise between mobility and stability in the musculoskeletal system. For the two movement examples given, consider the effects of cumulative strain when lowering and raising the body in movement (Figure 17.5 A and B).

Analysis of the basic movement pattern of the trunk, involved in lowering and raising the body, helps to demonstrate points raised in the previous sections. There is considerably more stabilising muscle work involved in lowering the body in the manner identified in Figure 17.5A, which is predominant in much human movement, i.e. the straight leg, stoop forward method, than muscular effort which produces movement. Because of the movement of the body weight forward in relation to the base, with no lowering of large parts of the body, i.e. flexion of the lower limbs, the primary requirement is that of stability to prevent overbalancing of the increasingly unstable body. In Figure 17.5B, lowering is initiated by relaxation of the knees, hips and spine to allow segmental 'collapse' into the base of support.

Analysis of movement in Figure 17.5A is given in Table 17.1. Note which muscles fulfil the roles of mobility and, in particular, stability. Many of the muscles providing stability would not be considered primarily as stabiliser muscles anatomically, e.g. the hamstrings, rectus femoris, gastrocnemius, tibialis posterior, tibialis anterior, and so on. All these muscles are long muscles with tendinous insertions required for primary mobilising actions during gait and propulsive actions.

A question arises. If these muscles are required to work excessively in a fixator role, does this compromise their ability to work optimally when required as mobilisers? It has been established that there is a training effect on muscles as a result of their activity, and that this can lead to recruitment changes and the selectivity of muscle fibre recruitment

(Goldspink & Williams, 1981). It may be argued that this is unlikely except perhaps in elite athletes in whom such compromises may inhibit optimal performance. However, if conflict between mobility and stability occurs over a sustained period, there may be a more subliminal effect which may be a major contributor to cumulative strain. Furthermore, does the overuse of mobiliser muscles as fixators impact upon those more associated with stabilisation, e.g. erector spinae?

It seems sensible to consider whether such a simple movement can be modified to reduce the potential conflict and to reduce the need for stability throughout the movement in so many joints.

Such an adjustment was advocated by McClurg Anderson in his movement training programmes in the 1940s and 1950s, and later by Vasey and Crozier (1982b). This adjustment suggests that the pattern of movement described below may be more efficient in terms of the stabilising muscle work required to lower the body.

The aim is to produce a movement pattern which is segmental in character, in which different parts of the body come into action successively so that gravity can assist movement while also minimising the need for stabilisation. To achieve this, the mechanical and physiological principles outlined here must be applied, the result being that joints maintained in the positions detailed in Table 17.1 should become part of the lowering and raising movement to prevent them being static.

The resulting basic movement pattern for lowering the body then becomes:
- Movement which begins near the base.
- Gentle relaxation and unlocking of the knees.
- Relaxation and flexion of the hips, and, sequentially, posterior rotation of the pelvis with associated flexion in the lumbar spine, while simultaneously widening the base in the direction of intended movement, usually with the toe of the front leg pointing in that direction.
- Relaxation, depression and protraction of the shoulder girdle together with movement of the head.

The manner in which the shoulders and upper limbs move depends on the objective of the movement. The key difference, however, between a top-heavy movement and a movement led by the base as described here, is that in the former movement, the initial bending action causes an increased concentration of pressure on the toes, thereby stimulating a postural reaction which leads to the stabilising work identified in Figure 17.5A. In a 'base' movement, the weight is taken down through the centre of the base as a result of unlocking the knees and hips in the right sequence.

Upward movement from this lowered position is initiated by the head in a lock action, and, segmentally, the shoulders, upper trunk, hips and knees return the body to its original position.

Figure 17.4 shows the influence of head position on trunk posture and therefore on the spinal ligaments and musculature. It also shows the position of the head which initiates good upward movement from a lowered position.

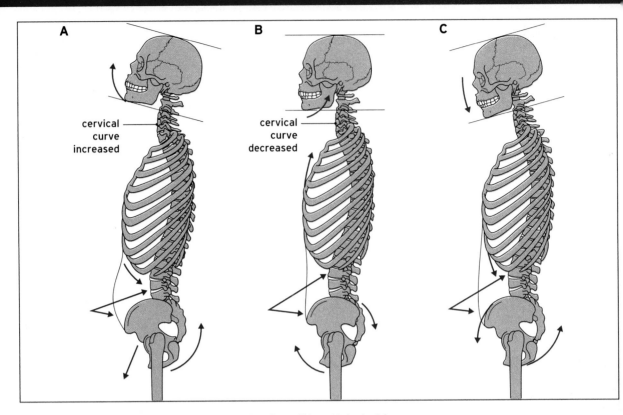

Figure 17.4 Influence of head position on trunk position. (Adapted from
McClurg Anderson, 1951.)

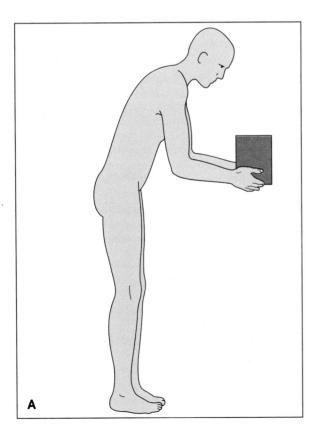

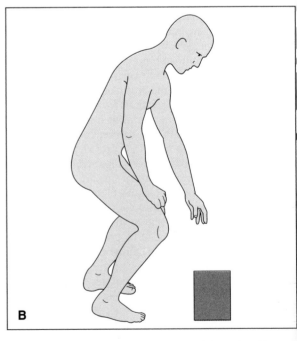

**Figure 17.5 A and B Two methods of lowering the
body to handle an object.**

REQUIREMENT FOR CONDITIONING IN MOVEMENT HABITS

Inherent in any approach to movement rehabilitation, i.e. where there is a need to change habitual movement patterns, is the preparation of the patient for change. To do this, thorough assessment of movement habits is required. Subsequent to this analysis, the patient is prepared for the change by 'conditioning' areas of the body using techniques that have three main objectives: firstly, to stretch soft tissues which adaptively shorten as a result of inefficient movement patterns; secondly, to increase sensory awareness of areas of the body which are most subject to misuse resulting from overstimulation of postural reflexes; and thirdly, as a result of increased sensory awareness, to prepare the patient for the employing of a new movement pattern.

It is important to attempt to counteract the effects of cumulative strain before attempting to alter movement patterns and habits. Change in movement habits may help to maintain a healthier state for the joints and soft tissues, but only once normal tissue extensibility has been restored.

Failure to recognise the need to prepare the patient for movement pattern rehabilitation in this way may merely contribute further to their problems. It is rather like encouraging a baby to walk before it has mastered control of its reflexes, resulting in a stiff, inefficient and unbalanced walking pattern. Crozier and Cozens (1995) suggest that the central core of their neuromuscular approach is the conditioning programme. This programme consists of both specific conditioning and patterning movements.

STRETCHING PROGRAMME

Initially, the main purpose of a stretching programme as part of a conditioning process to prepare for change, is to counteract the effects of cumulative strain. Look back at Figure 17.3 and consider the muscle groups which developed tension during the exercise. The muscles identified

Muscle analysis of movement		
Movement	**Muscles/structures involved**	**Primary function**
Flexion of the cervical spine	Initiated by sternocleidomastoid and the scaleni	Mobility
	Erector spinae working eccentrically to control against gravity (spinalis cervicis)	Mobility
	Erector spinae to maintain position	Stability, as centre of gravity falls in front of lordosis
Flexion of the thoracic and lumbar spines	Initiated by the abdominals	Mobility
	Erector spinae working eccentrically to control against gravity	Mobility
	Erector spinae to maintain position	Stability as centre of gravity anterior to lumbar spine
Flexion of the hips	Iliopsoas to initiate movement	Mobility
	Gluteus maximus and hamstrings working eccentrically to control against gravity	Mobility
	Gluteal muscles and hamstrings to maintain position	Stability as centre of gravity anterior to the hip joint
Extension of the knees	Quadriceps femoris maintaining position of knees	Stability
Dorsiflexion of ankle	Probably occurs as body weight moves forward, controlled by eccentric activity in the posterior crural muscles then maintained by interplay between anterior and posterior crural muscles	Stability
Pronation of the subtalar joint	Occurs as a result of body weight moving forward, controlled by interplay between tibialis anterior and posterior and the peroneii	Stability
Extension of the toes	Occurs as body weight moves forward, lumbricals prevent buckling of toes and interossei help to maintain balance together with interplay between the long toe flexors and extensors	Stability

Table 17.1 Muscle analysis of movement.

here are also included in a group of muscles identified by Janda (1983), which are commonly found to be shortened; these are listed below. Perhaps there is an indication here of a reason why adaptations in muscle length occur in certain muscle groups.

Those muscles most commonly found to be shortened anteriorly include the:
• Pectoralis major.
• Finger flexors of the hand.
• Iliopsoas.
• Adductors of the thigh.
• Rectus femoris.
• Tensor fasciae latae.
• Gastrocnemius and soleus.

Those muscles most commonly found to be shortened posteriorly include the:
• Levator scapulae.
• Upper part of the trapezius.
• Erector spinae.
• Quadratus lumborum.
• Piriformis.
• Hamstrings.

Stretching movements which will be effective in counteracting the effects of cumulative strain must therefore be specific in character and directed at these target muscle groups.

The body has a natural tendency to indicate to itself the type of stretch required. For example, after sitting in front of a computer screen for some time, it is instinctive in many people to extend the arms, chin and chest backwards over the back of the chair. This should form the basis of corrective stretching, as it is a movement which stretches the anterior musculature which is prone to shorten (see exercise above).

As well as considering the anatomical sites of the soft tissues which tend to become adaptively shortened, it is important to consider how these muscles become subject to cumulative strain. Normal movements, and particularly those associated with top-heavy patterns, produce increasing stiffness of the muscles attaching the limbs to the girdles and spine, as these are the muscles which constantly stabilise the bases of the limbs.

Specific stretching programmes to counteract the effects of cumulative strain need to stretch muscles to increase their elastic components, and this must be done slowly. It is also essential to consider the need to stretch fascial connective tissue, and therefore the best method with which to effect this stretch.

UPPER LIMB STRETCH

Try the following exercise (Figure 17.6). Sit comfortably with the arms free to move. Raise the point of your shoulder as high as possible. Slowly bring the hand up in front of the shoulder with palm inwards. Move the shoulder backwards (and feel it naturally becoming depressed) while extending the elbow, wrist and fingers. For a second, very gently squeeze the shoulder and hand away from the body, raise the chin, and slowly press the chest upwards and forwards. Relax and allow the limb to return to its resting position. Try the exercise bilaterally.

As you perform this exercise (Figure 17.6), feel the comfortable stretch on the anterior musculature. Note the inclusion of the shoulder girdle in the movement, which prevents the trapezeii acting as stabilisers. This is a fundamental fault in many stretching programmes for the upper limbs.

This exercise can be repeated in different ranges of abduction/elevation to stretch different components of the anterior musculature. Note that the stretch position

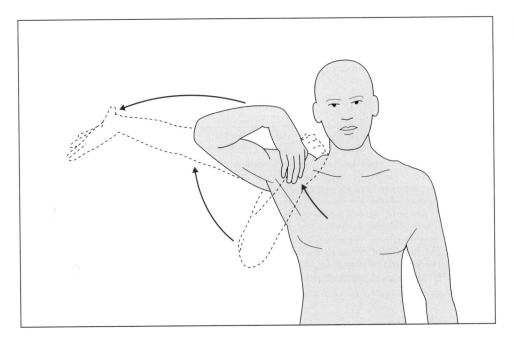

Figure 17.6 Upper limb stretch.

is similar to the upper limb Tension Test 2 advocated by Butler (1991) for neural tension of the median nerve.

As with all stretching programmes, movements such as this need to be conducted approximately 4–5 times consecutively, with normal breathing control. The tendency to hold the breath while performing stretching movements, particularly in the upper limbs, counteracts their effect, as some of the muscles being elongated will be signalled to work to raise the shoulder girdle. Clearly, this is in conflict with the objective of stretching them, and tends to aggravate cumulative strain in the neck, shoulders and upper chest.

The example given is just one, but note how it complies with the principles of efficient movements described on page 233. This exercise may be useful to reinforce the principles of movements of the upper limb generally.

In lying, the same principle applied to the stretching movement—i.e. moving the proximal parts first, easing the hip and knee away from the trunk, stretching the distal parts last, with the ankle moving into dorsiflexion to stretch the calf—allows a good stretch to be induced in the whole of the lower limb. In the case of individual muscles which are more extremely shortened, more specific stretching exercises can be used, but total limb stretches should always be used in addition, as fascial stretch is essential if elasticity is to be facilitated. The fascial arrangements in the limbs require full limb movements to induce stretch on these tissues.

MOVEMENT PATTERN CHANGE

In an attempt to demonstrate the logic of the neuromusculoskeletal environmental interactions concept, the basic movement pattern in the trunk should be considered in the context of back pain.

The segmental nature of the 'efficient' movement described above is its key to reduce inappropriate stabilising muscle work. Yet even when the spine is mobile, it requires some guiding stability as it moves segmentally. Lumbar segmental stability has received much attention recently (Jull et al., 1993; Jull & Richardson, 1994; Richardson et al., 1995). Lumbar segmental stability is provided by osseous, ligamentous and muscular structures, but it is the muscles of the local system, with their direct attachments to the lumbar vertebrae, that have the greatest capacity to affect segmental stiffness (Crisco & Panjabi, 1990). Muscle control in this area is therefore of considerable importance in determining appropriate segmental movement. It seems that both the multifidus and the transversus abdominis muscles are important in this regard (Richardson & Jull, 1996).

Dysfunction of the transversus abdominis muscle has been demonstrated in patients with low back pain by the use of electromyelographic experiments (Hodges & Richardson, 1995). This has led to the development of a rehabilitation concept which focuses on active stabilisation of the lumbar spine by reversing the dysfunction of the multifidus and transversus abdominis muscles (Richardson & Jull, 1996).

At a later stage in the rehabilitation of the trunk musculature, using this concept, it is suggested that isometric exercise for the deep lumbar muscles can be combined with dynamic functional exercise.

It would seem that McClurg Anderson's ideas about the importance of segmental mobility in functional movement, and the ideas put forward by Jull & Richardson regarding lumbar segmental stability, may be mutually useful in considering a prevention and rehabilitation strategy for low back pain. Firstly, there is a need to ensure that local muscle control is appropriate. Jull & Richardson advocate a specific exercise programme to facilitate control in identified dysfunctioning muscles (Richardson & Jull, 1996). This, they suggest, should be combined with dynamic functional exercise (which they do not describe).

However, it seems sensible to stress the importance of a regimen of movement exercises to facilitate appropriate control of muscles in the lumbar region. Such a programme of conditioning stretches should satisfy several needs, namely, to:

- Restore normal length to adaptively shortened muscles and fasciae.
- Ensure an awareness of movement through the sensory system, as well as developing direct muscle control.
- Facilitate and condition particular movements in preparation for the re-education of functional movements which are advocated as more efficient in reducing cumulative strain. In particular, sensory awareness and good control of pelvic tilt is essential.
- Further develop sensory awareness to encourage change in the basic pattern of movement used in lowering and raising actions.
- Apply basic actions to change the basic movement pattern in the trunk, fundamental in human movement, e.g. sitting to standing, standing to sitting, pushing, pulling, lifting, and so on.

Jull & Richardson's concept was developed scientifically, and the ideas of McClurg Anderson were developed more anecdotally, yet both concepts have much in common. Perhaps the strength of the neuromusculoskeletal environmental interactions concept is its vision of the overall problem in human movement, namely, the tendency to misuse the postural reflex system with the result that muscle imbalances occur.

And so, in the prevention and treatment of back pain, and movement analysis and re-education, using the principles of the neuromusculoskeletal environmental interactions concept seems to be compatible with the conceptual basis of the muscle imbalance theorists, and, as such, merits academic attention. Its value is strengthened by virtue of the fact that it is a means of educating patients about the biomechanical, kinesiological and neurophysiological basis of movement in relation to its objectives, and as such is a patient-centred approach. Its essence can be taught at varying levels of depth and breadth, and it is therefore potentially useful for all patients irrespective of intellectual capability.

The principles of the neuromusculoskeletal environmental interactions concept, in terms of movement analysis and re-education, can also be applied to any painful area of the body. A simple consideration of biomechanics, kinesiology and neurophysiological principles, and how they impact on the resulting group action of muscles, allows the clinician to consider whether a predominant movement pattern may contribute to cumulative strain. This allows for modification, following a stretching regimen and movement pattern change as described.

CONCLUSION

The role of muscles in the genesis of some musculoskeletal disorders has received increasing attention in recent years. This signifies a healthy return to a wider assessment of the origin of pain in the neuromusculoskeletal system, after decades in which many physiotherapists paid excessive attention to an arthrogenic and discogenic view. Some musculoskeletal disorders are of course solely evident in muscular, tendinous and ligamentous tissues.

This chapter outlines a specific approach to the prevention of, and therapeutic intervention in, painful disorders of the musculoskeletal system, which has evolved over many years. It is founded on the work of McClurg Anderson (1951), and integrates knowledge of how muscles react to the displacement of the centre of gravity of the body (and its parts) and how they are subject to control by the CNS. It is called the neuromusculoskeletal environmental interactions concept.

This concept advocates a wider approach to the causation, prevention and rehabilitation of some musculoskeletal disorders, which may lead to a better fundamental understanding. The roles of movement patterns and muscular overuse in the development of cumulative microtrauma are suggested as a mechanism by which adaptive shortening in muscles may occur. It seems likely that changes in muscle function play an important role in the development of many painful disorders of the musculoskeletal system. It is held that the assessment and analysis of disorders of the musculoskeletal system, drawing upon knowledge of the interactions between the human body and its environment, is essential to build a complete picture of causal factors. The same knowledge leads to clinical management decisions about prevention, treatment and rehabilitation strategies. It is important that this knowledge is used to develop rehabilitation strategies. So often, assessment of movement patterns is neglected, resulting in the re-education element being missing, so that full rehabilitation of the patient is incomplete. The basic therapeutic approach to musculoskeletal disorders should begin with a thorough analysis of movement patterns; then, with the information gained, more efficient patterns of movement developed in the context of the patient's interaction with an environment which includes gravity. This is the essence.

The ideas contained within this neuromusculoskeletal environmental interactions concept need more scientific appraisal in relation to each musculoskeletal disorder. Further scrutiny of these ideas will result in better rehabilitation strategies in the prevention and treatment of disorders of the musculoskeletal system. The concept has implications for orthopaedic and medico-legal practice.

ACKNOWLEDGEMENTS

I would like to thank Emeritus Professor RG Burwell, The Centre for Spinal Studies and Surgery, and Department of Human Morphology, Queens Medical Centre, Nottingham, UK, whose advice and commentary on this text have been invaluable and Marie Donaghy, senior lecturer, Queen Margaret College, Edinburgh, UK, for her encouragement and for providing me with copies of much of Tom McClurg Anderson's original work.

REFERENCES

Adams M, Hutton W. Gradual disc prolapse. *Spine* 1985, **10**:524-531.

Adams M, Dolan P, Hutton W. Diurnal variations in the stresses on the lumbar spine. *Spine* 1987, **12**:130-137.

Butler DS. *Mobilisation of the nervous system.* Churchill Livingstone; 1991:153-156.

Crisco JJ, Panjabi MM. Postural biomechanical stability and gross muscular architecture in the spine. In: Winters JM, Woo SL-Y, eds. *Multiple muscle systems.* New York: Springer Verlag; 1990:438-450.

Crozier L, Cozens S. *Efficient handling and moving: a neuromuscular approach.* Moves Education Services: Basic course notes; 1995.

Goldspink G, Tabary JC, Tabary C, Tardieu C, Tardieu G. Effect of denervation on the adaptation of sarcomere number and extensibility to the functional length of the muscle. *J Physiol* 1974, **236**:733-742.

Goldspink G, Williams PE. Development and growth of muscle. In: Gubba F, Marechall G, Takaes O, eds. *Mechanisms of muscle adaptation to functional requirements. Advances in Physiological Sciences.* Oxford: Pergamon; 1981:87-98.

Hodges PW, Richardson CA. *Neuromotor dysfunction of the trunk musculature in low back pain patients.* Washington: Proceedings of the World Confederation of Physical Therapy Congress; 1995.

Jull GA, Richardson CA. Rehabilitation of active stabilisation of the lumbar spine. In: Twomey LT, Taylor JR, eds. *Physical therapy of the lumbar spine,* 2nd ed. Edinburgh: Churchill Livingstone; 1994:251-283.

Jull G, Richardson C, Toppenburg R, Comerford M, Bui B. Towards a measurement of active muscle control for lumbar stabilisation *Aust J Physiother* 1993, **39**:187-193.

McClurg Anderson T. *Human kinetics and analysing body movements.* London: Heinemann; 1951.

McClurg Anderson T. Human kinetics and good movement. *Physiotherapy* 1971, **57**:169-176.

Nachemson A. The influence of spinal movements on the lumbar intradiscal pressure and on the tensile stresses in the annulus fibrosus. *Acta Orthop Scand* 1963, **33**:183-207.

Ortengren R, Andersson GBJ. Electromyographic studies of trunk muscles with special reference to the lumbar spine. *Spine* 1977, **2**:44-52.

Pecina MM, Bojanic I. *Overuse injuries of the musculoskeletal system.* CRC Press; 1993.

Pitt-Brooke JCL. The relation of movement patterns to muscle length and strength in health and dysfunction: the case for a wider approach to musculoskeletal disorders. *Clin Anat* 1995, **8**:152.

Richardson CA, Jull GA. Muscle control—pain control? What exercises would you prescribe? *Man Ther* 1996, **1**:2-10.

Richardson CA, Jull GA, Richardson BA. *A dysfunction of the deep abdominal muscles exists in low back pain patients.* Washington: Proceedings of the World Confederation for Physical Therapy Congress; 1995.

Sherrington C. *The integrative action of the nervous system.* Cambridge: Cambridge University Press; 1947.

Stubbs DA, Baty D, Buckle PW, *et al. Report: back pain in nurses. Summary and recommendations.* University of Surrey: Robens Institute; 1986.

Vasey J, Crozier L. A move in the right direction. *Nursing Mirror* April 28, 1982a:42-47.

Vasey J, Crozier L. Get into condition. *Nursing Mirror* May 5, 1982b:22-28.

Vasey J, Crozier L. At ease. *Nursing Mirror* May 12, 1982c:28-31.

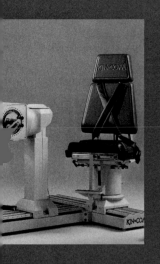

18 K Jones

ISOKINETIC DYNAMOMETRY

CHAPTER OUTLINE

- The isokinetic dynamometer
- Principle of isokinetic systems
- Modes of operation in the isokinetic dynamometer
- Programme facilities of the dynamometer
- Sources of error in isokinetic dynamometry

- Disadvantages of isokinetic exercise
- Advantages of isokinetic exercise
- Evaluation parameters
- Uses of isokinetic dynamometry in the clinical setting

INTRODUCTION

Isokinetic dynamometry, originally described by Hislop & Perrine (1967), is a relatively recent tool used in rehabilitation. Although comparatively expensive, a number of dynamometers are being purchased for research and treatment purposes, and many are being installed in physiotherapy departments in both the academic and clinical environments.

Originally patented by Cybex (Ronkonkoma, New York) in 1962, there are now several other dynamometers available, such as the Kin-Com AP (Chattanooga Group, Hixon, TN), Lido and Biodex, all of which enable the measurement of static and dynamic muscle strength.

The dynamometer is capable of providing objective and quantifiable strength data in static (isometric) situations, and it also has the advantage of providing similar information for dynamic muscle contraction.

The early dynamometers were known as passive systems, i.e. they were only capable of measuring the torque or force generated during a concentric (shortening) and an isometric (static) contraction. Active systems are more recent, and although they can still operate passively, they are now able to quantify eccentric muscle contraction. This ability has since focused much attention on the investigation of delayed onset of muscle soreness.

THE ISOKINETIC DYNAMOMETER

The Kin-Com AP (Figure 18.1) is a typical example of an isokinetic dynamometer. It consists of a chair and dynamometer which are both capable of rotating about 360° in the transverse plane. Additionally, the dynamometer of the Kin-Com is also able to rotate vertically. This latter feature enables the patient to be positioned in a number of ways. For example, it is possible, with practice, to set the patient up to allow exercise of the shoulder joint complex in one of the two functional diagonal patterns of movement, namely that of flexion, abduction and lateral rotation (Voss *et al.*, 1985).

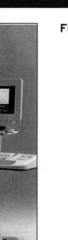

Figure 18.1 Kin-Com AP.

PRINCIPLE OF ISOKINETIC SYSTEMS

The same design principle is common to all dynamometers. Each consists of a fixed axis with a rotating lever arm attached to a moveable head (Figure 18.2).

The lever arm is driven either hydraulically or electrically, and accommodates the movement generated by the patient contracting muscles in such a way that the distal limb segment moves through the joint range at a constant angular velocity. However, this does not take place until the patient's limb exceeds the preset angular velocity which has been programmed into the machine by the physiotherapist.

MODES OF OPERATION IN THE ISOKINETIC DYNAMOMETER

Modern machines are capable of testing and exercising muscles in a wide range of exercise modes: passive, isometric, isotonic and isokinetic. These can be combined to provide a tailor-made exercise regimen to suit the individual.

PASSIVE MODE

When operating in the passive mode, the velocity remains constant and no voluntary force is required by the patient to initiate the movement. It is a useful mode in which to start to familiarise the patient with the machine. The motion obtained in this mode can be likened to that achieved using a continuous passive motion (CPM) machine to maintain postoperative range of movement after, for example, a total knee replacement. Additionally, it is a useful mode to begin motor relearning, as required, for example, after an anterior cruciate ligament repair. When progression is necessary, active assisted movement can be incorporated into the passive mode.

ISOMETRIC MODE

During isometric exercise, the muscle contracts without shortening or lengthening. As the force of contraction increases, there is an increase in the tension generated by the muscle, but there is no change in muscle length and there is no visible joint movement. Isometric exercise is also called 'static' exercise.

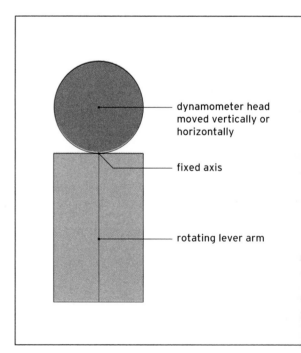

dynamometer head moved vertically or horizontally

fixed axis

rotating lever arm

Figure 18.2 Diagrammatic representation of a dynamometer.

The isometric mode on the dynamometer allows the physiotherapist to programme a series of isometric hold angles throughout the patient's available range of motion. For example, the quadriceps muscle may be weak towards the inner range. Strength here is essential for a normal gait. It may also be weak at 90° of knee flexion. Strength here is important to assist with rising from sitting. These two areas of weakness may be improved using one programme specifically designed for the patient.

The physiotherapist is able to train the quadriceps at these specific angles by presetting these as hold angles before starting the exercise. The machine passively moves the patient's limb to the first preset angle (90°) of knee flexion and instructs the patient, via a screen prompt, to contract the quadriceps isometrically for a predetermined time, e.g. 5 seconds. The machine then instructs the patient to relax, and the limb is allowed to reposition or is moved passively to the next hold angle in inner range and the process repeated.

ISOKINETIC MODE

The concept of isokinetic exercise involves training or testing muscle strength under conditions of constant angular velocity. The isokinetic dynamometer can be programmed to fix the speed of movement of the exercising muscle throughout its exercising range of movement. In this mode, the angular velocity of the lever arm will remain constant, unlike during isotonic exercise, where it is variable and controlled by the patient (see below). The external load applied to the moving segment remains consistent with the maximum capacity of the muscle throughout the range of either concentric or eccentric contraction.

ISOTONIC MODE

The term 'isotonic' (iso = same, tonic = tension) is somewhat of a misnomer, and is therefore best regarded only as a 'working definition', because muscle tension never remains constant throughout range as implied.

During functional activity, the tension varies as the muscle alters its length through the available range, and the muscle develops its maximum tension at only one point in range. This point is usually identified in the habitual functional range for that specific muscle. Most muscles tend to develop maximal tension when approaching mid to inner range, since it is in this range that they tend to function in normal daily activities.

During the isotonic mode on the dynamometer, the patient selects the exercise velocity and thus it may vary across the range. The muscle tension may also vary through the available joint range and will be weakest at the extremes of range and greatest in mid range.

PROGRAMME FACILITIES OF THE DYNAMOMETER

In addition to providing the contraction modes described above, dynamometers allow the physiotherapist to select several other parameters such as the velocity at which the exercise should take place, the range of movement in which it should be performed, the number of repetitions required, and the moment/force threshold values and damp setting. The important ones are described below.

VELOCITY

The exercise velocity is measured in degrees per second. Current dynamometer velocities range from 1° to 500° per second. Although a velocity of 300° per second seems very fast when exercising on a dynamometer, it is in fact much slower than the velocities generated in many sporting events. For example, velocities of 6180° per second have been recorded in top-flight baseball pitchers (Perrin, 1993). Also, an isokinetic velocity is not functionally normal, since no muscle contracts through range at constant velocity; rather, it varies according to the task in hand. For example, when reaching to pick up a glass, the triceps extends the elbow initially relatively quickly before the biceps provides the braking force as the glass is approached.

Angular velocities on current machines are classified into three categories: slow (1° to 60° per second), intermediate (60° to 240° per second) and fast (over 240° per second). The most usual clinical testing and training velocities range between 30° and 240° per second.

Force generation at these different velocities varies substantially. In a concentric contraction, greatest force is generated at the slowest angular velocities, and least force at the fastest velocities. But this pattern is not repeatable for an eccentric contraction, where force generation in the lower limb has been shown to decrease, increase or remain constant (Cress et al., 1992) when the velocity is increased.

RANGE OF MOVEMENT

The exercising range of movement can be controlled by programming the desired start and stop angles into the dynamometer computer. Mechanical stops positioned slightly beyond these programmed values are also an additional safety feature on some machines. All systems, however, do have a patient-controlled cut-out switch which can be operated immediately should the software control mechanism fail or the patient for some other reason, perhaps because of pain, need to stop exercising.

EXERCISE REPETITION

The number of repetitions can easily be programmed to suit individual requirements. For example, it is possible to design an exercise programme which consists of five isometric holds, each performed at a different joint angle, followed by a full-range isokinetic contraction repeated concentrically and then eccentrically three times; the whole sequence then being repeated after a short rest.

MOMENT/FORCE THRESHOLD VALUES

All dynamometers have torque limits, i.e. the maximum amount of resistance that they can provide. If exceeded, an error message and/or alarm is activated.

SOURCES OF ERROR IN ISOKINETIC DYNAMOMETRY

Three main sources of error which lead to inaccurate information are reported within the literature and summarised as:
- Failure to take into account the effect of gravity which may assist or resist limb motion (Winter *et al.*, 1981).
- Torque overshoot.
- Malalignment of the biological and mechanical axes, and failure to stabilise the patient on the dynamometer to ensure localisation of the movement to the joint undergoing testing or treatment.

CORRECTING FOR GRAVITY

The gravitational effect on limb movement should be noted, especially when performing an isokinetic evaluation (Winter *et al.*, 1981).

Obviously, movements which are tested in the horizontal plane counterbalance gravity and therefore there will be no gravitational error. However, in movements in the coronal or sagittal plane, the limb and dynamometer are either resisted or assisted by the force of gravity. Torque measurements tend to be overestimated in muscles assisted, and underestimated if opposed by gravity (Perrin *et al.*, 1992).

Modern dynamometers provide an in-built software option which enables correction of gravitational errors.

TORQUE OVERSHOOT

Torque overshoot is a phenomenon which occurs in all dynamometers. When a patient starts to perform an exercise against a preset load, there is a tendency for a greater effort to be produced than that required. This causes an initial excessive acceleration of the limb segment above the preset velocity. To counteract this, the dynamometer attempts to introduce a deceleration force. The result is a sudden peak in the torque readings in the first few hundredths of a second at the onset of the movement. This is known as torque overshoot.

Damping of the signal and damping of the resistance have been incorporated in dynamometers to minimise the effects of torque overshoot. Damping of the signal effectively omits the first few hundredths of a second of the torque data. Damping of the resistance involves the gradual introduction of a breaking force until the preset isokinetic velocity is reached. 'Ramping' is the time taken for this breaking force to occur.

Several disadvantages are associated with damping. These disadvantages, summarised by Jones & Barker (1996), are that:
- The measurement of angle-specific torque is confounded by the damp setting, as the accuracy is dependent upon the amount of the damp setting.
- Damping may eliminate some aspects of the torque signal.
- Changes in the analogue scale due to damping are not known and are therefore unquantifiable.

Preload is a system similar to damping and is available on certain machines. A preload allows the limb to be pre-accelerated to its terminal isokinetic velocity and is introduced before active movement of the limb segment occurs (Jensen *et al.*, 1991).

The effects of damping and preload in the clinical context have yet to be evaluated.

DISADVANTAGES OF ISOKINETIC EXERCISE

The disadvantages of isokinetic exercise are that:
- Learning to use the dynamometer takes time. Ideally, a member of staff should be assigned to use it regularly so that expertise is developed. However, unless in a specialist rehabilitation clinic, this would be considered a luxury. Dynamometers are also relatively expensive for the average physiotherapy departmental budget.
- The isokinetic mode involves segment movement occurring at a constant angular velocity, but normal functional movement does not take place at such fixed velocities (Dvir, 1991).
- Malalignment of the biological and mechanical axes of rotation will not produce a true reflection of muscle performance (Rothstein *et al.*, 1987). This is compounded when complex joints are involved. For example, if it is assumed that a typical isometric quadriceps contraction produces 30 newtons (N), then a 2 cm error in alignment will produce an 8% difference in muscle performance, as demonstrated by the simple calculation:

$$30 \text{ N at } 25 \text{ cm} = 7.5 \text{ Nm},$$
$$\text{but } 30 \text{ N at } 23 \text{ cm} = 6.9 \text{ Nm},$$
$$\text{therefore the error} = 0.6 \text{ Nm} = 8\%.$$

- Testing of a maximal voluntary contraction (MVC) in continuous mode can result in artificially high concentric curves immediately after an eccentric contraction. This is because elastic energy is stored during the eccentric phase and released at the start of the concentric phase. The eccentric contraction is in effect providing a facilitatory stretch for the concentric contraction via the stretch reflex mechanism.

ADVANTAGES OF ISOKINETIC EXERCISE

Isokinetic dynamometry:
- Is safe to use because during concentric exercise it applies no extra load to the limb, and any resistance encountered by the musculature is a function of the force applied by the patient to the apparatus (Newton's third law).
- Provides an objective and quantifiable measure of concentric, eccentric and static muscle strength.
- Allows multiple training capabilities through its isokinetic, passive, isometric and isotonic modes.
- Provides efficient loading of muscles and joints through range, thus minimising potential for injury.
- Provides a method of assessing strength which is not limited to the weakest point in the range. The resistance accommodates to the muscle strength through range.
- Enables isokinetic exercise to be performed. This does not require the same degree of skill and co-ordination to

stabilise a free weight as does isotonic exercise. Consequently, it may reduce the risk of muscle and joint strain which can result from efforts to control a weight in an 'open', i.e. unconstrained, environment as is the case in isotonic exercise (Osternig, 1986).

Can identify muscle weakness at a certain point in range. Specific targeting of this range during treatment may reduce time spent undergoing rehabilitation.

May indicate structural integrity of the evaluated joint and its supporting structures.

Enables standard communication of muscle strength data between professionals.

EVALUATION PARAMETERS

Human movement involves exertion of force on the bony body levers. It is brought about by muscle contraction and culminates in a rotation of body segments about their joint axes.

Several parameters are used to describe exercise outcomes when using isokinetic dynamometry. An explanation of each is provided below.

TORQUE

Torque is the ability of a force to produce rotation. Some dynamometers measure torque directly, while others measure force at the point of application of the load cell. If the load cell is located on the lever arm, the dynamometer will measure force; if positioned at the axis of rotation in the dynamometer head, it will measure torque.

Torque is calculated using the formula:

torque = force measured at the load cell × moment arm.

If the force on the moment (lever) arm is perpendicularly applied, and the distance from the axis of rotation to the point of application is known, it is possible to convert force to torque using the above formula.

All dynamometers can display torque information graphically, which can be useful for analysis. Additionally, most provide a facility to download (usually in ASCII format) onto a floppy disk to enable detailed analysis.

Torque can be analysed in three ways: as peak, average peak and average torque.

Peak Torque

This is the highest point on the isokinetic curve.

Average Peak Torque

This is perhaps a more representative indication of patient performance since it is the average of a number of peak values taken over several consecutive torque curves. For example, a patient performs three consecutive concentric contractions, and for each contraction a torque curve is produced. The peak torques from each of these contractions are then summed and averaged to provide one value. This is known as the average peak torque.

Average Torque

This is measured using the entire tracing of one or several consecutive isokinetic curves. The advantage of obtaining averaged values is that artefacts due to deceleration of the limb and lever arm might have overall less effect than they would on the peak values (Perrin, 1993). To obtain comparative average values during consecutive evaluations, it is important to ensure that the range of motion through which the limb is tested remains constant.

Torque Ratios

Torque values obtained in the isokinetic mode are often expressed in terms of ratios for agonist to antagonist muscles or for comparisons between contraction types of the same muscle (Albert, 1991). However, the use of ratios is somewhat controversial due to lack of standardisation of the gravity correction procedure and the ratio calculation. Normative ratio values are so far unavailable for any muscle group, although torque ratios for the hamstrings and the quadriceps are the most frequently reported, with ratios of between 0.43 and 0.90 cited for these muscles (Albert, 1991).

WORK AND POWER

The calculation of the area under a single isokinetic torque curve is representative of the work done by the muscle group, and is defined by the SI unit of measurement known as the joule (only true for graph of moment versus angle and not for moment versus time). Average power is the work done divided by the time taken to perform the contraction. Measured in watts, it is the average rate of doing work.

All of the parameters described above can be evaluated at slow, intermediate or fast angular velocities.

USES OF ISOKINETIC DYNAMOMETRY IN THE CLINICAL SETTING

There are three main uses of dynamometry in rehabilitation: evaluation of static and/or dynamic muscle strength, treatment and research.

ISOKINETIC EVALUATION

An evaluation provides quantitative information on the nature of muscle contraction. For example, a patient may have been sent to the physiotherapy department complaining of continued weakness in the anterior thigh muscles after a partial rupture of this group 6 months previously. Despite intensive exercise therapy, this has failed to respond.

Evaluation in this instance may provide valuable information concerning the specific point or points in range which are still demonstrating diminished strength. Targeting of these areas using exercise therapy and/or dynamometry will be possible after evaluation.

Performing an Isokinetic Evaluation

A number of factors will influence how this is carried out, such as:
- Diagnosis.
- Age of patient.
- Rehabilitation status.
- Muscle group(s) to be tested.

When carrying out an evaluation, it is important to calibrate the system. This can be achieved easily, since recent machines have in-built calibration facilities. To ensure reliability and validity of the evaluation outcome, care should be taken to accurately align the axes of rotation of the limb and dynamometer and to standardise the patient testing position.

Isokinetic Lower Limb Evaluation

The following evaluation methodology is described in Jones (1996).

1. Assess the patient by both subjective and objective examination.
2. Familiarise the patient with the isokinetic dynamometer.
3. Explain the test aims.
4. Ensure that the patient warms up without the dynamometer, e.g. stretches, cycle ergometer.
5. Position and stabilise the patient accurately on the dynamometer.
6. Test the contralateral limb first.
7. Align the joint and dynamometer axes of rotation as closely as possible.
8. Use gravity correction if testing in a gravity-dependent position.
9. Select the test type, e.g. concentric/eccentric for knee extensors.
10. Select the test velocity, e.g. 30° per second.

11. Warm up on the dynamometer using the 'warm up mode.
12. Perform the maximal test at the chosen velocity, e.g. perform three concentric/eccentric repetitions with overlay facility, with a 30-second or 1-minute res between repetitions.
13. Record test details to ensure replication on retest.
14. Retest at the same time of day as the original evaluatio was performed.

Results of the Evaluation

An example of an evaluation result carried out on a Kin Com AP is shown in Figure 18.3.

The graph should be examined carefully to ensure tha basic information, such as patient name, date and tes details, is correct. In addition:

- Ensure that if carrying out a concentric evaluation a curves reflect a common pattern.
- Ascertain whether the data are raw or averaged. In othe words, does the graph demonstrate a single test or is the averaged curve from a series of tests?
- Note the position of the peak torque. This should be coin cident with the maximal biomechanical advantage for th joint in the normal subject. If it occurs slightly before th maximal biomechanical advantage, it may indicate tha the patient has produced a highly motivated and aggres sive attempt; if slightly behind, it may indicate less mot vation or concern over giving a maximal effort during th evaluation.

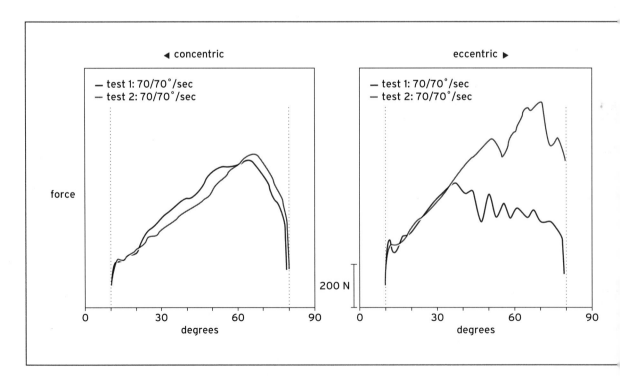

Figure 18.3 An isokinetic lower limb evaluation. (Reproduced by courtesy of Chattanooga UK, Oxford.)

The amplitude of the curve gives an indication of the force/velocity generating capacity of the tested muscle group. Comparisons should be made with the other side to establish whether the evaluation is abnormal. The coefficient of variation, which is often reported at the base of the graph, will give an indication of the reproducibility if carrying out a test in overlay mode. For example, if three maximal concentric contractions of the quadriceps are performed and averaged, the coefficient of variation indicates how closely all have approximated to a hypothetical optimum MVC. Tests with coefficients of variation of below 10% are generally acceptable as a true reflection of the patient's MVC (Sapega, 1990).

The peak eccentric force (tension) should always be larger than the concentric force on the normal evaluation. Gross abnormalities, such as pain inhibition, are often identified as breaks in the normal evaluation curve. However, as yet, specific diagnosis with curve analysis is not considered to be accurate (Dvir, 1991).

Advantages of an Isokinetic Evaluation

The advantages of an isokinetic evaluation are that it:

Provides a baseline measurement from which to progress and evaluate therapy.

Provides information about muscle imbalance.

Provides information on the precise point in range where pain or weakness is present.

Can be used to localise treatment to a specific point in range.

Reliability of Isokinetic Devices

The following factors described by Albert (1991) have all been shown to affect the reliability of results obtained in an isokinetic evaluation. These are listed by Jones (1996) as:

- Machine calibration.
- Joint axis alignment with that of the dynamometer.
- Gravity correction (Winter et al., 1981).
- Stabilisation of joint to be tested.
- Patient position and level of stabilisation.
- Design of protocol.
- Physiotherapist commands.
- Visual feedback from screen.
- Patient co-operation.
- Patient fatigue.
- Psychological state of the patient.

It should be noted that many of the reliability studies have been confined to the lower limb, and so currently there is a need for similar studies on other joints, particularly those of the upper limb (Walmsley & Pentland, 1993). Reliability is generally good, with intra-reliability (same subject tested on different days on the same machine) better than inter-reliability (same subject tested on two different machines on the same day). Some of the reasons for this have been attributed to differences in positioning and stabilisation of the patient, physical differences between the isokinetic machines, and differences in the method in which raw data are manipulated.

Validity

For a tool to be valid, it should be capable of measuring what it is supposed to measure, and the measured quantity should be relevant. Dvir (1995) cites several aspects of validity in respect of isokinetic dynamometry. These are summarised in Table 18.1.

Dvir (1995) suggests that isokinetic test findings are valid for specific dysfunctions, but states that inferences

Explanation of validity of isokinetic evaluation	
Type of validity	**Explanation/definition**
Content validity	Are the parameters measured relevant to muscle performance?
Construct validity	Does isokinetic testing measure strength?
Convergent	Do isokinetic findings display expected patterns, e.g. of changes with age?
Discriminant/divergent	Are tests good at distinguishing muscle performance from confounding factors, e.g. pain?
Criterion-referenced validity	Do isokinetic test results correlate well with external criteria or outcomes?
Concurrent	Do findings match existing situations, e.g. functional capacity, such as walking?
Predictive	Can isokinetic testing predict future outcomes, e.g. injury or progress?

Table 18.1 Explanation of validity of isokinetic evaluation.

cannot be generalised. To this end, he stresses the need for more validity-oriented research.

An area which has received criticism in the past, regarding validity, is that of the effect of gravity during evaluation procedures (Winter *et al.*, 1981). Failure to take into account that gravity can resist or assist during an evaluation, depending on patient position, can produce invalid data. In response to this criticism, a gravitational correction factor has now been incorporated into the recent dynamometers.

TREATMENT

Following an evaluation, the dynamometer can be programmed with a tailor-made treatment regimen for the patient. The programme should be reassessed regularly and the patient progressed accordingly.

Progression largely depends on patient capability, but a basic guide is provided below for a patient who is using the dynamometer for the first time and requires to progress through all modes.

1. The patient should initially be acclimatised to the dynamometer in the passive mode using slower velocities. Such velocities facilitate motor learning and make the patient feel secure on what can be perceived as a daunting piece of apparatus.
2. Active assisted exercise can be incorporated into the passive mode when the patient has become familiarised with the dynamometer.
3. A number of isometric holds at different points within the range can then be added at points of known weakness which have been identified at evaluation. The isometric exercise mode is also useful if pain is present during voluntary movement.
4. The isokinetic mode is incorporated and allows dynamic contractions to take place in a finely controlled loaded situation.
5. Isotonic exercise is the final addition to the treatment programme since this approximates to normal function. In this situation, isotonic contractions approximate to, but cannot replicate, normal function. The advantage, however, is that they occur in a controlled and protected environment. This possibly facilitates a standardised replication of the motor programme which closely approximates to that of the unconstrained functional activity.

Exercise Protocols in the Clinical Setting

In light of the above, it is possible to design and tailor a progressive exercise programme on the isokinetic dynamometer to suit the individual. However, standard rehabilitation programmes are now becoming available for the treatment of specific conditions. The most popular condition for which programmes have been designed involves rehabilitation after injury and repair of the anterior cruciate ligament.

Isokinetic Exercise using the Diagonal Functional Movement Patterns

Until recently it was impossible to set up a patient to exercise in one of the more functional diagonal body planes described by Voss and colleagues (1985). All available exercise positions were defined according to the sagittal, coronal or transverse planes of movement, i.e. the anatomical planes. However, manufacturers have begun to design isokinetic machines with dynamometers which are capable of spinning 360° in the transverse and vertical planes of movement. This addition allows the incorporation of the functional diagonals into the exercise programme.

Muscle Fibre Type and the Selection of a Treatment Velocity

An important consideration in the selection of a treatment programme is the relative contribution made to the contraction by the different muscle fibre types. Slow twitch—slow oxidative (SO)—fibres have motor units which respond at lower thresholds, and have low conduction velocities and long twitch contraction times. Fast twitch—fast glycolytic (FG)—fibres have motor units which respond at higher thresholds, and have higher conduction velocities and short twitch contraction times.

From this description it would be expected that at slow angular velocities slow twitch fibres would be recruited and at fast velocities the fast twitch fibres would primarily function. However, current theories favour the recruitment of both fibre types irrespective of exercise velocity (Rothstein *et al.*, 1987). Additionally, while there is a distinct order of recruitment in the concentric contraction, i.e. slow to fast twitch, recruitment in an eccentric contraction seems to be more selective, favouring the type IIB (FG) fibres (Korvanen *et al.*, 1984).

Importance of Visual Feedback in Isokinetic Exercise

The advent of computer technology has enabled the incorporation of visual feedback into isokinetic systems, where the patient is able to see the torque curve on the screen as they are performing an exercise or evaluation.

Results from a study which compared an evaluation of an MVC of the quadriceps when the patient was able to see the monitor, with those when the monitor was positioned out of sight, demonstrated significantly greater forces in the former situation (Carlson *et al.*, 1992). These results suggest a need for consistency in either excluding or including visual feedback during testing.

During treatment, the aim of an exercise programme is to gain strength as quickly and as safely as possible. It is probable, in view of the above findings, that the incorporation of visual feedback will decrease rehabilitation time. It should be remembered, however, that not all pathologies subjected to isokinetic regimens require or are capable of attaining high force output.

RESEARCH

The isokinetic dynamometer is being used increasingly as a research tool for quantifying static, concentric and latterly, eccentric muscle contraction. Many studies have focused on the lower limb, while few have examined isokinetic capabilities in relation to the upper limb. There is also minimal information on isokinetic dynamometry in disability, particularly relating to the quantification of spasticity. With the increasing demands for, and installations of, these machines the scope for research in these fields is vast. Of particular note, and mainly with the advent of the active dynamometer, researchers now have the ability to examine the characteristics of the eccentric muscle contraction. Important aspects relating to this area are summarised below.

Non-contact soft tissue injuries tend to occur during the eccentric phase of a muscle contraction, (Garrett, 1986). Unlike a concentric contraction where muscle fibre recruitment is sequenced from SO (type I) to FG (type IIB) muscle fibres, eccentric contractions are known to selectively recruit type IIB fibres first. It is these fibres which show highest damage in a non-contact soft tissue injury, and therefore it is important to tension these fibres appropriately, to ensure maximal rehabilitation (Albert, 1991). This can be achieved using the dynamometer or by prescribing resistive exercise which specifically targets the damaged muscle group.

It has recently been cited in the literature that joints which have poor eccentric capacity (shock absorption) tend to be predisposed to osteoarthritis (Marks, 1993). It is possible, therefore, that patients with osteoarthritis could benefit from rehabilitation-specific eccentric contractions (Duncan et al., 1989). However, one of the disadvantages of eccentric exercise is that of delayed onset of muscle soreness. This is characterised by pain, muscle swelling, loss of active range of movement, decreased peak torque and elevated electromyelographic activity. Its cause is not known, but several theories have been addressed. These include the build-up of lactic acid, selective damage of the Z bands which are weakest in the type IIB fibres, the occurrence of tonic muscle spasms, connective tissue damage in type IIB fibres, and an increase in tissue fluid.

REFERENCES

Albert M. *Eccentric muscle training in sports and orthopaedics*. Edinburgh: Churchill Livingstone; 1991.

Carlson AJ, Bennett G, Metcalf J. The effect of visual feedback in isokinetic testing. *Isokinet Exerc Sci* 1992, **2**:60-64.

Gress NM, Peters KS, Chandler JM. Eccentric vs concentric force-velocity relationships of the quadriceps femoris muscle. *J Sports Phys Ther* 1992, **6**:82-86.

Duncan PW, Chandler JM, Cavanaugh DK, *et al.* Mode and speed specificity of eccentric and concentric exercise training. *J Sports Phys Ther* 1989, **11**:70-75.

Dvir Z. Clinical applicability of isokinetics: a review. *Clin Biomech* 1991, **6**:133-144.

Dvir Z. *Isokinetics: muscle testing, interpretation and clinical applications*. Edinburgh: Churchill Livingstone; 1995.

Garrett WE. Basic science of musculotendinous injuries. In: Nicholson JA, Hershman EB, eds. *The lower extremity and spine in sports medicine*. St Louis: CV Mosby; 1986:42.

Hislop H, Perrine JJ. The isokinetic concept of exercise. *Phys Ther* 1967, **47**:114-117.

Jensen RC, Warren B, Laursen C, Morrissey MC. Static pre-load effect on knee extensor isokinetic concentric and eccentric performance. *Med Sci Sports Exerc* 1991, **23**:10-14.

Jones K, Barker K. *Human movement explained*. Oxford: Butterworth Heinemann; 1996.

Korvanen V, Suominen H, Heiddinen E. Mechanical properties of fast and slow skeletal muscle with special reference to collagen and endurance training. *J Biomech* 1984, **17**:725.

Marks R. Muscles as a pathogenic factor in osteoarthritis. *Physiotherapy Canada* 1993, **45**:251-259.

Osternig LR. Isokinetic dynamometry: implications for muscle testing and rehabilitation. *Exerc Sports Sci Rev* 1986, **14**:45-80.

Perrin DH. *Isokinetic exercise and assessment*. Leeds: Human Kinetics Publishers; 1993.

Perrin DH, Hellwig EV, Tis LL, Shenk BS. Effect of gravity correction on shoulder rotation isokinetic average muscle force and reciprocal muscle group ratios. *Isokinet Exerc Sci* 1992, **2**:30-33.

Rothstein JM, Lamb RL, Mayhew TP. Clinical uses of isokinetic measurement. *Phys Ther* 1987, **67**:1840-1844.

Sapega AA. Current concepts review: muscle performance evaluation in orthopaedic practice. *J Bone Joint Surg* 1990, **72A**:1562-1574.

Voss DE, Ionta NK, Myers BJ. *Proprioceptive neuromuscular facilitation*, 2nd ed. Philadelphia: Harper and Row; 1985.

Walmsley RP, Pentland W. An overview of isokinetic dynamometry with specific reference to the upper limb. *Clin Rehabil* 1993, **7**:239-247.

Winter DA, Wells RP, Orr GW. Errors in the use of isokinetic dynamometers. *Eur J Appl Physiol* 1981, **46**:397-408.

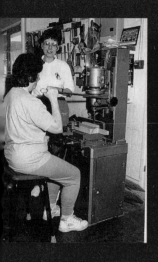

19 G N Smith
RETURN TO FITNESS

CHAPTER OUTLINE

- **Aims of rehabilitation**
- **Assessment and categorisation**
- **Stages of rehabilitation**
- **Early stage**

- **Intermediate stage**
- **Late stage**
- **Pre-discharge stage**

AIMS OF REHABILITATION

By definition, rehabilitation is the restoration of function. To rehabilitate is to bring back to a previous normal condition. Obviously, in some circumstances this is not totally true, as the injury or illness may preclude the patients from returning to their previous normal condition; although this should be the ideal goal where possible.

The ultimate functional requirements of the patient should be of paramount concern when planning rehabilitation programmes. Clearly defined aims must be identified and adhered to. The overall and specific aim for rehabilitation should be to return the patient to full functional fitness in the shortest, safest, possible time. Note the emphasis on shortest, safest, possible time; also, the requirement to return the patient to full functional fitness.

To achieve this aim, it is imperative that the physiotherapist and practitioner understand the functional requirements of the patient. For example, what is a professional footballer required to do when he returns to full activities? It is not the playing of the game that is recognised as work, rather the training to play. This training has to be undertaken on a daily basis, with changing climatic conditions, over a 10-month period each year. An understanding of what this patient will have to return to is a priority for anyone wishing to treat and rehabilitate professional soccer players.

Likewise, what is it that a labourer or bricklayer is expected to do in order to return to work safely and effectively? Whereas professional sportsmen do not have to 'work' while they are rehabilitating, self-employed builders do. A physiotherapist involved in rehabilitating this type of patient must therefore be aware of the patient's needs and, where possible, assist the patient accordingly.

Similarly, some patients may have sedentary occupations but perform at an elite level of sporting excellence. The physiotherapist needs then to identify the priority, and plan the rehabilitation programmes accordingly. While this type of patient can return to work earlier, the need to train and perform as an elite sportsperson may actually be the specific priority. Identifying the patient's needs, and planning a realistic rehabilitation programme around their everyday activities, will demonstrate understanding and empathy with their situation, thus gaining their trust and co-operation.

Physiotherapists and practitioners working in a rehabilitation environment must have a clear understanding of the occupational requirements of their patients. In sport, this is known as having 'sports-specific knowledge.' In an industrial or occupational rehabilitation setting, specific knowledge and understanding of the functional demands of the industry or occupation are cardinal considerations. Without this knowledge, understanding and empathy, it is very difficult to rehabilitate patients back to unrestricted activities safely and effectively.

ASSESSMENT AND CATEGORISATION

Before planning any rehabilitation programme, it is necessary to assess and categorise the patient. The assessment needs to be a thorough clinical and objective procedure. Adequate time must be allocated to allow the physiotherapist to perform these assessments, especially with new patients. While there will always be continual ongoing assessments of the patients in the programmes, the initial assessment of the new patient is probably one of the most important components of the actual rehabilitation procedure. It must therefore be treated as such.

At the end of the examination and assessment, the physiotherapist should have identified all of the patient's problems. It is these problems that then give the aims of the programme from which the means can be identified. Rehabilitation is about solving problems. Patients present with a series of problems that preclude them from returning to either full functional fitness or to ultimate levels of occupational competencies. It is only by identifying these problems that a realistic and appropriate rehabilitation programme can be planned.

At the end of the assessment it is also necessary to establish a 'contract of agreement' between the physiotherapist and the patient. This is achieved by identifying what the patients perceive as their 'main problem' at that time. If their perception of the main problem is unrealistic for their level of ability, it is necessary for the physiotherapist to modify this perception to a more realistic level. For example, if the patient sees their inability to play sport or return to the factory floor as their main problem when they present with a painful, swollen, knee joint that necessitates them using walking aids, their expectations must be reviewed. If it is not, then everything that is achieved during the rehabilitation programme will be seen as negative until such time as the patients return either to playing sport again or working on the factory floor. It is hoped that this will be the ultimate result, but in some circumstances these goals may never be achieved.

Therefore, if the physiotherapist can renegotiate the perception of the main problem to that which is achievable, and modify the problem as the programme progresses, then the patient's attitude will be more positive. For example, with the patient described above, if the physiotherapist can persuade them to see that the pain and swelling is the main problem, and that with the reduction and alleviation of these symptoms their quality life would be improved. Hence, these symptoms should be treated as the priority. This would then enable the patient to progress to full weight bearing without the use of walking aids, then on to running and, hopefully, through a progressive programme, to their ultimate goal, i.e. a return to unrestricted activities. As each problem is overcome, the patient remains positive and confident, and the physiotherapist has a compliant and motivated patient to work with.

Also, following the comprehensive assessment, it is necessary to categorise patients to the level of rehabilitation they should be assigned. It may also be necessary to categorise and classify the patients into occupational and sociological groups. This will then allow patients of a similar background, culture, humour and language to work together and motivate each other. Likewise, patients with similar disabilities can work together provided they are at a comparable level of recovery and within the same stage of the rehabilitation programme. This bonding or subgroup culture will have a positive effect on the motivation of members within the group, and assist the physiotherapist responsible for overseeing the rehabilitation programmes of each member within the group.

However, where the patient does not easily fit into either an occupational subgroup or rehabilitation stage, neither should be imposed on the patient. If they are, the group dynamics will be affected and the benefits lost. The patient will feel that they are imposing and do not belong. Thus, feeling uncomfortable, their motivation and recovery are affected. Similarly, the members of the group on which the outsider has been imposed, feel that there is an intrusion and their salutary group dynamics are lost. Thus, wherever possible, consideration should be given to patients with differing occupational or cultural backgrounds or at different stages of the rehabilitation programme, so that these patients are not allocated to an inappropriate group. If, however, all patients referred to the rehabilitation unit come from diverse backgrounds or are at varying levels of the rehabilitation programme, the group will become mixed and will form its own group dynamics and therefore be effective. When an individual enters a group with a dissimilar background and culture, problems arise; hence the reason for many occupational groups and organisations in the past establishing their own rehabilitation centres—for example, the armed forces, the police force, the fire service, miners' unions and football associations, to name but a few. It is the philosophy of rehabilitating and treating patients from similar occupational and cultural backgrounds that has made these centres so successful.

STAGES OF REHABILITATION

There are four main stages of rehabilitation into which patients can be classified and categorised. These stages are:
- The early stage.
- The intermediate stage.
- The late stage.
- The final functional pre-discharge stage.

Each stage has its own specific criteria for recognition of, and progression from. Likewise, while patients may be grouped into functional or occupational categories and stages of rehabilitation, their programmes should be individualised to their needs.

In each of the first three stages of the rehabilitation programme, there are three aims which must be achieved. These aims are:
- To provide a progressive exercise and treatment programme for the injured limb(s), ensuring that recovery is established and maintained.

- To provide a programme of exercises to maintain or improve the mobility, strength and general fitness of the unaffected limbs, as well as cardiovascular fitness, without prejudicing the recovery of the injured limb.
- To ensure that the rehabilitation and exercise programmes are carried out with the maximum attention to safety and effectiveness.

As the patient progresses through each stage of rehabilitation, the emphasis on the first two aims will alter accordingly, whereas awareness and heed of the third aim will need to increase as the programme becomes more dynamic.

EARLY STAGE

This stage of rehabilitation can be generalised as the period where the injured limb is non-weight bearing. It has also been described as the time from injury to almost full pain-free activities. In the lower limb, it corresponds to the time when the patient is completely non-weight bearing on the injured/affected limb. With upper limb injuries, it is the time when the injured part may or may not be supported, and cannot, under any circumstances, have any weight bearing or resisted forces applied through it.

The early stage is often regarded as being the easiest to control and monitor. In the main, this is because with lower limb injuries, most activities are undertaken with the patient lying or sitting on a mat or plinth, therefore the activities are less dynamic. The patient with upper limb injuries will also need to undertake their exercises in a static or non-weight-bearing position. This will then ensure that there is no likelihood of over-enthusiastic participation in dynamic activities.

It is, however, often the hardest of the rehabilitation stages to plan and prepare for, as the physiotherapist must continually be aware of the patient's problems and disabilities. It is always the physiotherapist's responsibility to ensure that the patient's recovery is not placed at risk. At no time during this stage in the rehabilitation process should any competitive activities be introduced which may involve physical contact.

In the early stage of rehabilitation, mobilisation and flexibility exercises should be commenced as soon as possible. These exercises can be active or passive, and always performed within the limits of pain and discomfort and without weight-bearing forces being applied through the injured limb. Specific strengthening exercises for the injured limb should be started as early as possible, again within the limits of pain and discomfort. They should also be predominantly isometric. The emphasis in rehabilitating the injured limb should be on controlled, progressive exercise programmes which will increase the range of movement and strength of the injured limb without exacerbating the injury or being detrimental to its recovery. The other limb and the remainder of the body, however, can be subjected to an aggressive exercise programme, provided no adverse stresses or strains are placed upon the injured part. This will help to ensure that cardiovascular fitness is maintained (or improved),

as well as the strength and mobility of the non-affected parts of the body. The physiotherapist must therefore strike a balance between working the patient to the maximum that the disability will permit and ensuring that the injured limb is allowed to recover without provoking further problems to it, or detrimentally affecting the recovery pattern.

Besides undertaking specific individual exercise programmes, the patient undergoing early rehabilitation for lower limb injuries can participate in static quadriceps exercises or non-weight-bearing class activities. The patient with upper limb injuries can participate in group activities provided that no external forces are applied to the injured limb and that the programme does not include any dynamic activities that will increase the risk of external forces and torsional stresses being applied to it. Non-weight-bearing competitive group activities can be included during this stage of rehabilitation. These will often help to address the patient's competitive instincts as well as promoting the group dynamics described earlier.

Activities such as sit-down volleyball and sit-down cricket are suitable and appropriate for this stage of the rehabilitation programme. While the least active of the rehabilitation stages, it is the one that requires total awareness and concentration by the physiotherapist. It is the time that both the physiotherapist and the patient must be mindful of risk situations and the possibility of re-injury due to the most trivial of circumstances.

The patient may progress from early rehabilitation to the intermediate stage when:
- Weight-bearing forces can be gradually applied through the limb in a partial weight-bearing manner—with fractures, this is usually at the stage of clinical union.
- For knee injuries/problems, the injured joint has no effusion and the patient is pain free and able to flex the joint to 90°. The patient must also have the ability to extend the knee in a controlled manner from 90° to full extension without pain.
- For other joints, the patient has at least two thirds of the normal, functional and anatomical movement of that joint, with no pain or persistent swelling. In reality, there may be some slight swelling in injured joints which does not inhibit the patient from achieving the necessary two thirds of normal movement. In these circumstances, patients can be allowed to progress to the next stage of rehabilitation providing that the swelling does not become worse with increased activities or the range of movement does not become reduced with loading. It should also be noted that any braces, external splintage or crutches must not be discarded at this time. In fact, they are often more appropriate as the patient progresses to more dynamic activities in the next stage.

It is often very difficult to predict the length of time the patient will remain in the early stage of rehabilitation. It is only when the criteria for moving through to the intermediate stage have been established that patients can be allowed to progress with their rehabilitation programme.

In some cases, where the injury is fairly minor, the patient may only remain in the early stage of rehabilitation for a few days. However, the patient who has had major reconstructive surgery, fractures or multiple injuries, can only be allowed to progress when all of the criteria have been met. This may often take many weeks, and in some circumstances, months. It is therefore essential that the physiotherapist clearly outlines to the patient the criteria for progression to the next stage of the rehabilitation programme, rather than giving time guidelines; hence the importance of establishing a problem-solving approach to the planning of rehabilitation programmes.

INTERMEDIATE STAGE

This stage is when the patient with a lower limb injury progresses from non-weight-bearing through partial weight-bearing to full weight-bearing activities. The patient with upper limb problems will evolve progressively to the stage when they have full joint mobility and muscular control over the injured arm.

For the patient with lower limb problems, this is also the time when walking re-education programmes are included. The patient should also be advised to continue with the use of crutches and/or walking sticks until such time as they have a normal gait pattern. Patients will frequently discard walking aids too early, thus subjecting the limb to abnormal stresses before a correct walking pattern has been achieved. This will then exacerbate problems, which can result in either re-injury or other associated minor problems. Patients should be advised that the use of walking aids will assist in re-educating normal gait patterns, and must be retained. At this point, it is also worth stressing that correct instructions in the use of walking aids is a very important part of the physiotherapist's role at the beginning of the intermediate stage of rehabilitation. Time spent ensuring that patients are able to use crutches/walking sticks correctly will be beneficial in the later stages of the programme. Helping them to understand the importance of using the walking aids will also help to prevent repetitive minor trauma to the recovering joints by the incorrect usage or early discard of the equipment. Patients must, therefore, be taught correct partial weight-bearing patterns with their crutches or walking sticks. They must also be instructed in sitting down, standing up, walking up and down stairs (using either two sticks, or one stick and a bannister—if such is available) and getting in and out of a car. It should also be stressed that using two crutches in the early partial weight-bearing stage is far more effective and efficient than trying to use one stick/crutch only. Likewise, when the patient progresses to using one stick, they should be educated and informed as to the rationale of holding the stick on the non-affected side and not on the side of the injury, as is common practice.

During the intermediate stage of rehabilitation, the physiotherapist should aim to meet the following overall objectives, namely:
• To regain full normal range of anatomical movement in all the joints of the injured limb. Active, passive and resisted ranges of movement should also be restored in all joints.
• To increase the strength of all of the muscles acting functionally over the joints of the injured limb. Strengthening exercise programmes should be progressed according to the general principles of overload. Increasing the resistance and number of repetitions will improve strength, whereas high-repetition, low-resistance exercises will improve endurance. In the later stages, power can be developed by modifying the speed through which the exercises are performed.

The above objectives can be met by the patient progressively working from non-weight-bearing through partial weight-bearing to full weight-bearing exercises throughout the full range of joint movement that is available:
• To maintain and improve the general and cardiovascular fitness of the rest of the body. The specific activities to achieve this can be more dynamic provided that the injured limb is not subjected to any stresses and forces for which it is not prepared. Cycling, rowing and swimming activities are excellent rehabilitation tools to use at this time.
• To maintain and improve the strength and co-ordination of the non-affected limb. In the early part of the intermediate stage, many of the activities will be similar to those undertaken in early rehabilitation. However, as the patient progresses, co-ordinated exercises using both limbs, as well as the whole body, can be incorporated. Bilateral, eccentric and concentric exercises should be performed, progressing from partial weight-bearing to full weight-bearing activities as the patient's abilities improve.
• To restore and re-educate normal patterns of gait for patients with lower limb injuries.
• To restore and re-educate bilateral and symmetrical patterns of normal movements for patients with upper limb injuries.

Clearly, patients who are given good walking re-education programmes will achieve normal gait patterns much earlier than those who are not. Patients will also tolerate increased weight-bearing activities through the affected limb much easier if part of this programme is undertaken in a swimming/hydrotherapy pool. This will enable patients to walk in varying depths of water, progressively affecting the weight being taken through the injured limb, and allowing them to establish correct walking patterns in this medium. The deeper the water, the less the effect of the body weight, and vice versa; a practical application of hydrostatic physics. For the patient who has had serious multiple injuries to the lower limb, this is frequently the most effective way of re-educating correct walking patterns which cannot be reproduced on dry land owing to the patient's fear of taking weight through the injured limb.

In restoring and re-educating bilateral and symmetrical patterns of normal movement for the upper limbs, the physiotherapist is advised to identify the patient's dominant limb. If it is this limb that has been injured, the patient will be far more willing to use it in performance of necessary daily activities of living. If, however, it is the non-dominant limb that has been injured, the patient will require far more encouragement to exercise this part of the body, as it is not needed for normal daily activities of living, hence the necessity for bilateral, symmetrical exercise programmes.

The patient with a lower limb injury should not participate in any competitive or dynamic activities which involve full weight bearing or require rotational forces to be applied through the injured leg. Also, the patient with upper limb problems should not be permitted to take part in any dynamic or competitive activities where external and uncontrolled forces can be applied to the injured arm. During this stage both types of patient will, however, become involved in more dynamic activities and engage in programmes that require bilateral resisted exercises. These exercises should always remain within the control of the patient. Excessive enthusiasm in competitive games can often be attributed as the main cause for either re-injury or further injury to the patient in the intermediate stage of rehabilitation. Therefore, whenever competitive activities are introduced, these should be controlled and refereed assertively. Competitive activities do have an important role to play and must not be totally excluded from this stage of the rehabilitation programme.

For the physiotherapist, the intermediate stage of rehabilitation is far more dynamic than the early stage. It requires much more planning, control and attention to safety. Exercise regimens must be progressive and beneficial to the recovery of the injured limb without provoking further damage or causing other injuries. In the early stage of rehabilitation, the patient is exercising in a static environment, whereas in the intermediate stage, greater movement is introduced. It is imperative that the physiotherapist is aware of all of the dangers, both intrinsic and extrinsic. Intrinsic dangers are inherent in the patient's over-enthusiasm to 'push themselves' in their exercise programmes; hence the need for comprehensive assessments with rigid guidelines and criteria being established. Extrinsic dangers are often attributable to:

- Too many people participating in the activities.
- Mismatch of the patient's capabilities during formal exercise classes.
- A lack of awareness by the physiotherapist to the environment in which the exercises are taking place; for example, the patient being expected to perform dynamic activities in a room that is either too small or cluttered with other patients and equipment. The greater the amount of movement required in rehabilitation, the larger the space needed. Thus, the group should become progressively smaller as the degree of movement required increases.

The criteria for moving from the intermediate stage through to the next part of the rehabilitation process are that:

- For lower limb injuries, the patient should have full range movement of all joints on the affected limb. These should also be pain free with no persistent swelling. It is also essential that the patient has a normal, full weight-bearing walking pattern and has reached the stage where they are ready to commence running. Without a normal pain-free walking pattern, running will prove difficult and potentially damaging. It should also be stressed that running does not form part of the intermediate stage of rehabilitation.
- For upper limb injuries, the patient should have bilateral and symmetrical movements of all of the joints in both limbs. There should be no restriction of movement due to pain or lack of muscle control. The patient must also be able to perform controlled bilateral functional weight-bearing exercises without resorting to trick or compensatory movements.

The actual time spent in the intermediate stage of rehabilitation depends upon the individual patient. Before moving on to the more advanced and dynamic later stages, the patient must meet the established criteria. Obviously, the patient with minimal injuries will progress through the intermediate stage fairly swiftly. It is, however, the stage that forms an important bridge between early and late rehabilitation, and one that has specific criteria to adhere to. Too often, especially with sportspersons, the patient is progressed from early non-weight-bearing/partial weight-bearing exercises through to running, without any recourse to gait re-education.

The patient who has sustained more serious injuries will take much longer to progress through the intermediate stage of rehabilitation. With such patients, the physiotherapist must be completely in control and totally aware of the safety implications. Patients frequently become more frustrated during the intermediate stage than at earlier stages of rehabilitation. This is usually due to the fact that while intermediate rehabilitation is more dynamic, with development of a greater level of fitness towards the end of the stage than was apparent when commencing rehabilitation, the patient is still very restricted in their physical capabilities. Frustration and impatience often take over during this stage, with the result that the patient endeavours to progress to a running programme before they are anatomically, physiologically, pathologically or functionally able. Responsibility lies with the physiotherapist to ensure that, at all times, the patient is aware of their limitations and of the resultant complications and problems that could occur if they become too impatient. This specifically applies to patients with lower limb injuries.

Similar problems also affect patients with upper limb injuries. Towards the end of this stage of rehabilitation, they may have normal ranges of movement and the ability to participate in controlled dynamic activities, but if they progress too quickly, they may be unable to meet the extra demands placed upon them. Re-injury or further injury would then occur. When this happens, the responsibility lies with the physiotherapist and not the patient. Therefore, once again, the achievement of firmly established criteria, rather than the completion of specific periods of time, is the important factor for determining progression from this stage of rehabilitation to the next.

LATE STAGE

This is the most dynamic stage of rehabilitation to date. It is where the patient will undertake a much more aggressive and fitness-oriented programme of exercises compared with the earlier stages of rehabilitation. Far more emphasis will be placed upon general fitness. Likewise, the affected limb will ultimately be exercised without protection or limitations.

With a greater emphasis on more dynamic activities, the physiotherapist will require far more control and discipline of the group. Smaller practical groups are necessary. The physiotherapist must be able to control all aspects of the class or exercise session at all times, even if it is being undertaken in an outdoor environment. Also, while more energetic than the previous stages, it is still classified as 'a stage of rehabilitation'. Physiotherapists must not lose sight of the fact that they are dealing with patients recovering from injuries. They should also be aware that over-exuberance by the patient, combined with a lack of control from themselves, will result in problems that can be detrimental to the ultimate recovery of the patient. Clearly defined aims must be identified and adhered to. These are:

- To re-educate normal functional activities in the injured limb. Wherever possible, these should include the normal functional activities to which the patient ultimately will return.
- To increase the general functional fitness of the patient bilaterally and symmetrically. Once again, occupational and functional gross body movements are introduced progressively, the aim being to re-educate and develop the co-ordination and skills necessary for the patient to return to normal unrestricted activities. For the sportsperson, this may include a progressive programme of 'sports-specific' activities. As the patient becomes more confident and co-ordinated, further complex activities can be introduced. These may involve the use of equipment relevant to the patient's occupation or sport. Wherever possible, the performance of these activities should be carried out within the normal working or sporting environment to which the patient wishes to return.
- To prepare the patient for their return to normal unrestricted activities.

Allied to the overall aim of rehabilitation, it should now be clear why an understanding of the occupational/functional requirements of the patient is a necessity. Patients must be physically able to meet the demands that return to their normal unrestricted activities is going to place upon them. For example, if the patient's occupation is that of a factory worker who is required to stand for 7–8 hours per day, then the rehabilitation programme must prepare the patient adequately to do this. Undertaking 30 minutes of exercise in a hospital gymnasium will be insufficient. The patient requiring high levels of fitness and ability should undertake a programme of full day rehabilitation activities, wherever possible, on at least 2–3 consecutive days. The activities should also be similar to those that the patient will undertake when they return to work. This is often known as a 'work hardening programme'. These specific programmes prepare patients to return to a more physical and demanding occupational environment safely and effectively.

Again, it must be stressed that this phase of rehabilitation is still classified as part of the recovery process. The activities undertaken, while becoming more demanding and sports specific, should not cause re-injury or further problems. If there are indications of regression or problems, then this will be a confirmation that the patient is working at a level that is too advanced for them at that particular time. The aims should be to enable the patient to progress safely and effectively through this stage of rehabilitation, and to assist them in overcoming any physical, physiological or psychological problems they may have in respect to meeting the demands of their occupation or sporting activities.

The late stage of rehabilitation is also the stage that physiotherapists regard as relatively easy. This is not, and should not, be so. It requires far more planning and a greater understanding of the functional and occupational requirements of the patient than do any of the earlier stages. It is also the stage that requires a careful balance between general fitness-related activities and strengthening programmes for the injured limbs. Too often patients are subjected to respiratory distress before any benefit is achieved from the exercise programmes. This is frequently due to too much emphasis being placed upon running and vigorous activities, rather than specific functional strengthening programmes. There is, however, a need for fitness-related work. This will obviously need to be much harder than it was, as patients who have progressed from the earlier stages of rehabilitation will be generally fitter. There must, however, be a balance between activities that require cardiovascular fitness and those which are specifically functionally designed to strengthen the affected limbs.

It is also during this stage that the activities should be more sports/occupation-specific. Special attention must be paid to the biomechanics and techniques of performing these skills and activities. Unlike the earlier stages of rehabilitation, it is at this time the physiotherapist must concentrate on a 'total body' approach. In normal conditioning and training programmes, the participants work bilaterally. In rehabilitation, however, patients usually have one affected limb. Thus, during the early and intermediate stages, the emphasis will have been placed on rehabilitating the injured limb as a separate entity, while trying to maintain or improve the general fitness of the rest of the body. Emphasis will also have been placed upon working the injured limb on its own so that the non-affected limb was prevented from compensating for the deficiency and did not prejudice improvement and recovery. At the late stage of rehabilitation, there should be no differences between the injured and the non-injured limb—this will have been achieved progressively as the patient passed through the intermediate stage—and therefore bilateral activities can be undertaken. At this time the 'total body concept' can be utilised and the patient worked aggressively. If, however, it is identified that the patient has retained a residual deficiency between the injured and non-injured limb, the patient must be reclassified and 'backtracked' to the intermediate stage of rehabilitation. Likewise, if at any time during late rehabilitation patients experience pain, swelling or other problems, then they must be reassessed as to their eligibility for remaining at this stage of the programme. If necessary, they should be reclassified and taken out of this stage. It is suggested that if patients experience problems, physiotherapists should look to themselves and ensure that they have not been too enthusiastic or over-exuberant with their exercise programmes and regimens.

At the end of the late stage of rehabilitation, patients are still required to progress to one final phase before discharge. All too often it is the late stage of rehabilitation that is regarded as the final one. However, this should not be so. Even though it is dynamic and energetic, and patients undertake activities as close to normal life as possible, it is still part of the progressive recovery and rehabilitation process. It is also still a time when problems may present. The physiotherapist must, therefore, remain totally aware of this. Should problems occur, the patient will need to be reassessed and re-categorised.

During the late stage of rehabilitation, the physiotherapist must remain totally focused and willing to regress the patient if necessary. Patients should not be discharged to full unrestricted activities from the late stage of rehabilitation. They may, however, be able to participate in most of their daily activities, which in the case of sportspersons may involve approximately 75% of their normal training activities. However, before final discharge and classification as 'fit to return to unrestricted activities', all patients should progress to a final functional pre-discharge programme. This is especially important for occupations or activities that require high levels of general fitness and functional endurance, e.g. professional and elite sportspersons, the military, workers in heavy industry, miners, the police and firemen. Patients who requires lesser levels of functional and occupational fitness can be discharged from the late stage of rehabilitation, although this is obviously not ideal. However, if their fitness or occupational expectations are of a higher level than activities undertaken in the late-stage programmes, they must also be progressed through to the functional pre-discharge programme.

The criteria for progressing from the late stage of rehabilitation to the pre-discharge group should be that:
• The patient must have full, normal ranges of movement (active and passive) in all joints of the affected limb. Also, these ranges should not be affected after exercise. It is therefore required that the physiotherapist assesses active and passive joint ranges of movement before and after exercise.

• All movements should be of full range and pain free.
• There should be no persistent or residual swelling. Similarly, after exercise, there should be no evidence of developing swelling or effusions.
• There should be good proprioceptive function.
• The patient should have regained (or retained) a level of cardiovascular fitness similar to that present before the injury.
• The patient should have demonstrated, in a controlled environment, that they have retained or regained the necessary skills relevant to their occupational and/or functional requirements.

If there is doubt about any of the criteria above, then the patient should not be discharged or progressed to the next stage. Any deficiency should be identified and worked upon. Once again, the length of this stage of rehabilitation will be determined by the patient's ability rather than time.

Commonly, a reason for patients being unable to progress and cope with the pre-discharge stage is lack of fitness, rather than the non-recovery of the injured limb. This is usually an indication that general and cardiovascular fitness programmes have not been incorporated into the earlier stages of rehabilitation, hence the importance of ensuring that the patient is given exercise programmes to maintain, improve or restore cardiovascular fitness during these stages. Swimming, cycling, rowing and general circuit training are all activities that will help to achieve this.

Finally, as stated earlier, the late stage of rehabilitation is by far the most aggressive and dynamic of any of the stages encountered to date. It is also the period when many problems not previously identified can be exacerbated. The physiotherapist must look to identify these and deal with them accordingly. This may require re-categorising the patient and referring them back to the intermediate stage. This could be for exacerbation of a problem not related to the actual injury for which the patient is undergoing rehabilitation. It is far better to do this than to allow the patient to progress to the pre-discharge stage before they are physically, pathologically or physiologically prepared.

PRE-DISCHARGE STAGE

This is, sadly, the stage omitted from many rehabilitation programmes. It is a global problem and one that should be addressed forthwith. The pre-discharge stage is the one in which the physiotherapist makes the decision that the patient is 'fit to return to unrestricted activities' or not. It is the period of rehabilitation through which patients must do everything that will be expected of them when they return to their normal activities. It is also the time when any problems encountered or deficiencies identified mean that the patient must be re-categorised and reassigned to the late stage of rehabilitation. They must not be allowed to return to their normal activities.

The main aim for this part of the rehabilitation programme is to identify and expose any deficiencies that the patient may have. If the patient is able to participate successfully in everything they are asked to do during this stage, they can then be discharged 'to return to unrestricted activities' without any fears or doubts being expressed either by them or by the physiotherapist.

Unlike in the previous stages, the physiotherapist must try to provoke and identify any deficiencies that would be detrimental to the patient returning to their normal functional activities. Thus, if at any time during the session deficiencies are exposed and problems encountered, the patient must be referred back immediately for reassessment and re-categorisation.

Physiotherapists involved in the earlier stages of rehabilitation should not undertake the reassessment as they will have already achieved their aim. This reassessment should ideally be undertaken by the physiotherapist responsible for the patient in the late stage of rehabilitation. If this is not practical, then the physiotherapist taking the pre-discharge group should plan to reassess the patient at the end of that specific session and not during it. Time spent in reassessing one patient will disrupt the continuity of the session and also allow other patients to have an unscheduled rest period.

A pre-discharge programme should be lively and energetic. It should also correspond to the activities that patients require following final discharge. Sessions must be designed to imitate as closely as possible the occupational/functional requirements to which the patient is going to return. During each session, the patient must meet the following criteria before them being regarded as 'fit to return to unrestricted activities'. The physiotherapist must endeavour to determine positive answers to each of the following questions:

Has the Injury Recovered?

If the patient still has a limited range of movement, pain and persistent swelling, this indicates that the injury has not recovered, and therefore the patient should not be returned to full activities. If these signs and symptoms increase during or following a pre-discharge session, this is a positive indication that the patient still has pathophysiological problems which are exacerbated with the intensity of the activities. Such patients would, therefore, have further problems if allowed to return to their normal environment.

There may also be times when patients, coaches and managers will try to persuade the physiotherapist that these signs and symptoms would not prejudice the patients' return to full activities. In the short term this may be true. However, with clearly defined pathophysiological problems, patients are demonstrating that the injury has not recovered and therefore they are at risk of either further injury or exacerbation of the original problem. While it is agreed that some instability can be protected by strapping, taping and functional bracing, and that a degree of comparative muscular weakness is acceptable, such patients will still be at risk. Their functional performance will be affected, with the potential for putting both themselves and colleagues at risk. Pain, swelling and lack of movement are indications that the injury has not recovered. Therefore, the patient should not be progressed any further until such time as these are eradicated.

If, however, the answer to the above question is yes, then the next one is:

Does the Patient have the Physical (Aerobic) Fitness Necessary to Perform Everyday Tasks?

Aerobic fitness is defined as the ability to take in, transport and utilise oxygen. Aerobic exercise should be relatively comfortable and sustainable for between 20 minutes and several hours. It should be possible to carry on a conversation during moderate aerobic exercise. In everyday terms, it is the requirement for patients physically to cope with the demands placed upon them over a sustained period without undue fatigue. If attention has not been given to improving and maintaining cardiovascular and general fitness during the earlier stages of rehabilitation, then the patient will not be able to resume normal functional and occupational activities. For example, if the patient is a professional footballer, normal daily activities, i.e. training, will usually commence with a warm-up run. If the rest of the group perform at 55%–60% of their maximum ability during this warm-up, but the patient on returning to the group has to work at 80%–85% of their capacity to stay with them, then that patient is at risk. The moment members of the group move into their normal training activities and increase their work rate, usually to 75%–80% of maximum, the patient is immediately placed in an overload situation and will be unable to perform at the level required. This places the patient at risk of re-injury or further damage. This patient should not have been returned to full training as he did not have the required level of aerobic fitness to undertake his normal daily activities.

The objective, physiological testing of fit sportspersons, pre-competition and post-training, is a method of determining the benchmark to which the patient should return after injury or illness. If this has not been carried out previously, it should be undertaken at this stage. The following tests are commonly used in sport to assess aerobic fitness.

The 12-Minute Run

This is performed on a 400 m track. The patient runs/walks as far as they can in 12 minutes. The test has been performed on USA airforce personnel for many years, and is a suitable guide for general fitness. Fitness level norms referring to the distances that should be covered include:

- <1500 m (<3 laps), very poor.
- 1500–2000 m (4–5 laps), poor.
- 2000–2400 m (5–6 laps), fair.
- 2400–2800 m (6–7 laps), good.
- >2800 m (>7 laps), excellent.

This test can also be modified for the 'non-runner'. By using a bicycle and doubling the distances, comparative fitness levels can be established.

The 2400 m Test

Again, this test is performed on a 400 m track. The subject should run/walk six laps of the track as fast as possible. The time taken to complete the distance is noted. The normal indications and relevant levels of fitness are:

<8 minutes, excellent.
8–10 minutes, good.
10–12 minutes, fair.
>12 minutes, poor.

It is important to remember that the two tests described above usually last for approximately 12 minutes each. However, as described earlier, 20 minutes is now regarded as the minimum time for testing and reconditioning aerobic fitness. While less than the ideal time, these two tests are still commonly used as 'indicators' and are useful for patients requiring a reasonable level of general fitness. For sportspersons and those patients requiring higher levels of occupational fitness, the following two tests are more applicable:

The Timed 20-Minute Run/Cycle

The patient runs or cycles on a track or measured course for 20 minutes. The distance covered in that time is measured and recorded. The following gives an indication of comparative levels of fitness according to the distance covered:

Running

>5 km, excellent.
4–5 km, good.
3–4 km, fair.
2–3 km, poor.

Cycling

>10 km, excellent.
8–10 km, good.
6–8 km, fair.
4–6 km, poor.

The Progressive Shuttle Run Test

This test, designed by Ramsbottom and colleagues (1988), has probably become one of the most widely known means of assessing aerobic fitness objectively and simply. The test is a progressive and maximal running programme over a 20 m distance. Each level in the test lasts 1 minute, and there is a slight increase in the speed required to cover the distance during each progressive level. The test is controlled by a prerecorded tape; this is now commercially available. Initially designed to assess an individual's maximum oxygen uptake levels, comparative to those performed on a treadmill, the simplicity of the test has enabled it to be modified and used in all environments. Each level has a predetermined number of shuttles to complete, and provided that the participant maintains the running speed determined by the tape, they are demonstrating an ability to cope with the increasing demands being placed upon them. As soon as the individual fails to reach the turn at the same time as the audiotape 'bleeps', they are withdrawn from the test and the number of levels and shuttles completed is recorded. This then gives an objective level for the person to either equal or beat on subsequent testing.

While this test has only been commercially available for a limited period of time, there are already norms being established from it. In professional soccer within the UK, players performing in the premier league need comfortably to reach the later stages of level 14. This means that they will have been running for a continuous 14 minutes over the 20 m distance, turning each end of the track in time with the tape. At level 1 the time allowed for each 20 m shuttle is approximately 9 seconds, whereas at level 12 this will have reduced to 5 seconds. Although less than the 20 minutes usually recognised as being effective for measuring aerobic capacity, because the test is progressive and maximal it is accepted as a valid measurement of aerobic fitness.

The following can also be regarded as respectable norms, where:

• ≥Level 15, excellent.
• Level 13 or 14, very good.
• Level 12, good.
• Level 11, fair.
• <Level 10, poor.

As with all fitness testing, provided that each test is standardised and repeatable, it can be classified as objective. Utilising any of the above tests as an indicator for the return to unrestricted activities will give the necessary answers to assist the physiotherapist in making the right decision. Obviously, should more scientific tests be required, these can be performed in a human performance laboratory on a treadmill with a gas analyser unit. However, in a rehabilitation environment, this specificity is not usually required, and provided the tests are objective and relevant, they will give the necessary information as to the patient's aerobic fitness. It is therefore essential that the physiotherapist understands the physical requirements of the patient's occupation. It is also useful to have an indicator as to normal levels of fitness. If the patient is unable to attain these normal levels, they are not eligible for discharge and should be returned to the late stage of rehabilitation to work on general cardiovascular/aerobic fitness.

If the answer to the initial questions is yes, then ask:

Does the Patient have the Necessary Skills to Perform Daily Activities?

Whatever the occupation or sport, there is a requirement to perform skills. The longer a patient is away from normal activities, the greater is the risk of losing the necessary co-ordination and ability to execute these skills without having to concentrate excessively. Normally, skills contain reflex actions that are conditioned by hours of repetition. Without this repetition the ability to perform skills in a co-ordinated and reflex manner is lost. After any period of injury and disability, regardless of the length, a patient will progressively lose the physical ability to perform the skills in a co-ordinated manner, although subconsciously they may still feel able to do so. Similarly, where there has been injury with associated joint and muscle problems, the biomechanics of the skill-related activities will also have been affected. If, during the rehabilitation programmes to date, no attention has been paid to simple skill-related exercises relevant to the patient's occupation, the patient will be unable to perform the necessary functions required of their occupation at this stage. This would then put the patient at risk on their return to normal daily activities, as the problems would not have been identified and attended to, hence the necessity for any physiotherapist involved at this stage of the rehabilitation process to have relevant occupational- or sports-specific knowledge. In the sports environment, the physiotherapist should work alongside the coaches to understand what is required by patients on their return to full, unrestricted training. In an occupational/industrial environment, the physiotherapist should ensure that they know what is required by the patients when they return to their normal working activities. There is therefore a need for the physiotherapist to spend time in the workplace, identifying and familiarising themselves with the occupational skills with which the patients need to be competent. For any physiotherapist considering a career in sport, attendance on coaching courses would be extremely beneficial.

If the patient is unable to perform the necessary skills in a co-ordinated and competent manner during this stage of the rehabilitation process, they should be referred back to the late stage so that they can work specifically on these deficiencies. Also, if the patient has had inadequate proprioceptive re-education during the earlier stages of rehabilitation, the deficiencies in performance of the skills will be more dramatically evident in the pre-discharge sessions. This will also need to be addressed by referring the patient back.

If, however, the patient demonstrates a proficient level of skills at this time, then ask:

Does the Patient have the Necessary Anaerobic Fitness Required to Perform Normal Activities?

Anaerobic fitness is the ability to perform exercises or activities independent of oxygen. Glucose is metabolised utilising adenosine triphosphate (ATP) to produce the energy required. The limiting factor in anaerobic fitness is the production of lactic acid, the by-product of anaerobic metabolism. Sports, including squash, soccer and sprint events in athletics, and 'pressure' occupations, for example the police, require high levels of anaerobic fitness. They require an ability to perform short sharp bursts of activity independent of oxygen, and to recover and repeat the activity when called upon. This element of fitness is integral to being able to perform sports such as soccer, rugby, squash and hockey at the highest level.

Poor anaerobic fitness will result in an early production of lactic acid, which can cause muscle pain, vomiting and fatigue; symptoms that individually and collectively affect performance and the patient's ability to cope with the demands placed upon them. This is the reason why modern conditioning work for sport is based upon the concepts of interval training, specific to the requirements of the individual event or game. The police, armed forces, fire service and heavy industry are all occupations that require their employees to perform short sharp bursts of activity on a repetitive basis—the rate of repetition being determined externally rather than internally, i.e. the recovery period is enforced by circumstances, requiring individuals to have the ability to recover adequately to meet the demands placed upon them. Obviously, the consequences of being unable to meet these repetitive demands in sport are not as onerous as those within some of the other occupations mentioned, where a poor anaerobic fitness could result in serious or fatal accidents. Hence, anaerobic fitness is a component of fitness that is extremely important not only in sport but also in many occupations.

Once again, this is an element of fitness with which physiotherapists concerned with this stage of rehabilitation must be aware. It is even more important that they understand the specificity of this type of fitness relative to the sport, occupation or industry for which their patients are being rehabilitated. Once more, a knowledge of normal levels of fitness will assist in assessing patients and planning their rehabilitation programmes. At this stage it will also ensure that appropriate anaerobic tests are performed to determine the patient's capabilities. Wherever possible, these tests should be performed in an environment similar to the one to which the patient will be returning. For sports patients, these tests should be performed in either a training or competitive environment, and for industrial patients, in a simulated work environment. There is a formidable range of activities that can be utilised to test anaerobic fitness. However, all activities must be appropriate to the ultimate needs of the patient and relative to the activities to which they are returning.

Ideally, the physiotherapist dealing with occupation- or sports-specific patients should try to obtain baseline data from fit subjects to derive the 'norms' for the special tests in this part of the rehabilitation programme. This ensures that any decisions made are objective rather than subjective. Should the patient fail at any time to meet the demands placed upon them, i.e. by not recovering or not being able to perform the tests required, deficiencies will have been exposed. The patient should then be referred back to the late stage of rehabilitation so that they can work on increasing their anaerobic fitness before returning to the pre-discharge group at a later date. To expect patients to regain this element of fitness in their sport, training or normal working environment is usually unrealistic. As stated earlier, the potential for serious problems is greater if the patient is allowed to return to unrestricted activities with poor anaerobic fitness. They will not be able to cope with the demands placed upon them, putting themselves and colleagues at risk. It is also worth pointing out that it is not only the patient's ability to recover during the session that should be assessed, but also their condition the following day. If the exercises and activities have been excessive and the patient's body is unable to clear the acidosis, they may have muscular stiffness and pain the following morning. If they are then unable to clear these symptoms with submaximal exercise and to reproduce the previous day's session, they must be classified as unfit to return to unrestricted activities. In their normal working or training activities, the patient would be expected to perform on consecutive days, so if they lack the ability to recover to reproduce the activity levels of the previous day, they would be unable to meet the demands of normal unrestricted activities. This is why it is important, wherever possible, to schedule pre-discharge assessment sessions on 2–3 consecutive days so that this component can be assessed realistically. After all, it is pointless only being able to work without problems on 1 day and to require 2 days for recovery before repeating that work! This is a very important consideration and one that is all too frequently neglected or overlooked.

If, however, the patient demonstrates that there are no deficiencies in their anaerobic fitness, then ask:

Has the Patient Recovered Psychologically from the Trauma?

After a major trauma, patients can suffer a flashback, or *déjà vu*, if there are conditions similar to those from which the original injury or trauma was caused. This means that if the patient has sustained a serious injury from a major traumatic incident and similar circumstances arise in the future, the patient can experience a psychological 'flashback' syndrome. If this should occur at a crucial time during a sporting or occupational situation, the consequences could be serious. It is therefore imperative that within the pre-discharge stage of rehabilitation, activities are introduced to identify whether this is a potential problem area which needs to be addressed. If, for example, the patient sustained a fractured tibia and fibula from the direct violence of a tackle in football, then the first time similar circumstances arose, that player's performance and total attitude could be affected adversely. Similarly, if the patient suffered an occupational accident, then the first time they returned to that or a similar environment, their psychological wellbeing and performance could be affected adversely unless the physiotherapist understands and addresses the concept of 'post-traumatic stress'. These problems can only be negated in the later stages of rehabilitation if the physiotherapist is aware of the circumstances under which the patient's injuries were sustained. Similar activities are then introduced to erase potential psychological problems from the patient's subconscious.

In the case of miners involved in accidents underground, it is usually only on return to the work that psychological problems are identified. Normally, these patients show no physical or psychological problems in the rehabilitation environment; instead, the problems tend to recur on return to the surroundings in which the accident occurred. Furthermore, it seems that the greater the trauma, the more extensive the psychological problems that need to be negated.

In rehabilitation, the physiotherapist should have a knowledge of the mechanics of the injury and the environment in which it was caused. Then, within the late stages of rehabilitation, similar circumstances should be set up and the patient progressively taken through them. By repeating the activity and not experiencing similar problems, the patient's fears and worries can be overcome. However, if there are environmental considerations, such as the fear of going back underground, being in a car, or going into a particular sporting place, these elements should also be introduced as part of the rehabilitation programme. In rehabilitation, the aim is to help patients overcome their fears and problems, and assist them in realising that the chance of re-injury is unlikely.

In the pre-discharge stage of rehabilitation, the aim is to expose any deficiencies in this area and reproduce and highlight any subconscious or psychological fears of the patient. If these are exposed, then the patient must be returned to the late stage of rehabilitation to enable the physiotherapist to identify and overcome these problems. Hence, it is necessary for the pre-discharge programme to plan activities and sessions similar to those to which patients are aiming to return. The activities should also be undertaken in surroundings similar to those to which the patient will return. Also, timing should correspond to the normal as much as possible, in both length and time of day. For example, if the patient is a footballer who is required to train every morning, from 10.00 a.m. to 12 noon, the pre-discharge assessment sessions should be of a similar time and duration and on an outside football pitch. If, however, the patient is a factory worker who is required to start work at 7.00 a.m., then, wherever possible, this should be a criterion for planning the session. It is only when the patient undertakes these simulation sessions and activities that any real deficiencies will be identified and exposed. When patients have successfully completed this type of programme, their confidence and self-esteem are confirmed and enhanced. Patients are then able to return to unrestricted activities without any fears or problems.

Sadly, this is a component of functional rehabilitation that is frequently ignored. If missed, problems may not manifest until circumstances similar to those surrounding the original injury recur. This may not happen for a long time; however, when it does, the implications and resulting consequences can be serious. It is an area that must be addressed both in the formal rehabilitation programmes and in the pre-discharge assessment sessions, albeit in different ways. In the formal rehabilitation programmes, the patient is helped to overcome the associated anxieties, fears and worries, and in the pre-discharge assessment sessions, any residual deficiencies and psychological problems are identified and exposed. It is only by doing this that patients can be classified as having 'recovered psychologically' from their injuries and trauma.

If the patient has recovered psychologically on completion of treatment, then the physiotherapist will have positive answers to the questions:
- Has the injury recovered?
- Has the patient the necessary aerobic fitness to perform normal activities?
- Has the patient the skills necessary to perform normal activities?

- Has the patient the anaerobic fitness necessary to perform normal activities?
- Has the patient recovered psychologically from the injury or trauma?

If the answer to any of these questions is negative, the patient must be reclassified and referred back to the appropriate level of the rehabilitation programme so that the deficiencies can be worked upon and eliminated. If the answer to all the questions is positive, then the patient can be returned to full, unrestricted activities safely and confidently; in the case of the sports patient this would be the return to unrestricted training, and for the occupational or industrial patient this would mean the return to all normal, unrestricted daily activities, without fear and with confidence.

While the programme above typifies the aim of all physiotherapists concerned with rehabilitation, sadly, functional rehabilitation is a discipline being eroded and neglected. Regardless of the reasons, whether political, financial or educational, it is something with which all medical and paramedical practitioners should be concerned.

CONCLUSION

The principles of rehabilitation can be modified and applied to all categories of patients regardless of age, disability or background. Clearly, the more dynamic or physical the demands to be placed upon the patient, then the more comprehensive and intense the rehabilitation programme should be. Likewise, by applying the criteria defined in the pre-discharge stage, patients can be classified objectively and safely as fit. This should dispel any fears or worries the patient may have on discharge when only part of the rehabilitation process has been completed.

Economically and sociologically the demands placed upon limited rehabilitation resources will ultimately be reduced if patients are subjected to comprehensive programmes earlier. Too often the patient only receives a small part of the rehabilitation process, and is expected to undertake the remainder unsupervised. While this may seem reasonable for patients whose physical and psychological expectations are low, it is not acceptable for those requiring higher levels of occupational and industrial fitness. Unfortunately, patients who do require higher levels of occupational and industrial fitness still rarely receive a rehabilitation commitment compatible with their needs and expectations.

Rehabilitation is a major and important part of physical medicine. By definition, it is the restoration of function, and the return to the previous normal condition wherever possible. The ultimate aim should be to achieve this in the shortest, safest, possible time. By applying the principles above, and demonstrating integrity, commitment, dedication and a professional willingness to listen and learn, these aims can be achieved safely and effectively. The physiotherapist will also experience high levels of job satisfaction and professional pride.

Rehabilitation should be interesting and fun, both for patients and for practitioners. Hopefully, some of the main problems and pitfalls commonly encountered when planning rehabilitation programmes have been highlighted. This chapter has clarified the rationale for each stage of the rehabilitation programme, as well as identifying the criteria for the planning of those stages and the progress of patients through them. While not detailing specific programmes, an overview of the main principles and considerations have been given, which should enable the physiotherapist to develop their own individual autonomy within this exciting field of physical medicine. By applying the principles outlined, the physiotherapist will be able to plan rehabilitation programmes specific to the patient's needs, encompassing the patient's particular circumstances.

Patients present with problems. It is the physiotherapist's responsibility to identify these problems and to educate the patient to overcome them safely, effectively and comprehensively through the rehabilitation process.

FULL TIME REHABILITATION PROGRAMME - SAMPLE TIMETABLE

The key points are outlined in Table 19.1.

New Patient Assessments
Patients are assessed by the physiotherapist and doctor to identify the problems that will need to be addressed during the week's rehabilitation programme. Medical fitness is also determined, and patients classified according to their relevant rehabilitation level.

Individual Programmes
Patients are assigned their own specific programmes. These programmes will include designated mobilising, strengthening and proprioceptive exercises for their injured limbs. They will also include any therapeutic modalities required in addition to 'hands-on' physical therapy. The programmes are specific to the treatment and rehabilitation of injuries and injured limbs.

Circuit Training
These sessions form part of the general fitness programmes. Each circuit should be designed to allow the patient to work all of the non-injured parts of the body. Circuits should be modified according to the patient's disabilities. These circuits may be competitive, e.g. one versus one, two versus two, sports/occupational specific or designed to meet each patients individual needs. Where the physiotherapist is looking for quality, exercises in the circuit should have clearly defined goals and targets. Where 'fun' and hard work are required, circuits should be competitive. Different programmes should be used during each circuit training session to avoid boredom and repetition.

Remedial Games
Remedial games are used in rehabilitation programmes to assist in 'team building' and group dynamics. The sessions

	Monday	Tuesday	Wednesday	Thursday	Friday
Full-time rehabilitation programme - sample timetable					
Morning					
09.00-09.15	New patient assessments	Warm-ups	Warm-ups	Warm-ups	Warm-ups
09.15-10.30		Individual programmes	Bikes	Individual programmes	Bikes
10.30-11.00	**Break**	**Break**	**Break**	**Break**	**Break**
11.00-12.30	Individual programmes	Hydrotherapy, swimming	Individual programmes	Hydrotherapy, swimming	Individual programmes
Afternoon					
1.45-3.15	Circuit training	Individual programmes	Circuit training	Individual programmes	Reassessments 'Decisions'
3.15-3.30	**Break**	**Break**	**Break**	**Break**	
3.30-4.45	Remedial games	Remedial games	Remedial games	Remedial games	
4.45-5.00	Individual treatments	Individual treatments	Individual treatments	Individual treatments	

Table 19.1 Within the programme presented components are adjusted to the level of fitness of participants i.e. to intermediate and late stage.

also add an element of fun and camaraderie to the programmes. While the games are obviously fun, they are classified as exercise sessions and, as such, should help to restore confidence and general fitness. Every group member should be able to participate in the remedial games; the games must be appropriate to the group member with the greatest disability. In the early stages of rehabilitation, the games will be less dynamic than during the later stages. The physiotherapist must maintain control of the patients at all times during the remedial games. Appropriate remedial games for the different levels of rehabilitation include:
- Sit-down cricket.
- Sit-down volleyball.
- Carpet bowls.

The physiotherapist should not be limited by the patient's disabilities, and the patient should be able to adapt as required.

Individual Treatments
At the end of each day, the patient should be given a cursory assessment to ensure that none of the activities have provoked problems or exacerbated previous symptoms. This is a short session which allows the patient to be checked and treated before leaving rehabilitation for the day. It is also allows the physiotherapist to give advice and to instruct on activities during the evening.

Warm-Ups
Each day should start with a short warm-up period. The aim of this session is to prepare the patient for the day's activities. It is also an opportunity to assess the patient for any residual stiffness or problems caused by the previous day's activities. These warm-up sessions can be taken as exercise to music or as formal 'stretching' and loosening programmes. A combination of the two, alternated each day, is ideal and is more beneficial for both the patient and the physiotherapist.

Hydrotherapy or Swimming
The hydrotherapy or swimming pool can be utilised as:
- A medium in which to perform formal exercise programmes which may include walking re-education sessions.
- A medium in which to maintain and/or improve general fitness. These sessions will contain a combination of aerobic and anaerobic activities.
- A medium in which to play remedial games and meet the competitive needs of the patients, safely and effectively. Races, games and swimming activities can be incorporated.

Bicycles
Indoor and outdoor bicycles can be used in the rehabilitation programme to maintain and improve cardiovascular and general fitness. The programmes can include group

rides over long distances, e.g. 12–15 miles, aiming either for a time target or for improving aerobic fitness. Shorter sprint-type activities can be incorporated for anaerobic fitness conditioning. For patients in the early stages of rehabilitation, indoor static bicycles can be used and, where appropriate, single-leg activities on the non-injured limb should maintain or improve cardiovascular fitness.

Reassessments and Decisions

Patients are reassessed at the end of the week by the physiotherapist and doctor (if available). Reassessment should identify and confirm improvements, or deterioration, and allow the physiotherapist and the patient the opportunity for re-evaluation of problems. At the end of the session, a decision will need to be made about whether:

- The patient has now reached the stage where progression to the next part of the rehabilitation process can be permitted.
- The patient has not improved significantly, and further time at this rehabilitation level is required to consolidate recovery.
- The patient has been unable to cope with the demands of this stage of the rehabilitation programme, and symptoms and problems have exacerbated. The patient should therefore be reassessed for possible referral to an earlier stage of the programme.

It should be emphasised that patients are reassessed at the end of an intense period of work, and that the weekend will give an opportunity to recover from this. It is often appropriate to reassess the patient at the start of the following week, to confirm previous assessments and classification. Where patients are being discharged and are unable to return for full-time rehabilitation the following week, they should be given clear instructions and advice about continuing the programme at home. While this situation is obviously not desirable, unfortunately it often occurs. Advice and instructions to the patient should be written down, and a copy sent to the patient's doctor and/or physiotherapist.

PRE-DISCHARGE REHABILITATION PROGRAMME – SAMPLE TIMETABLE

The key points are outlined in Table 19.2.

PRE-DISCHARGE GROUP

Assessments and Re-evaluation

Patients referred to this group have met the criteria necessary for this final functional stage of the rehabilitation programme. The aim of the pre-discharge stage is to identify any deficiencies, so patients must have reached the point where they are able to cope with the demands that will be placed upon them. In the assessment session, the physiotherapist must determine that all injuries have recovered, and that the patient has successfully completed the late stage of rehabilitation before being passed on to this group. If at any time during evaluation the physiotherapist

believes that the patient is not ready to embark upon the pre-discharge programme, the patient should be referred back for further rehabilitation.

Bicycles

Outdoor bicycles are used in the pre-discharge stage for general fitness work. The session can be:

- Aerobic, i.e. long sustained work over a given distance. Distances can vary between 12 and 18 km. Patients must either complete the distance in a given time, or as quickly as they are able.
- Anaerobic, i.e. short, sharp, sprint activities, either individually or in pairs. Each sprint lasts no longer than 4 or 5 minutes and is followed by a fixed period of recovery before repeating the sprint. Five to 10 repetitions of the sprint would be appropriate.
- Competitive, e.g. team relays, paired activities or time trials.

Remedial Games

The remedial games sessions in the pre-discharge stage are obviously more dynamic than in the earlier stages but should still be tightly controlled. They are used for recreation and to build team spirit and group dynamics. Suggested games include volleyball, head tennis, rounders, bowls and badminton. Sit-down games can also be utilised in this stage, purely for fun and to assist the physiotherapist in controlling the group.

Walk or Run

Patients whose occupation or sport requires that they should run, should cover 6–10 km, normally at a sustained submaximal pace. Other patients should undertake walks of 4–6 km. It is also useful to introduce fartlek-type activities during this session. 'Fartlek' is a Swedish term meaning speed-play. It is a type of training where participants vary speed according to their mood as they run over a given course. Speed may be increased or decreased at given targets and for specific distances, although it is usual for the runner to determine individual points of change.

End-of-Day Assessments (Warm Down)

At the end of each day, specific time needs to be set aside to check the patient and ensure that none of the activities during the day have exacerbated any problems or exposed deficiencies. A gentle programme of warm-down exercises should be introduced from the second day. The specific stretching exercises should be identical to those performed in the warm-up session at the start of the day. Any significant differences in stretching ability during this session compared with the start of the day, could indicate fatigue and be the first sign that the patient is tiring and unable to cope with the demands of the programme. The physiotherapist must then reassess the patient during the warm-up session the following morning to ensure that flexibility has been recovered. If flexibility has not returned, it confirms that the patient has not recovered and is 'at risk'.

Pre-discharge rehabilitation programme - sample full-time timetable					
	Day 1	Day 2	Day 3	Day 4	Day 5
Morning					
09.00-09.15	Assessments Re-evaluation	Warm-ups	Warm-ups	Warm-ups	Warm-ups
09.15-10.15		Circuit training	Bikes (anaerobic)	Circuit training	Bikes (competitive)
10.15-10.45	**Break**	**Break**	**Break**	**Break**	**Break**
10.45-12.30	Bikes (aerobic)	Pre-discharge 'work hardening session'	Pre-discharge 'work hardening session'	Pre-discharge 'work hardening session'	Assessments 'decisions'
Afternoon					
1.45-3.00	Remedial games	Swimming	Remedial games	Swimming	
3.00-3.15	**Break**	**Break**	**Break**	**Break**	
3.15-4.45	Walk/run	Remedial games	Walk/run	Remedial games	
4.45-5.00	End-of-day assessments	End-of-day assessments (warm down)	End-of-day assessments (warm down)	End-of-day assessments (warm down)	

Table 19.2 An example of a treatment programme for patients in the pre-discharge phase.

Warm-Ups

Each day should commence with a warm-up session. The aims of this session are, firstly, to prepare patients for all the activities into which they are going to be entered during the day and, secondly, to assess their recovery from the previous day's programme. It is imperative that a specific programme of stretching exercises is performed in this session and that the physiotherapist monitors each patient individually and carefully. If the patient is unable to maintain the degree of flexibility shown in earlier sessions, this indicates that fatigue is present and the patient is at risk. Whereas the warm-up sessions in the main rehabilitation programme are 'fun', at this stage they fulfil an important assessment and monitoring role.

Circuit Training

The circuit training sessions are general fitness, non-specific activities. They should, however, be endurance based rather than strength training programmes. The emphasis is on general fitness work and 'fun' rather than specific conditioning.

Pre-discharge Work Hardening Session

These are the periods in a week where the patient is subjected to a hard, final functional occupational- or sports-specific programme, similar to the activities and environment to which the patient will return. It is a session during which the patient must cope with all the demands presented, and one during which any deficiencies exposed

will result in the patient's reassessment and re-categorisation. Wherever possible, the session should replicate the demands of the working environment.

Swimming

Swimming is used as a pleasant, recreational activity, and as a means of working the whole body. Water is a medium that gives both assistance and resistance to exercise. Sessions are used as an alternative to the other gymnasium- and training-related activities. They also provide a medium in which submaximal and maximal activities can be performed without placing unnecessary torsional weight-bearing stresses and strains through the joints of the body.

Assessments and Decisions

By the end of the week, all the patients are reassessed and decisions are made about what they should do next. All patients who reach this part of the week without the exposure of any deficiencies, can be classified as fit to return to unrestricted and normal activities. They are advised to allow 36 to 48 hours recovery before returning to these 'normal' activities. Anyone reaching this point can be discharged with confidence.

For those patients with exposed deficiencies or problems, a decision needs to be made as to whether they should return to an earlier stage of the rehabilitation programme or be reassessed after a period of rest. Exposure of deficiencies indicates that the patients have not completed their rehabilitation programme. This should be completed before the patients are referred back to the pre-discharge group. At this point it is worth emphasising that the pre-discharge stage of rehabilitation is concerned with assessing the patient's capabilities and abilities to return to normal activities, and is not part of the formal rehabilitative process. Patients who cannot cope with the demands of the programme must be referred back to the appropriate level of the rehabilitation programme.

Finally, it must be emphasised that patients ideally spend only 1 week in this group and never more than 2 weeks. If they have been progressed to this stage appropriately, then it will serve either to confirm their readiness to return to unrestricted activities or to expose any deficiencies remaining. Therefore, during the final assessment, a decision can be made. If the session is used by patients and physiotherapists as a rehabilitation stage, it will not achieve its aims. There is also the danger that patients who spends too long in this group will be exposed to more risks and the possibility of either re-injury or problems elsewhere. This is often due to the accumulative effects of the physical demands placed upon them during the programme. It is an assessment programme only, not a rehabilitation and training programme.

GENERAL READING

American Academy of Orthopedic Surgeons. *Athletic training and sports medicine*, 2nd ed. Illinois: American Academy of Orthopedic Surgeons; 1991.

Andrews JR, Harrelson GL. *Physical rehabilitation of the injured athlete*. Philadelphia: WB Saunders; 1990.

Brunkner P, Khan K. *Clinical sports medicine*. Sydney: McGraw-Hill; 1993.

Peterson L, Renstrom P. *Sports injuries: their prevention and treatment*. Chicago: Year Book Medical Publishers; 1986.

Prentice WE. *Rehabilitation techniques in sports medication*. St Louis: Mosby; 1990.

Roy S, Irvin R. *Sports medicine: prevention, evaluation, management and rehabilitation*. New Jersey: Prentice-Hall; 1983.

Sharkey BJ. *Physiology of fitness*, 3rd ed. Illinois: Human Kinetics; 1990.

Smith GN. Sports injury clinic. In: *Rehabilitation*. London: Pelham Books; 1987.

Torg JS, Vegso JJ, Torg E. *Rehabilitation of athletic injuries. An atlas of therapeutic exercise*. Chicago: Year Book Medical Publishers; 1987.

Wilmore JH, Costil DL. *Training for sport and activity*, 3rd ed. Illinois: Human Kinetics; 1993.

Wilmore JH, Costil DL. *Physiology of sport and exercise*. Illinois: Human Kinetics; 1994.

Zuluaga, et al. (1995) *Sports physiotherapy–applied science and practice*. Edinburgh: Churchill Livingstone; 1995.

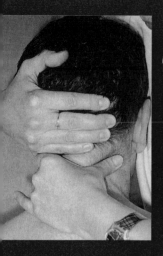

20 A Leigh

AN INTRODUCTION TO NAGs, SNAGs AND MWMs

CHAPTER OUTLINE

- Mulligan's approach to spinal and peripheral mobilisations
- The spine

- Special therapies
- Peripheral joints
- Possible theories

INTRODUCTION

Brian Mulligan is an innovative manual physiotherapist who has been prolific in developing many new physiotherapy techniques. These have evolved over the past 25 years and, because of their efficacy, have become very popular with manual physiotherapists and with patients.

Mulligan has proposed various theories to explain the effectiveness of these techniques and these are discussed below. A description of Mulligan's techniques are also given.

This chapter concentrates on the spine and the peripheral joints. Essentially, all the techniques used for both spinal and peripheral joint treatments fall under the two headings of passive accessory movements alone and passive accessory movements combined with active physiological movements.

MULLIGAN'S APPROACH TO SPINAL AND PERIPHERAL MOBILISATIONS

The following are common guidelines for treating the spine and peripheral joints:
- All techniques are repeated 6–10 times (Mulligan, 1995a).
- All techniques are painless.
- All techniques should provide immediate improvement in the level of pain and in the range of movement or function.

Where end-range stiffness is the sole or most significant problem, passive overpressure can be applied at the end of the active range without release of the accessory glide. This is also pain free and can be applied by the patient or the physiotherapist. Mulligan refers to this overpressure as 'the cream on the milk'.

Exercise, strapping, postural advice and patient self-management strategies are all important supporting procedures.

THE SPINE

There are four main technique concepts when dealing with the spine (Mulligan, 1995a). These are:
- Weight-bearing passive accessory movements applied on their own to the cervical and upper thoracic spine. They are called natural apophyseal glides (NAGs) and reversed natural apophyseal glides (RNAGs).
- Weight-bearing passive accessory movements combined with active spinal physiological movements. This technique is an accessory glide applied to a spinal segment with a concurrent active physiological movement that is sustained at the end of range. Mulligan believes this affects the apophyseal joints and therefore is a sustained natural apophyseal glide (SNAG).
- Passive accessory movements applied to the spine combined with active physiological movements of the limbs. These include mobilisation with movement (MWM) for pain of spinal origin (PSO) referred to the limb. For pain

referred to the upper limb, it is called spinal mobilisation with arm movement (SMWAM); similarly, for pain referred to the lower limb, it is called spinal mobilisation with leg movement (SMWLM).

- Special therapies. These include techniques applied for headache, vertigo and dizziness. Also to be included under this heading is a technique Mulligan has called cervical positional SNAG.

Mulligan treatments for acute wry neck and the technique of fist traction are not included in this text.

SELECTION OF APPROPRIATE SPINAL LEVEL

The choice of level for application of the treatment technique is achieved by a number of recognised methods, used singly or in combination. The choice takes account of the symptom area ('dermatome'), the areas of movement restriction and the accessory joint feel.

Symptom Area ('Dermatome')

It is understood that the area displaying symptoms frequently does not fit with true dermatomal area determinations, (previously damaged nerve root or pressure applied to dorsal root ganglion), but more often arising from non-dermatomal somatic structures. For Mulligan, however, the use of dermatome guidelines is an initial point of reference, and several areas will be palpated for dysfunction and the most effective result. For example, for pain present over the shoulder girdle and deltoid, possibly mobilise C3/4 segments. The palpation technique is the same as the treatment technique.

Areas of Movement Restriction

This involves the recognition of hypomobile areas that could feasibly be the source of the symptoms.

Accessory Joint Feel

Although the possible range of movement that can be produced is important, it is the quality of the through range and end-of-range feel that more significantly guides the manual physiotherapist towards suspecting fault at one or more levels.

FACTORS COMMON TO ALL TECHNIQUES WHEN APPLIED TO THE SPINE

When techniques are applied to the spine, there are certain factors common to those techniques. These are that:

- The techniques are applied along the facet plane, i.e. along the orientation of the spinal facet joint. The angle of application of the technique is different for each level of the spine, and even differs on either side of the spine. For example, at the C2/3 level, the facet plane is horizontal, whereas at T5/6, the facets are angled more acutely. If the technique is appropriate and applied correctly, however, it will be a painless procedure which will improve the patient's signs and symptoms.

- Techniques are applied centrally to the spine as well as unilaterally. Benefit is gained from minor adjustments of the inclination of the applied pressure, e.g. caudally/cranially or medially/laterally. In general, central techniques should be applied initially, progressing to unilateral techniques. In any treatment session, the selection of central or unilateral techniques is based on the patient's response, i.e. is the effect within the physiotherapist's expectations for the present clinical situation?

- The techniques are applied with the patient either sitting or standing.

- The maximum grade of pain-free mobilisation is used. Generally, this is a large range, approximately equivalent to Maitland mobilisations of grades II–III (Maitland, 1986). It is possible to apply the treatment using Maitland's guidelines (Maitland 1986). In the author of this chapter's experience, it is also possible to successfully extend the mobilisations and apply them as combined movements (Edwards, 1984, 1992).

NATURAL APOPHYSEAL GLIDE

This technique is applied directly to a selected cervical or upper thoracic segment; C2–T2/3, or C2–T4 if control can be maintained. It is a mid-to-late range, pain-free oscillatory technique applied centrally over the spinous process or unilaterally over the facet joint. For the C5/6 segment, for example, when applied centrally, mobilisation of the C5 segment on the C6 segment produces a flexion or posterior gapping force; when applied unilaterally, mobilisation of the inferior facet of the C5 segment on the superior facet of the C6 segment produces a flexion or unilateral posterior gapping force on the side of the application.

Physiotherapist's Position

The physiotherapist's arm is cradled lightly around the patient's head at the level of the upper jaw, taking care not to block the patient's breathing or crush the skull (Figure 20.1 and Figure 20.2A). The fifth finger of the cradling arm is placed around the spinous process of the vertebra at the level chosen for treatment. For example, where the problem is identified at the level of C5/6, the fifth finger is placed around the spinous process of C5 for a central mobilisation (see Figure 20.2A). The physiotherapist's trunk is used to control the patient's position. (Consideration should be given to the patient's comfort in this close positioning.)

Patient's Position

The patient sits in an optimum position for posture and comfort and, where possible, the plinth height is altered to enable the physiotherapist to implement treatment. If the patient displays an antalgic posture, the positioning and application of the technique should accommodate this posture and not try to correct it. As the antalgic posture improves with treatment, the positions of the patient and physiotherapist, and the techniques, are adjusted accordingly.

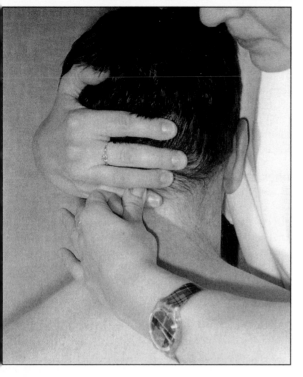

Figure 20.1 Starting position for the NAG.

Physiotherapist's Action

Pressure is applied to the middle interphalangeal joint of the fifth finger of the cradling arm (see Figure 20.1 and Figure 20.2B). This pressure is usually applied by a suggested 'flick grip', although there are a number of other methods, for example, using the hypo- or hyperthenar eminence. The technique is applied to the facet plane of the chosen vertebral segment. Movement of the patient is resisted by the physiotherapist's trunk.

REVERSED NATURAL APOPHYSEAL GLIDE

The principles of practice and guidelines for use for the NAG are appropriate for the RNAG. The only difference is the site of pressure application for the mobilisation.

For the C5/6 segment, the fifth finger of the cradling arm is again placed around the spinous process of C5. The mobilisation, however, is applied to C6. In this case, C6 is moving up under C5, or C5 is moving relatively backwards over C6. This movement causes an extension or compression of the C5/6 segment. Unilateral mobilisations are applied in a similar way, i.e. over the C6 articular pillar in this example.

INDICATIONS FOR USE

The decision to use the NAG or the RNAG is based on the more frequent success of the NAG. Mulligan suggests

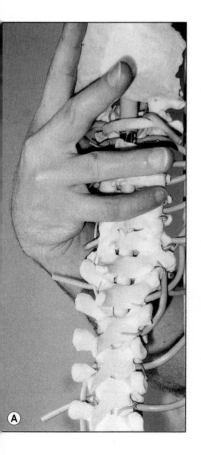

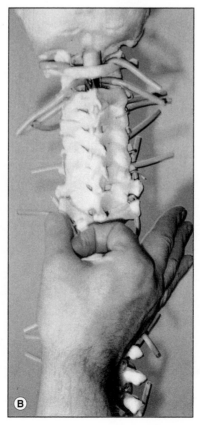

Figure 20.2 Application of the NAG technique. Position of (**A**) the fifth finger of the cradling arm and (**B**) the flick grip in position for the technique.

that eight out of 10 patients respond to the NAG, the remaining two patients requiring the RNAG. It is possible to apply the technique with respect to the movement dysfunction, i.e. a NAG for a flexion (stretch) dysfunction and a RNAG for an extension (compression) dysfunction (Edwards, 1992).

Both techniques are applied to patients with acute, subacute or chronic conditions. They are also valuable techniques for the reduction of the soreness that follows treatment using SNAGs or manipulations (high-velocity thrust).

SUSTAINED NATURAL APOPHYSEAL GLIDE

SNAGs can be applied centrally or unilaterally to all spinal joints between C2 and L5. These techniques are passive accessory movements combined with an active physiological movement. This combination of movements is unique in manual therapy. Following assessment, treatment is applied to restore lost range of movement and to reduce the pain provoked by active movement. The patient is instructed to perform the painful, restricted movement chosen for treatment, and the appropriate central or unilateral technique is selected. Almost invariably, there is more than one movement requiring treatment.

Clear instruction is required regarding the speed of performance, the need to sustain the end position, and the commands given, i.e. 'go', 'hold' and 'return'. Most importantly, patients must perform the forward and return movements actively. Self-treatments can be taught, but are not included in this text.

Physiotherapist's Position

The physiotherapist stands behind the patient, with their feet and body positioned to perform the accessory glide effectively (Figure 20.3A). The physiotherapist's thumbs are positioned over the spinous process of the vertebra at the chosen level for central mobilisation, or over the articular pillar for unilateral mobilisation. For example, for the level of T8/9, pressure is applied to the spinous process or articular pillar of T8.

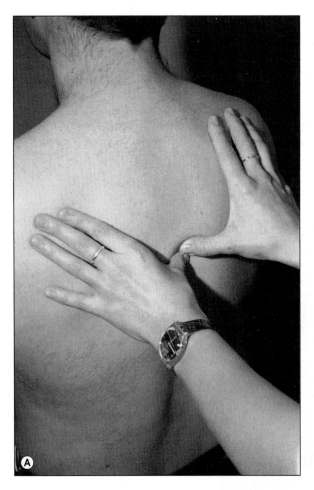
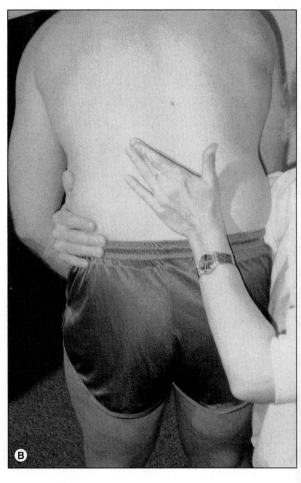

Figure 20.3 Starting position for the SNAG when (A) sitting and (B) standing.

Patient's Position

The patient can be sitting or standing. In the seated position, the patient may need to be stabilised on the couch using a seatbelt. The technique can be applied quite strongly, and the patient should be positioned carefully to facilitate localisation of the technique. The seatbelt may be used when applying thoracic or lumbar SNAGs in standing, or the physiotherapist may use their trunk to stabilise the patient's position (Figure 20.3B). The choice of position is based on that which will promote the best effect for the patient and be most effectively controlled by the physiotherapist.

Physiotherapist's and Patient's Action

On the command 'go', the patient performs the required physiological movement in the manner taught, e.g. thoracic rotation and lumbar flexion. Simultaneously, the physiotherapist performs a central or unilateral accessory mobilisation at the chosen level. The SNAG is performed to the end of the pain-free range and sustained for 1 or 2 seconds. The patient is then asked to return actively to the starting position. It is important that the physiotherapist encourages the accessory movement along the line of the facet joint, to achieve the end of the available range. This necessitates the physiotherapist moving their body with the accessory movement. The starting position and movement of the physiotherapist are important in producing a pain-free glide.

Accuracy in treatment is essential. It may be observed that the thoracic spine remains relatively still, while the lumbar spine or hip joints may be areas most readily used in the patient's compensated or 'normal' movement patterns. Therefore, movement should be encouraged where it is lost, not where the patient habitually moves. The thoracic spine is notoriously absent from our body image.

MOBILISATION WITH MOVEMENT FOR PAIN OF SPINAL ORIGIN

These are accessory movements applied to the spine, with physiological movements of the limbs (SMWAMs, SMWLMs) performed simultaneously (Figure 20.4A and B). These techniques are used when symptoms displayed

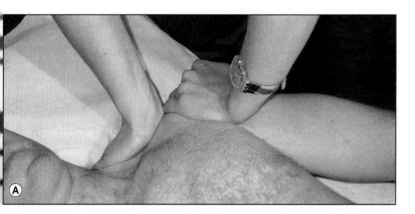

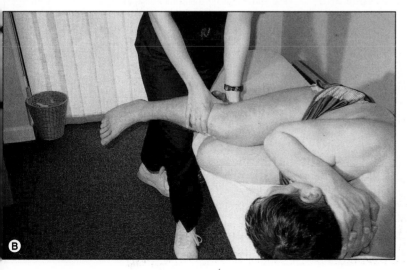

Figure 20.4 (A) Upper limb MWM for PSO (spinal mobilisation with arm movement). (B) Lower limb MWM for PSO.

in the limb are suspected to have been referred from the spine. There may also be pain in the spine or it may be felt in the limb alone. These techniques may also be applied if there are 'light' neurological symptoms or symptoms believed to be related to altered neurodynamics (Butler & Gifford, 1989, 1994; Butler, 1991; Shacklock, 1995). As with all spine-based treatments, the choice of level can be based on dermatome segmental referral, appropriate accessory feel—and response—or the subjective or objective immediate improvement or worsening seen on application of the technique. Figure 20.4A and B shows an example of the technique applied to a joint in the upper and lower limb respectively. Self-treatments can be taught but are not included in this text.

Physiotherapist's Position
The physiotherapist stands behind or to one side of the patient.

Patient's Position
The patient can be sitting or standing.

Physiotherapist's Action
A lateral (transverse) glide to the spinous process of a chosen spinal segment is applied, usually away from the side of limb symptoms. The pressure is maintained while the patient performs the physiological symptomatic movement, e.g. a painful arc during shoulder abduction or pain during a straight leg raise. The symptoms and quality of the movement should improve immediately. It is then possible to show the patient how to perform the treatment at home. If the mobilisation away from the side of the symptoms does not work, then a lateral glide towards the symptoms can be attempted. Several segments above and below the suspected level should be investigated to identify the most useful and effective level for treatment. In isolated situations, two levels require a lateral glide. These may be applied in the same or in opposite directions.

Patient's Action
The patient is directed to perform exactly the physiological movement that is hypomobile or responsible for symptom production. Instruction should, as with the spinal SNAG, include the commands that will be given and the expected response to the treatment.

SPECIAL THERAPIES

TECHNIQUES APPLIED FOR HEADACHE
These include four techniques—one performed by the patient and the remainder by the physiotherapist. The techniques are only applied when the patient has a headache, and should, as with all Mulligan treatments, bring rapid relief, otherwise the technique should be abandoned.

The four techniques are:
- The headache SNAG.
- The reversed headache SNAG.

- Fist traction.
- Upper cervical traction.

The reader should note that self-treatments are excluded from this text, as are the techniques of fist traction and upper cervical traction.

Headache SNAG
Physiotherapist's Position
This is the same as for the NAG. The technique is applied to the C2 segment. C2 moves anteriorly under C0/1 (Figure 20.5A).

Patient's Position
This is the same as for the NAG.

Physiotherapist's Action
The biceps or the forearm of the cradling arm should now act as a fixator to movement of the head. When performing the NAG for C3–T2/3, the cradling arm does not resist the movement of the head. The headache SNAG is applied centrally or unilaterally to C2 with great care, moving slowly to the end of the range, and sustained for at least 10 seconds. The technique is not a true SNAG in that there is no active physiological movement, but it is sustained. The technique may also be applied where 'woolly' sensations are complained of in the head, or where there are low-grade symptoms which have no overt neurological or arterial source. The overriding remit is that the pain or symptom reduces during the application and the patient derives benefit from the treatment.

Mulligan has proposed several techniques that are successfully applied to the upper cervical spine for a variety of neuromusculoskeletal-based symptoms. It should still be a prerequisite that the patient has no confirmed vertebral artery signs that are due to arterial disease, or severe mechanical dysfunction or sensitivity. It is advisable that the upper cervical spine ligament stability tests are performed before treatment (Aspinall, 1990; Beeton, 1995). There is always a need to apply these techniques with extreme care and to be wary of potential situations where instability may be present, e.g. in Downs syndrome and rheumatoid arthritis.

Reversed Headache SNAG
This technique is the reverse of the headache SNAG. C1/2 is fixed and C0 glides forward and is sustained at the end of the range (Figure 20.5B). It is important that considerable care and sensitivity is used when applying this technique.

Physiotherapist's Position
With the reversed headache SNAG, the hand of the cradling arm cups the occiput. The other hand grips the upper cervical spine using a lumbrical grip so as to restrict movement from the joints of C1–3. It must still be comfortable.

Patient's Position
This is the same as for the NAG.

Physiotherapist's Action

The hand of the cradling arm applies an anterior draw pressure so that the occiput moves forward on the relatively fixed cervical spine. The end position is maintained for a few seconds.

TECHNIQUES APPLIED FOR VERTIGO AND OTHER VERTEBRAL ARTERY SIGNS

It should be standard practice to examine the vertebral artery and upper cervical spine ligament stability when faults are suspected to arise in C0–4, particularly when there has been any trauma, e.g. whiplash. Positive signs are a contraindication to manipulation (high-velocity thrust), and great caution should be employed if mobilisation is considered a viable option. However, Mulligan has developed successful methods of mobilisation for symptoms that arise from dysfunction of the C0–3 complex. Vertebral artery signs or complaints of a 'woolly head' can be treated successfully using techniques applied to C2 or to the C1 transverse processes. Mulligan (1995a) has reported successful alleviation of the persistent reflux experienced by one patient on rotation of the head.

The mechanism of symptom production could feasibly arise through vertebral artery compromise, but there is also considerable evidence to suggest that the anatomy and neurophysiology of the C0–3 segments are a potential source of headache and vertigo (De Jong *et al.*, 1977; Bogduk, 1986, 1989; Dwyer, 1990). The joints of the C0–3 complex synapse within the trigeminocervical nucleus (TCN) with shared nuclei of the cranial nerves. Links also exist with the vestibulocochlear nerve, and thus balance may be impaired or auditory dysfunction may occur. Therefore there is a rationale for the treatment applied to this region to alleviate a variety of symptoms including headache and others which are more difficult to explain, e.g. toothache, sinusitis, tinnitus and swallowing difficulties.

It is emphasised that the symptoms arise as a neuromusculoskeletal-based response, and not for any other reason. As with all these techniques, the application should be pain free and should produce an immediate improvement. Self-treatments are not included in this text, but can be taught.

The vertebral artery and vertigo techniques are performed as SNAGs on C2 or the transverse process of C1. They are applied centrally, contralaterally (opposite the pain or sign) or occasionally ipsilaterally (same side as the pain or sign). Six repetitions are usual, and it is normal for one to four treatments to be required. Stating an order of efficacy does undermine the need to treat and respond within the context of the individual patient and condition,

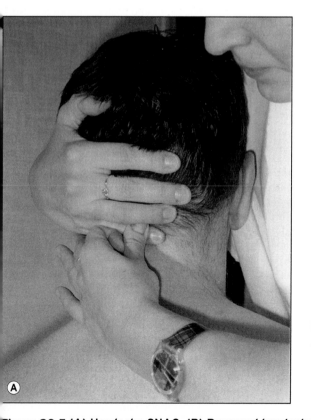 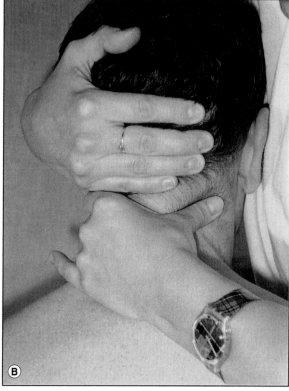

Figure 20.5 (A) Headache SNAG. (B) Reversed headache SNAG.

however, with these techniques it is common for the following order to be tried:
1. Central C2 SNAG.
2. Contralateral C1 SNAG.
3. Ipsilateral C1 SNAG.
4. Contralateral C2 SNAG.

An ipsilateral C2 SNAG is also a possible option.

Extension and rotation are the most commonly encountered movements producing symptoms; however, the movement generating the symptoms is the one chosen for attention.

These techniques can be used with great success when C1/2 restriction of movement is the problem with no untoward symptoms. Congenital fusion of the C0/1 and C1/2 segments, though not common, should be borne in mind when examining this area.

Cervical Positional SNAG

This technique is a true SNAG, i.e. an accessory glide combined with a patient-activated movement. It seems most successful in the middle-aged patient with some degeneration at the C5/6 and C6/7 levels. The movement that responds best has been found to be rotation. Mulligan is currently using only rotation as the SNAG movement.

Physiotherapist's Position
The physiotherapist stands behind the patient.

Patient's Position
The patient sits.

Physiotherapist's Action
For the C6/7 level, place the distal phalanx of the left thumb on the left of the C7 spinous process, and the right thumb on the right of the C6 spinous process. By applying a concurrent lateral glide toward the midline, both thumbs effectively generate a rotation to the right of C6 at the C6/7 level (it is recognised that other actions occur simultaneously at adjacent segments).

Patient's Action
At the same time as the accessory movement is produced, the patient rotates their head to the right (assuming this is the painfully restricted movement), and the end of range achieved may then be overpressed by the patient. The overpressure should increase the range of pain-free movement, otherwise it is not applied.

PERIPHERAL JOINTS

There are two main concepts regarding peripheral joints. These are:
• MWM i.e. passive accessory movements combined with active physiological movements. These may also include the addition of end-range overpressure performed by the physiotherapist, the patient or a person chosen by the patient to assist in the home programme.

• Pain-release phenomena (PRP). These comprise three passive techniques using stretch, glide and compression respectively, and one patient-active technique. All the techniques can be shown to be useful in a patient's home programme.

Firstly, the concepts will be described and the rules of application of the techniques for treatment of the peripheral joints given. Specific examples will then be described for the upper and lower limb for PRP and MWM treatments.

There are two rules that should be followed: the concave or convex rule and the joint plane rule. These are based on concepts put forward by Kalternborn (1980). Both will help in deciding the direction of treatment and in achieving pain-free application of a technique.

CONCAVE OR CONVEX RULE
This rule is applied to give the physiotherapist a guide as to the direction in which to apply the accessory glide.

If the moving joint surface is concave, e.g. the articular surface of the tibia during non-weight-bearing flexion, the mobilisation is in the direction of movement of the lower leg, e.g. an anteroposterior pressure on the anterior of the tibia for flexion. The reverse is true for a convex surface, e.g. the humeral head. The mobilisation is in the opposite direction, i.e. if the arm is abducting from the side, the accessory mobilisation is a caudal glide on the superior aspect of the head of humerus. For the shoulder, it is more common for anteroposterior and posteroanterior accessory glides to be used for all physiological movements.

JOINT PLANE RULE
The direction of the accessory movement should be at a right angle to the joint treatment surface (Figure 20.6). This avoids the joint surfaces potentially becoming wedged together.

The many treatment options for every joint and structure cannot be described fully in this section. The aim here is to outline the concepts that are applied, to give examples, and to leave the physiotherapist to experiment. The possibilities are almost endless, and although Mulligan documents an enormous array of techniques—in writing (Mulligan, 1995a and b) and on video— there is undoubtedly more to discover. The variations of individual patient presentations may require the physiotherapist to make occasional changes to the standard techniques to effect an improvement. However, the basic techniques correctly applied following the concept guidelines, normally produce very satisfying results.

BASIC CONCEPTS
The MWM is unique in the world of manual therapy. All MWM techniques have the same expectations as with the spinal techniques, i.e. they are painless to apply and, if indicated and applied correctly, produce immediate results.

MWMs are the peripheral joint equivalent to a SNAG for the spinal joints. The difference lies in the application of the accessory movement. With the SNAG, the accessory movement is applied in the direction of the active movement and along the facet plane. With MWM, the accessory movement is applied at right angles to the joint line and is designed to correct a 'positional fault'.

Examples of MWM accessory movements include:
- Medial or lateral glide e.g. hinge joints. These may be applied with a seatbelt or with manual pressure, depending on which provides the best control and comfort.
- Posteroanterior and anteroposterior glides, e.g. to ball- and-socket joints, adjacent metacarpal or metatarsal joints.
- Rotation, e.g. to the carpometacarpal joint of the thumb.
- Compression, e.g. to the patellofemoral joint.

The accessory movements can be applied with minor changes of angles of application, or combined to produce the most effective technique. Strapping is frequently used to maintain improvement after treatment and, combined with self-management strategies, provides an innovative and exciting way of treating the peripheral joints.

A general rule is that if the pain is on the lateral side then a lateral glide is applied, and, correspondingly, a medial glide is used to alleviate pain on the medial side. It is well known that the knee and elbow joints are far more complex than the label 'hinge joint' implies. However, they frequently respond very well to simple glides. This obviates the need to apply complex mechanical knowledge, and they can be effectively considered under the rather simplistic term of hinge joint.

Where the expected glide produces no change to the condition, another technique should be tried; e.g. lateral glide, to posteroanterior and anteroposterior glides or lateral glide to medial glide.

The glide must be sustained while the active movement is repeated for three sets of 6–10 repetitions. With more acute conditions, the physiotherapist may use as little as one set of three repetitions. The most common causes for lack of success in treatment are that the

sustained accessory movement is released or the joint plane rule is breached.

Once an improvement has been effected, it is wise to stop until the next visit or the patient's response is more clearly known. The use of overpressure to the active element of the technique is frequently used to produce the final resolution of a condition, although this is not always necessary. Overpressure can be applied by the patient or physiotherapist.

The most significant and/or painful movement, or key objective sign (e.g. a weight-bearing movement, pulling a plug from a wall) is used in combination with an accessory glide. Some examples are given later but these may include a lateral glide of the elbow during elbow extension for 'tennis elbow' or lateral elbow pain syndrome.

The wrist joint most commonly responds to a lateral glide. Rotation is usually a second choice or it can be used combined with the lateral glide.

The reader should not rely on test or examination results alone as this will inhibit or close therapeutic vision or knowledge base; as for all treatments and current neuromusculoskeletal understanding '... it ain't necessarily so' (Grieve, 1986). This reminds us that what we know is little and may be incorrect, and that dogma is not acceptable.

Pain-release Phenomena (PRP)

There are four techniques within this section:
- A joint stretch, e.g. quadrant stretch—hip or shoulder, hip and shoulder (Maitland, 1986), and capsular stretch—hip or shoulder (Cyriax, 1985).
- A joint compression, e.g. to the great toe, patellofemoral joint (Maitland, 1981).
- A joint glide, e.g. a posterior glide of the shoulder.
- A static resistance PRP treatment technique, e.g. active wrist extension.

They are painful to apply, but the pain reduces over the duration of the application. Again, they are repeated 6–10

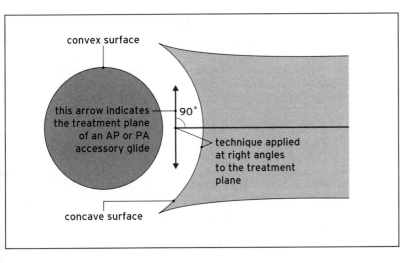

Figure 20.6 The joint plane rule.
AP: anteroposterior,
PA: posteroanterior.

times, and the symptoms and the objective or functional signs are improved on retesting.

All knee problems require the technique to be applied for 25 seconds. Techniques applied to other areas all require 20 seconds.

These techniques are used almost entirely in the treatment of chronic conditions. However, a 5-second pain-relief rule can be applied for more acute conditions, providing relief is achieved in that time. It would not be recommended that PRP are tried within the first 48 hours of the onset of an acute injury or condition.

The amount of resistance to be used is the most difficult thing to gauge when applying PRP. Physiotherapists new to the techniques would be advised to apply a pressure that takes only a few seconds for the pain to disappear before then trying a stronger pressure.

Key guidelines to follow with MWMs and PRP are that the physiotherapist produces a minor change in the sustained alignment of one bone to another or one joint surface to another, while the patient performs the 'painful' action or function (MWM). If this results in relief from pain and an increase in range, then the correct glide has been chosen. Minor alterations in the angle or force, or a change to a different glides may be necessary to improve the patient's response.

The techniques described below are by no means the whole range of Mulligan techniques; however, they provide an insight into the application. Thoughtful, careful and accurate investigative handling may provide the physiotherapist with 'new' and surprising results. It is possible to combine MWMs with PRP, and an example will be given for the elbow. The physiotherapist is requested at all times to keep an open mind and to be receptive to subtle handling changes producing successful resolution to a situation.

Taping for ideal position and patient self-treatment strategies are important elements of the treatment process in all the examples detailed in Table 20.1.

Examples of application in treatment include:
- A basic hinge joint MWM for the elbow. This will also be described with overpressure, and finally as a combined MWM/PRP.
- A weight-bearing MWM and a weight-bearing PRP for the knee.
- An MWM for an 'inversion sprain'.
- An MWM for 'plantar fasciitis' for the mid-tarsal joint.
- MWM used with a neurodynamic technique for the shoulder.

Basic Hinge Joint MWM for the Elbow

This example assumes the patient requires a lateral glide for the right elbow for painful or limited extension.

Physiotherapist's Position

The physiotherapist's hold should be as close to the elbow joint line as possible. The left hand supports and provides fixation to the outer aspect of the upper arm, while the right hand holds the ulnar aspect of the lower arm. The physiotherapist's thumbs lie parallel to each other and to the anterior elbow joint crease. The physiotherapist's forearms should also be in the same plane as each other, and this should enable the wrist to be held straight.

Patient's Position

The patient should be supine or sitting. The lower arm is supinated as far as possible.

Physiotherapist's Action

The right arm produces a lateral glide of the lower elbow joint complex on the fixed humeral section. This is painless

Examples of techniques available	
Joint/structure	**Potential treatment examples**
Hinge joint (simple or complex), e.g. elbow, knee, finger, wrist	Mobilisation with movement (MWM) with medial/lateral glides plus resistance plus overpressure (OP), pain release phenomena (PRP), tape for ideal position and self-treatments, combined PRP and MWM
Compound joints, e.g. shoulder, hip, carpal, tarsal, patellofemoral	MWM with anteroposterior (AP) glides, MWM plus seat belt traction, plus resistance, plus OP, PRP, tape for ideal position and self-treatments, combined PRP and MWM
Soft tissues, e.g. lateral (medial) elbow pains, inversion ankle sprain	MWM with medial/lateral glides and AP glides, plus resistance, plus OP, PRP, tape for ideal position and self-treatments, combined PRP and MWM
Special examples, e.g. neurodynamic techniques, sesamoid pain	MWM with medial/lateral glides and AP glides using the appropriate neurodynamic movement, plus OP, PRP, tape for ideal position and self-treatments, combined PRP and MWM

Table 20.1 Examples of techniques available.

and is held while the patient performs the required physiological activity, e.g. extension of the elbow.

Patient's Action
The patient performs elbow extension 6–10 times with the glide held.

To achieve full range, passive overpressure can be added by the patient, carer or another physiotherapist. Some changes of the physiotherapist's and patient's position may be required to enable the patient's arm to be passively extended.

Combined MWM/PRP for the Elbow
The technique described is useful in lateral elbow pain, e.g. tennis elbow, and can be adapted for an upper limb neurodynamic technique.

The physiotherapist's and patient's position and the physiotherapist's action remain as above, i.e. the appropriate glide to the elbow is maintained— in this example, a lateral glide.

Patient's Action
With the combined MWM/PRP, the patient's forearm is in pronation with the wrist extended and elbow fully extended (there should be no pain). Resisted wrist extension or middle finger extension is held for 20 seconds (as with all PRP some pain may be experienced).

With the upper limb neurodynamic technique, the wrist is actively flexed, with the forearm in pronation and the elbow in extension. Shoulder depression and/or abduction may be added to the starting position. Wrist flexion is repeated 6–10 times.

Weight-Bearing MWM for the Knee
A lunge movement is used to treat a painful loss of weight-bearing left knee flexion. This technique could be applied in the same way for pain or loss of movement within a specific part of the range of a squat action. In this example, a lateral glide is described.

Physiotherapist's Position
The physiotherapist may need to use a seatbelt strap to produce an effective glide, but this is dependent on the size of the patient. The padded belt is wrapped around the distal knee joint line of the patient and around the waist or trunk of the physiotherapist, who is in a half- kneeling stance. One hand is placed on the lateral side of the left knee distal to the knee joint, the other on the patient's hip to provide stability for the patient during the lunge action.

Patient's Position
The patient adopts a lunge position with the foot of the affected leg on a gymnasium stool or a chair, positioned before the beginning of the painful range.

Physiotherapist's Action
The physiotherapist leans back on the seatbelt while providing counterpressure on the lateral aspect of the knee joint. This should produce a pain-free lateral glide.

Patient's Action
The patient is instructed to lunge as deeply as possible over the left knee and then to return to the starting position for the required number of repetitions. Counterpressure applied by the physiotherapist will allow a controlled lunge. This should now render the action pain free.

The technique is repeated 6–10 times. The glide is released either between lunges or at the end of the series of repetitions.

Weight-Bearing PRP for the Knee
Physiotherapist's and Patient's Position
The physiotherapist's position is the same as for the weight-bearing MWM, except in this example the seatbelt is not needed. The physiotherapist's left hand (for the patient's left knee) is placed over the patella, and the right hand is used to stabilise the patient's hip during the lunge action. The patient's position is the same as for the weight-bearing MWM.

Physiotherapist's and Patient's Action
The patient slowly lunges forward until the onset of pain. Compression is applied to the patella by the physiotherapist marginally to increase the pain; the lunge and the compression are held. The pain should disappear within 25 seconds. An altered incline of medial or lateral glide to the patella may increase the effectiveness of the technique. The patient's action is the same as for the weight-bearing MWM.

MWM for an 'Inversion Sprain'
This technique is applied when there is loss of inversion, with or without pain. It can be applied during the acute or chronic stage following an inversion injury. It is often assumed that in the light of there being no bony injury, the lateral ligament/capsule has been damaged.

Patient's Position
The patient should be supine, with the knee supported and semi-flexed.

Physiotherapist's and Patient's Action
Since 1992, Mulligan and other physiotherapists worldwide, have found that the application of a backward glide of the fibula during active inversion produces a pain-free action with increasing range of inversion. During the backward glide of the fibula, the tibia is fixed by the physiotherapist's other hand.

The explanation for this is that there is a positional fault of the fibula, which has been drawn forward during the 'sprain', the lateral ligament remaining intact at least the anterior talofibular ligament and the calcaneofibular portions of the lateral ligament, (O'Brien, 1998).

MWMs for 'Plantar Fasciitis' for the Mid-tarsal Joint
The term 'plantar fasciitis' has been the source of some mystery and debate. The diagnosis of plantar fasciitis is

more of an umbrella term covering several possible causes. It can appear and disappear without or despite attempts to alleviate it.

The mid-tarsal joints are one potential source of dysfunction. They comprise the talocalcaneonavicular joint and the calcaneocuboid joint. Pain may occur through positional faults within the mid-tarsal complex and may be due to a number of causes, e.g. through tightness in the posterior crural muscles, a tight tendocalcaneus or subtalar joint dysfunction.

Subtalar joint dysfunction may be due to an altered pronation phase (extended pronation or delayed supination), faulty pronation through eversion of the rear foot (rear foot valgus) or reduced pronation due to rigidity of the foot. These faults may occur in the mid-tarsal joint as the initial point of breakdown of function or as the result of dysfunction in the gait cycle anywhere within the kinetic chain, usually when the kinetic chain is closed.

The MWM for the mid-tarsal joint can be applied as a non-weight-bearing technique or in a controlled weight-bearing position. Anecdotally (and logically), the weight-bearing version proves more successful, and this will be described.

Physiotherapist's Position
The physiotherapist sits or kneels facing the stool supporting the patient's foot.

Patient's Position
The affected foot is placed on a stool. It should be placed with the medial border of the foot close to one edge of the stool.

Physiotherapist's Action
The physiotherapist provides medial, lateral, anteroposterior or posteroanterior glide to the mid-tarsal joint. Anecdotal information indicates an oblique lateral or anteroposterior glide (an oblique downward motion) to the navicular, regularly affords more relief. This should not, however, negate other combinations.

Patient's Action
The patient performs a partial weight-bearing pronation or supination of the subtalar or mid-tarsal joint. In other words, an attempt is made to collapse and reform the medial longitudinal arch. Care must be taken not to increase weight bearing beyond the ability of the physiotherapist to control the accessory movement.

The glide is held for 6–10 repetitions, or can be released during each action.

MWM Combined with a Neurodynamic Technique for the Shoulder
Neurodynamic techniques (Butler & Gifford, 1989; Butler, 1991; Shacklock, 1995) are adjuncts to assessment and treatment of pain and dysfunction syndromes. The central issue is that healthy mechanics and physiology of the nervous system enable pain-free postures and movements to be achieved. The understanding of pathodynamics requires the understanding of the relation of pathophysiology to pathomechanics, encompassing the complexities of pain science, inflammation and repair, and relates to the stage of a disorder, for example, improving. This usually indicates, in simple terms, an increasingly familiar pattern of signs and symptoms, and suggests pathomechanical dominance.

However, when a clinical situation seems to reveal a 'positive' neurodynamic test, the basic guidelines for MWM treatments can be applied and seemingly alter the test results.

It is understood that MWMs affect the mechanical interface of the nervous system, so it could be argued that either the MWM has released some 'tension' rendering the neurodynamic test negative or that the mobilisation has positively affected the previously positive test.

The description of the treatment is not meant to inflame opinion in any direction or to disparage the significant enlightenment in physiotherapy thinking that both concepts have stimulated.

The MWM technique described is for the left shoulder, and it is assumed that the reader is familiar with upper limb neurodynamic tests. A modified upper limb test for radial nerve bias is used within this example. The patient's arm is held with the elbow fully extended, shoulder medially rotated, forearm pronated and wrist flexed. The cervical spine is in a neutral position and the shoulder girdle is held depressed. Abduction is the sensitising additional movement.

Physiotherapist's Position
The physiotherapist stands at the patient's head, facing towards the patient's feet.

Patient's Position
The patient is supine on the couch, with the arm in the starting position described above.

Physiotherapist's Action
The physiotherapist's right thigh applies suitable shoulder depression while the right hand applies an anteroposterior glide to the humeral head. Medial rotation of the shoulder, elbow pronation and wrist flexion are held by the physiotherapist's left hand.

Patient's Action
The patient performs pain-free abduction of the shoulder. All the usual guidelines apply.

POSSIBLE THEORIES

Mulligan has two main theories to account for the success of the spinal and periperal joint techniques:
• Positional faults – leading to maltracking
• Normal movement memory restoration

POSITIONAL FAULTS LEADING TO MALTRACKING
Positional faults are for the most part not visible on X-ray films or scans, yet the correction of suggested positional

faults produces a response amazingly quickly, regardless of the length of time the dysfunction has existed.

NORMAL MOVEMENT MEMORY RESTORATION

Movement is a series of automatic activities that are learned during growth and development; these patterns can be consciously modified. Pain and dysfunction produce abnormal movement patterns that may become learned and part of automatic actions.

It is normal for us to recognise familiar people, even at some distance, by their gait; similarly, we soon detect differences in the way they are moving when there is pain or dysfunction.

Mulligan suggests that re-educating normal actions with the addition of accessory glides enhances the ability to regain many of our more automatic movements in everyday life.

RELIEF OF PAIN AND DYSFUNCTION BY MANUAL THERAPY

Many ideas have been put forward to suggest how manual therapy produces relief of pain and restoration of function. For example:

- Both 'protective' spasm and inhibition of normal muscle function due to pain may produce altered joint biomechanics and imbalance in the normal co-ordinated group action of muscles. The net effect is a potential increase in pain, malalignment and inefficient activity. It must be realised that the mechanisms of pain production and body responses are extremely complex. They are intimately linked with multiple chemical interactions throughout the neuromusculoskeletal system, and are also affected by both emotional and social factors (Melzack et al., 1996).
- Movement occurs about an axis of rotation. The axis moves along a known path, and this alters when there is trauma, degenerative joint disease or altered muscle function (Sahrmann, 1992).
- Reduction in normal joint range (hypomobility) could be through scar shrinkage which produces altered joint function.

However, as mentioned previously, the method by which manual therapy produces results is still unclear (Difabio, 1986; Lee et al., 1996).

CONCLUSION

Criticism could be levelled at Mulligan's claims and lack of reasoning as to why certain repetitions are suggested. He is happy that the results speak for themselves. It is quite a relief to practise the 'art' of physiotherapy without the intense drive to prove the how's and why's. There is a need to improve our handling and palpation skills and not subdue them beneath a need for scientific sanction. Our patients and their pain do not always conform to science and logic.

Mulligan, like all of us, does desire the proof of skills, and we are obligated to show clear clinical reasoning and ultimately contribute to the proof of our skills. However, during the course of busy schedules and caseloads, quick 'little miracles' lighten the day and may add directly to answering some important questions.

Anecdotal information is not science: however, it is difficult as a manual physiotherapist not to consider visual evidence of a patient's response when there is an instantaneous relief from pain and a greater range of motion with specific improvements that last! There are, however, explanations for the efficiency of other manual techniques which are also applicable to the Mulligan approach. Although 'the answer' to how manual therapy relieves pain through movement remains elusive (Korr, 1978; Farfan, 1980; Wyke, 1985; Zusman, 1994), this should not undermine new conceptual frameworks in manual therapy or deter those seeking to improve knowledge.

It suffices to say that Mulligan's techniques provide a quick and exciting way of achieving occasionally miraculous results. Although they do not work in all cases, the ease and speed of application makes these methods an effective first port of call for manual therapy. Mulligan has shown that these techniques frequently work, but he would be the first to encourage educated and logical adaptation where necessary.

REFERENCES

Aspinall W. Cinical testing for craniovertebral hypermobility syndrome. *J Sports Ther* 1990, **12**:47-54.

Beeton K. Instability in the upper cervical region. Clinical presentation; radiological and clinical testing. *Manipulative Ther* 1995, **27**:19-32.

Bogduk N. Cervical causes of headache and dizziness. In: Grieve G, ed.: *Modern manual therapy of the vertebral column*. Edinburgh: Churchill Livingstone; 1986, 289-302.

Bogduk N. The anatomy of headache. In: Dalton M, ed.: *Proceedings of the headache and face pain syndrome*. Brisbane: Manipulative Physiotherapists Association of Australia; 1989, 1-16.

Butler DS. *Mobilisation of the nervous system*. Edinburgh: Churchill Livingstone; 1991, 185-201.

Butler DS, Gifford L. The concept of adverse mechanical tension in the nervous system. *Physiotherapy* 1989, **75**:622-636.

Butler DS, Gifford L. *The clinical biology of aches and pains. Pre-conference course note*. Edinburgh: Manipulative Association of Chartered Physiotherapists Conference: muscles and nerves on the move; 1994.

Cyriax J. *Illustrated manual of orthopaedic medicine*. London: Butterworths; 1985.

De Jong PTVM, De Jong JMD, Cohen B, JongKees BW. Ataxia and nystagmus induced by injections of local anaesthetics in the neck. *Ann Neurol* 1977, **1**:240--246

Difabio RP. Clinical assessment of manipulation and mobilisation of the lumbar spine. A critical review of the literature. *Phys Ther* 1986; **66**:51-54.

Dwyer A, Asrill C, Bogduk N. Cervical zygopophyseal joint pain patterns. *Spine* 1990; **15**:453-457.

Edwards BC. Movement patterns. In: Bower KD, ed.: *Proceedings of the MTAA conference on manipulative therapy*. Perth: Manipulative Physiotherapists Association of Australia; 1983:54.

Edwards BC. *Manual of combined movements*. Edinburgh: Churchill Livingstone; 1992, 102-106.

Farfan HF. The scientific basis of manipulative procedures. *Clin Rheum Dis* 1980, **6**:159-177.

Grieve GP. *Modern manual therapy*. Edinburgh: Churchill Livingstone; 1986.

Kalternborn FM. *Mobilisation of the extremity joints*. Bokhandel, Oslo: Olaf Norlis; 1980.

Korr I. What is manual therapy? In: Korr I, ed. *The neurobiologic mechanisms in manipulative therapy*. London: Plenum Press; 1978:229.

Lee M, Steven GP, Crosbie J, Higgs RJED. Towards a theory of lumbar mobilisation—the relationship between applied manual force and movements of the spine. *Man Ther* 1996 **1**:67-75.

Maitland GD. The hypothesis for adding compression when examining and treating synovial joints. *Journal of Orthopaedic and Sports Physical Therapy* 1980 **2**:7-14 .

Maitland GD. *Vertebral manipulation*, 5th ed. London: Butterworths; 1986.

Melzak R, Wall PD. *The challenge of pain: a modern classic*, 2nd ed. London: Penguin; 1986.

Mulligan BR. *Manual therapy—NAGS, SNAGS, MWMs etc.*, 3rd ed. Wellington, New Zealand: Plane View Services; 1995a.

Mulligan BR. Spinal mobilisations with leg movement (further mobilisations with movement). *J Man Manipulative Ther* 1995b; **3**:25-27.

O'Brien T, Vinenzino B. A study of the effects of Mulligan's mobilisation with movement for lateral ankle pain: a case study design. *Manual Therapy* 1998; **3**:78-84.

Sahrmann S. *Advanced diploma in orthopaedic manual therapy. Course notes*. Auckland, New Zealand; 1992.

Shacklock M. Neurodynamics. *Physiotherapy* 1995; **81**:9-16.

Wyke BD. Articular neurology and manipulative therapy. In: Glasgow EF, Twomey LT, Scull ER, Kleynhams AM, Idczak RM, eds. *Aspects of manipulative therapy*. Edinburgh: Churchill Livingstone; 1985.

Zusman M. Manipulative therapy and mechanical pain. *Manipulative Ther* 1994; **26**:22-28.

INDEX

movement patterns 230-3, 239
Mulligan's approach to spinal and peripheral
   mobilisations
      common guidelines 271
      factors common to all techniques when
         applied to spine 272
      theories about mechanism 282-3
multiple myeloma 12, 129
multiply injured patient 28
muscle
      activity, gait analysis 153-154
      avulsion fracture 16
      belly, palpation 200
      bulk 200
      contractile/tendinous element 235
      coordination of action 233
      fibres 252
      fixator 233
      imbalance 231
      ischaemia, fracture-related 26-27
      isotonic 233
      length, normal 200
      movement analysis 239
      observation 198
      shortening 230-1, 239-240
      soreness, delayed onset 253
      strength 200
      testing 200
      work 214
muscular dystrophies 176, 182
myelodysplasia 177
myelography (radiculography) 55-56

N
natural apophyseal glide (NAG) 271, 272-273
Neer outcome method 119
nerve root 199
      compression on myelography 56
      pain 168, 191, 192, 208
neurapraxia 27
neurodynamic tests 199, 282-283
neurofibromatosis 146
neurological tests 199
neuromuscular skeletal environmental
   interactions (NMEI)
neuromusculoskeletal environmental
   interactions (NMEI)
      balance in movement 234
      biomechanical considerations 231-232
      conditioning in movment habits 239
      cumulative strain 230-231
      environmental interactions 235-236
      events that may lead to cumulative strain
         231
      historical review 229-230
      kinesiological considerations 233
      movement pattern change 241-242
      neurophysiological considerations 233
      preventing musculoskeletal injury 236-238
      spinal mobility 231-233
      stretching programme 239-241
neuropathy, diabetic 196
neurotmesis 27
nucleotomy 58

O
obesity 195
objective examination
      active movements 200-201
      analysis of findings, see case history
         analysis
      functional activities 198
      guidance for novice physiotherapist 197
      muscle testing 200
      neurodynamic tests 199
      neurological testing 199
      observation 198

other related joints 199
      passive movements 201
      reflection on findings 197-198
      soft tissue palpation 200
      swelling 199
objectivity of condition 211
ochronosis 14
Ollier's disease 11
Ortolani manoeuvre 136
ossification 3
osteoarthritis
      of elbow 103
      of hip 63-64
      intertrochanteric osteotomy 62
      of knee 68
      and osteoporosis 130
      pathology 12
      of shoulder 97
osteoarthrosis 26
osteoblastoma, benign 9
osteoblasts 3, 7, 121-122
osteocalcin 122
osteochondral drilling 82
osteochrondomas (exostoses) 11
osteoclastoma (giant cell tumour of bone) 12
osteoclasts 3, 7, 121, 122
osteocyte 121
osteogenesis imperfecta 4, 127, 145
oesteoid (unmineralised bone) 121
osteolysis
      broken cement causing 65, 66
      wear particles causing 66
osteoma 9
osteomalacia 7, 122
osteomyelitis 4-6
osteonectin 122
osteopenia 17, 123
osteophytes 12
osteoporosis
      abdominal surgery 195
      and age 204
      and arthritis 130
      calcium supplements 127
      in children 126
      complications 130
      definition 123
      and diabetes 196
      and diet 127-128
      diseases associated 126
      economic sequelae 124
      fractures 7, 123
      heparin-related 127
      immobilisation and 17, 126, 129
      incidence and prevalence 123-124
      investigations 125
      kyphosis 7, 130, 177
      male/female ratio 124-125
      mechanical consequence 130
      in men 7, 129
      pain relief 130
      pathology 3, 6
      postmenopausal women 128-129
      and pregnancy 127
      quality-of-life 124-125
      risk factors 123
      vitamin D supplements 127
      in young adults 7
osteosarcoma 7, 9, 9-10
osteotomy
      Bombelli 64
      Chiari 64, 138, 140
      Coventry 69
      definition 61
      Dunn's 144
      femoral 64, 81, 141, 145
      Ganz peri-acetabular 63
      general principles 61

osteotomy (cont'd)
      of hip 62
      indications 61
      intertrochanteric 62
      of knee 68-69
      McMurray 62
      pelvic 63
      postoperative care 64
      Salter 63, 138
      subtrochanteric 144
      transverse 63
      Wagner technique 64
Oswestry Disability Index 54, 59-60, 222
overpressure 199, 201, 279
overuse injuries 230

P
Paget's disease of bone 7-8, 122, 128
pain
      antalgic postures 198
      body chart 191-192, 208, 221
      characteristic features 208
      clinical features related to pathology 209
      day 194
      differential diagnosis model 21
      discogenic 165, 166, 168, 169, 232
      fractures 23
      medication taken by patient 195
      morning 194
      of muscle ischaemia 25, 26-27
      nerve root 168, 191, 192
      night 194
      nonverbal response 201
      onset of 196
      patient's face showing 195
      peripheral nerve 192
      referred 191
      and resistance 201
      and sleeping conditions 194
      sociocultural effects on 208
      variability 192
      visual analogue 193, 222
pain chart 191-192, 208, 221
pain clinics 28
painful arc 89, 92
pain-release phenomena (PRP) 278, 279-281
pain of spinal origin (PSO) 271-272
pamidronate 129
pannus 13
paraplegia 39, 43
parathyroid adenoma 7
parathyroid hormone (PTH) 7, 122
patellectomy 70
patellofemoral arthritis 70
patient
      attitude to problem 208
      illness response 204
patient-physiotherapist relationship 191, 197,
   204
Pavlik harness 137
pelvic fractures 17
pelvic region, localised lesions 195-196
Perdriolle method (spinal curvature) 179
peripheral nerve 27, 192, 200
Perthes' disease 140-142
Petrie (broomstick) plasters 142
physiotherapy
      ankle
         arthrodesis 85
         arthroscopy 85
         replacement 85-86
      cerebral palsy patients, surgery 159-162
      coxa vara 146
      developmental dysplasia of hip 138-140
      elbow replacement 106, 118-119
      fractures 27
      hip

A NEW, DYNAMIC TEXTBOOK THAT EVERY STUDENT SHOULD OWN...

ORTHOPAEDIC PHYSIOTHERAPY

Written by an expert team, this innovative new book provides a clear and comprehensive insight into the basic concepts of orthopaedics, specific orthopaedic conditions and the full range of physiotherapy treatment approaches during rehabilitation.

OTHER TITLES IN THE SERIES:

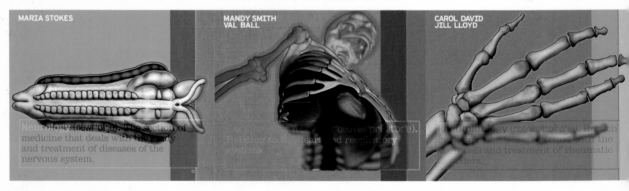

NEUROLOGICAL PHYSIOTHERAPY

MARIA STOKES

Neurology (new rol'ə). The section of medicine that deals with the study and treatment of diseases of the nervous system.

CARDIOVASCULAR/ RESPIRATORY PHYSIOTHERAPY

MANDY SMITH
VAL BALL

Relating to the heart and respiratory systems

RHEUMATOLOGICAL PHYSIOTHERAPY

CAROL DAVID
JILL LLOYD

Rheumatology (roo'mətol'ə'jē). English branch of medicine concerned with the diagnosis and treatment of rheumatic disorders.

ISBN 0-7234-2592-2

Mosby

9 780723 425922